Complete Review of

Gynecologic Oncology

With Recent Updates

Sharmila Arun Babu
MS Obstetrics and Gynecology (JIPMER), MBA (HM)
Additional Professor and Head
Department of Obstetrics and Gynecology
All India Institute of Medical Sciences (AIIMS)
Mangalagiri, Andhra Pradesh, India-522 503

Peepee Publishers and Distributors (P) Ltd.®

Complete Review of Gynecologic Oncology

Published by
Pawaninder P. Vij and Anupam Vij

Peepee Publishers and Distributors (P) Ltd.
Head Office: 160, Shakti Vihar, Pitam Pura, Delhi-110 034 (India)

Correspondence Address:
7/31, First Floor, Ansari Road, Daryaganj
New Delhi-110 002 (India)
Ph: 41512412, 23246245, 9811156083
e-mail: peepee160@yahoo.co.in
e-mail: peepee160@gmail.com
www.peepeepub.com
join us on facebook.com/pp.publishers

First Edition: 2020

ISBN: 978-81-8445-279-2

Dedicated to

My parents for their unconditional support and blessings

My teachers for teaching me the ABCs of medicine

My husband, Dr. Arun Babu for inspiring and motivating me

My kids Akshaya and Akash for sacrificing their share of time with me

Editor

Dr. Kantamani Bala Teja, MS ENT, MCh (Head and Neck Surgery)

Dr. Kantamani Bala Teja has done his MBBS from Dr. PSIMS & RF and Postgraduation from ASRAM Medical College. He is actively involved in UG & PG teaching and has special interest in various aspects of medicine. He has both national and state publications in his subject of concern.

Editorial Assistance

- **Dr. Padmapriya**, Resident in Pathology, Andhra Medical College, Visakhapatnam, Andhra Pradesh
- **Dr. Gaurang Narayan**, CRRI, IGMCRI, Puducherry
- **Dr. Balakrishnan Ramanan**, CRRI, IGMCRI, Puducherry

PREFACE

It gives me immense pleasure in bringing out this book **'Complete Review of Gynecologic Oncology–With Recent Updates'** which is aimed at complete, concise coverage of all the major topics in the field of Gynecologic Oncology. Gynecologic Oncology is rapidly evolving with several developments and innovative approaches in the last decade. This book is designed for medical students, residents and practitioners of Obstetrics and Gynecology who aim to quickly glance and capture the concepts of 'Gynecologic Oncology'. This book will also be a valuable source of information to all the students preparing for various postgraduate and 'Gynecologic Oncology' super speciality entrance examinations.

The chapters are presented in a concise format with bulleted points for better understanding and retention of the content. The book contains the most up-to-date information available on treatment of gynecologic cancers with an exclusive 'Recent Updates' paragraph at the end of all chapters. This book also contains Practice MCQs for those who are preparing for entrance exams. Extreme care has been taken to provide accurate information and the entire content is based on standard reference textbooks and latest evidence-based guidelines. I would like to emphasise that this book is specially designed for rapid revision and understanding of the concepts in the field of Gynecologic Oncology and readers are requested to refer to standard textbooks for more detailed information.

I would like to extend my sincere thanks to my publishers, Mr. Pawaninder Paul Vij and Mr. Anupam Vij, Peepee Publishers and Distributors (P) Ltd., New Delhi, India and their entire team for bringing out this book. I express my sincere thanks and gratitude to my husband, Dr. Arun Babu for all his valuable inputs and suggestions. I also thank all my past and present colleagues, students and my patients for their support.

I sincerely hope that this book will be of immense value and will fulfil the needs of all readers. Any feedback/criticisms regarding the book are welcome. Please write to the author at sharu_jipmer@yahoo.co.in. For updates about the book, please visit facebook page http://www.facebook.com/sharmila.author

Sharmila Arun Babu
MS Obstetrics and Gynecology (JIPMER), MBA (HM)
Additional Professor and Head
Department of Obstetrics and Gynecology
All India Institute of Medical Sciences (AIIMS)
Mangalagiri, Andhra Pradesh, India-522 503

ACKNOWLEDGEMENTS

Shri Vijayan, Cash Officer (Retd.), SBI, Puducherry

Smt. Sagoundala, Under Secretary (Retd.), Government of Puducherry

Shri Thirunavukkarasu, Government School English Lecturer (Retd.), Puducherry

Smt Sampurnam, Principal (Retd.), SSVHSS, Puducherry

Shri Srinivasan@Babu, PWD, Puducherry

Mr. Rajkumar, System Engineer, Apple, CA, USA

Mr. Dhinesh Shankar, EC Software, Chennai

Shri KV Raghavulu

Smt. KP Lakshmi

Shri Bhanuteja

Smt. K Lakshmi

Dr. Deepthi Alla, Dr. Rajesh, Dr. Rakesh, Dr. Ram Prasad, Dr. Kishore, Dr. Praveen, Dr. Mahesh, Dr. Venkateswarlu, Dr. Pawan, Dr. Ashok and Dr. Sathish

&

My sincere thanks to:

Dr. Mukesh Tripathi, Director, AIIMS, Mangalagiri

Dr. Joy A Ghoshal, Dean, AIIMS, Mangalagiri

Dr. Rakesh Kakkar, Medical Superintendent, AIIMS, Mangalagiri

CONTENTS

CHAPTER 1

MOLECULAR PATHOGENESIS AND GENETICS IN GYNECOLOGIC CANCER

INTRODUCTION

- Cancer comprises more than 200 diseases and is responsible for deaths in both developed and developing countries
- Cancer is the result of **accumulation of molecular alterations that change the normal characteristics of cells**
- **Altered cells attain distinctive features** such as variation in cell structure, diminished property of cell adhesion, capability to synthesize new enzymes, which helps their progeny to divide and sustain, even in the presence of normal surrounding cells which can inhibit their growth
- These alterations lead to **malfunctioning of the control system** that otherwise prevent overgrowth and uncontrolled proliferation of the cells.
- Tumors can be classified as **benign and malignant tumors**
  - **Benign tumors** are **slow-growing** expansive masses that remain confined to their original location and **do not invade** surrounding normal tissues or spread to distant body sites. However, a few of them can have malignant potential
  - **Malignant tumor** has the potential to **invade the neighboring normal tissues and spread to other sites of body by circulatory or lymphatic spread termed as metastasis**
  - Benign tumors can be removed by surgical intervention, but malignant tumors are often resistant to such localized treatments
- **Cancer can be classified into three main types based on the cell of origin-carcinomas, sarcomas, leukemia's and lymphomas**
  - The cancers of **epithelial cells are known as carcinoma**s–constitutes **90%** of all human cancers which includes cancers of breast, colon, lung, pancreas and prostate
  - The cancers from connective **tissues** like **muscle, bone, cartilage and fibrous tissue** are known as **sarcomas** and are rare tumors
  - The cancers, which arise from blood-forming cells and cells of the immune system, are known as **leukemia and lymphoma** respectively, account for about **8%** of human cancers
- Tumors can be divided **according to the tissue of origin such** as lung or breast carcinomas
- Tumors can be divided **according to the type of cells involved** like fibrosarcomas arise from fibroblasts, osteosarcoma arise from bones etc

History and Theories of Cancer

- The term **carcinoma was coined from the Greek word *'carcinos'* (which means 'crab'** which might denote the finger-like protrusions from a cancer cell) by Greek physician Hippocrates
- Later, Roman physician, **Celsus termed it *cancer, which* is the Latin word for 'crab'**
- Greek physician **Galen** described the phrase ***'oncos'* for tumors**
- The world's **oldest recorded case** of cancer was that of **breast cancer** reported in ancient Egypt in 1500 BC
- From the primeval, physicians are clueless over the cause of cancers and several theories have been put forth
- **The earliest theory was Hippocrates' Humoral theory** where he proposed that the human body has four humors (body fluids) specifically blood, phlegm, yellow bile and black bile and the imbalance in these fluids can result in cancer

- Later, it was replaced by **Lymph theory**, which proposed that cancer is the result of body fluid known as lymph that comes out of the blood
- In 1838, German pathologist **Johannes Muller** put forth the **theory of Blastema** where he proposed that budding elements (blastema) are responsible for development of cancer and proved that cancer is composed of cells and not lymph
- Later, **parasite theory** was accepted till 18th century that assumed that cancer was contagious and spread by parasite infection
- **Trauma theory** proposed trauma to be the cause of cancer
- **Virchow** (1821–1902) proposed **chronic irritation theory,** where he stated that chronic irritation is responsible for cancer and determined that cancer cells originates from other cells and considered that cancers "spread like a liquid"
- in 1860**, Karl Thiersch**, determined that **cancers metastasize** by the spread of malignant cells and not by the means of any unidentified fluid
- **Identification of oncogenes and tumor suppressor genes in the 20th century has revolutionized the understanding of cancer**
- **Proto-oncogenes** are genes that normally regulate cell division and degree of differentiation of cells**.** Mutations of certain **proto-oncogenes** alter the normal cells to grow in unregulated manner to become cancer cells
- **Tumor suppressor genes** are normal genes, which control cell division, DNA repair and apoptosis. Any deregulation in these genes can cause cancer

Characteristics of Cancer Cells

- Accumulation of mutations and genetic changes can result in normal cells acquiring distinct characteristics to transform into cancer cells
- **Cancer cells**
  - Have less requirement for growth factors to sustain growth and proliferation
  - Show trait of anchorage independence
  - Do not stop dividing after a predetermined number of generations
- **Hanahan and Weinberg** defined the properties of cancer cells as **"Hallmarks of Cancer"** that include the following (Figure 1.1)
  - Sustained proliferative signaling
  - Evading growth suppressors
  - Resisting cell death
  - Facilitating replicative immortality
  - Inducing angiogenesis
  - Activating invasion and metastasis
  - Genome instability
  - Energy metabolism reprogramming
  - Evading immune destruction

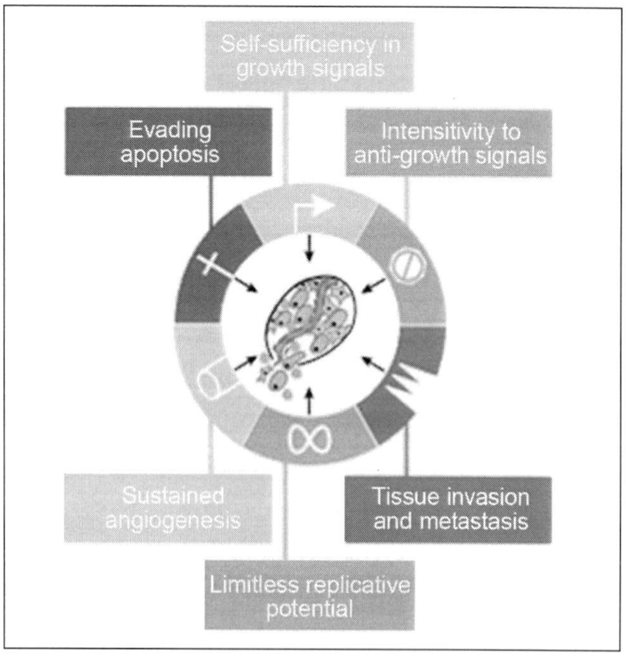

Figure 1.1: Weinberg fundamental principles of cancer

Causes of Cancer

- Predisposition of an individual to cancer is the **outcome of environmental (carcinogens) as well as genetic factors**
- A substance that causes cancer is known as **carcinogen**
- The concept of environment is used to define all non-genetic factors such as diet, lifestyle and infectious agents, which are responsible for approximately 80–85% of human cancers
- Environment can expose a person to **possible carcinogens** such as **asbestos, air pollution, tobacco smoke, radon, arsenic and chlorination by-products**

- **Lifestyle factors** such as **smoking and alcohol usage, obesity, diet, physical inactivity and reproductive and hormonal factors can serve as the basis of cancer and can be targeted for primary prevention**
- It is now well established that same extent of DNA aberrations or mutations in oncogenes and tumor suppressor genes in various species can result in different cancers due to presence of numerous polymorphic tumor susceptibility genes
- Recent data also imply that susceptibility to **"sporadic" cancers** in humans is attributed to **multiple polymorphic host genes** with relatively weak effects. This implies that, in addition to hereditary familial cancer syndromes, **sporadic cancers are also under strong genetic control**
- The genotype of an individual at a particular locus, can either increase or decrease their susceptibility to develop the pathology in response to environmental agent exposure

Molecular Alterations in Cancer

- Cancer is a multistage process that involves aggregation of multiple genetic alterations, regulated through different genetic predisposition as well as external factors
- **Mutator phenotype hypothesis** postulated that cancers arise because of mutations in genes that maintain genetic stability in normal cells. It is now well established that **cancer is the result of series of molecular alterations at the genetic and epigenetic level of cells that regulate cell proliferation consequently leading to uncontrolled cell growth. The** various genetic and molecular aberrations leading to gene mutations can be detected by molecular studies
- In majority of the cases, the molecular aberrations leading to tumorigenesis affect two different subsets of genes: **Proto-oncogenes (growth promoting genes) and tumor suppressor genes (growth inhibitory genes) that** normally regulate cell proliferation, apoptosis and repairing of damaged DNA

Proto-oncogenes

- Regulates cell growth and cell division **in a positive fashion**
- If any aberrations occur in these genes, it becomes an oncogene and promotes the development of cancer by increasing the encoded protein activity or high expression of the normal gene
- **Proto-oncogenes needs one mutational events for its gain of function (Dominant gene)**. Hence, **only one copy of the altered gene is sufficient for cancer promotion**

Tumor suppressor genes (antioncogene)

- **Suppresses cellular growth, proliferation and** helps in preventing cancer by keeping cell growth under control
- Tumor suppressor genes have the **opposite effect of oncogenes**, hence referred to as **antioncogenes**
- The tumor suppressor genes **needs two mutational events (point mutation, deletions) for its loss of function (act as recessive genes)**
- **Common tumor suppressor genes and their chromosome location are : RB1 (13q), p53 (17 p), BRCA1 (17q), BRCA2 (13q), WT1 (11q)**

Categories of mutations identified in cancers

- **Oncogenes are activated by** point mutation, overexpression, amplification, translocation, oxidative stress, epigenetic modifications (micro RNA, CpG island methylation, histone modification, chromatin remodeling), **chromosomal changes** such as terminal deletion, deletion, insertion, duplication, inversion, reciprocal translocation, Robertsonian translocation, ring chromosome, isochromosome and **Nucleotide changes** such as nucleotide deletion, insertion and substitution.
- Mutations in oncogenes change a single amino acid and lead to gain of activity that stimulates proliferation **(e.g., KRAS).** These mutations are **dominant** and **not dependent on changes in the other copy of gene**
- Mutations in tumor-suppressor genes **(e.g., *PTEN*)** and DNA repair genes **(e.g., *BRCA1*)** are generally small base insertions/ deletions or single base changes that cause **stop codons.** These lead to **truncated protein products that are nonfunctional. Loss of tumor-suppressor activity is usually dependent on deletion of other copy of gene**
- Several oncogene products (**HER-2/neu, K-ras, C-myc, P21**) and tumor suppressor gene products **(p53, p16)** are currently being investigated as independent **prognostic markers**

- **DNA Copy Number Changes - Deletion of one or both copies** of a tumor-suppressor gene due to genomic instability leads to loss of a gene product **(e.g., *RB1*); Gain of additional** copies of an oncogene leads to increased activity **(e.g., *HER-2/neu*)**
- **Aneuploidy**–Aneuploidy with gain or loss of complete chromosome is common in many cancers **(e.g., high-grade serous ovarian cancer)** and likely plays a role in cancer development and progression
- **Epigenetic alterations–Hypermethylation of CpG islands** in **promoter region of tumor-suppressor genes** may lead to gene inactivation **(e.g., *MLH1*); Loss of promoter methylation** in genes that stimulate proliferation may provide an oncogenic stimulus **(e.g., *IGF2*)**; Changes in acetylation of histone proteins that coat DNA may play a role in carcinogenesis
- **Aberrant gene splicing**–Genes may have alternative splice forms that produce messenger RNAs and proteins that have altered activity
- **MicroRNA's–Small noncoding RNAs** can affect gene expression by binding to messenger RNAs and blocking their translation. **Altered micro RNA expression** plays a role in development and behavior of cancers
- **Examples of genetic damage in cancers are given in Table 1.1**

Table 1.1: Examples of genetic damage in cancers

Type of genetic damage	Examples
Germline alterations	
High-penetrance genes	*BRCA1, BRCA2* (breast, ovarian cancers)
	MLH1, MSH2 (Lynch syndrome)
Low-penetrance genes	SNPs associated with various cancers
Exogenous carcinogens	
Ultraviolet radiation	*TP53* mutations in skin cancers
Tobacco	*TP53* mutations in lung cancers
Viruses	HPV inactivation of RB and *TP53* in cervical cancers
Endogenous DNA damage	
Cytosine methylation and deamination	*TP53* mutations in many cancer types
DNA Hydrolysis	Various genes
Spontaneous errors in DNA synthesis	Various genes
Free radical production due to oxidative stress	Various genes

Note

- *Normal cells are capable of undergoing division only a finite number of times, before becoming senescent*
- *Cellular senescence is regulated by a biologic clock related to progressive shortening of repetitive DNA sequences (TTAGGG) called telomeres that cap the ends of each chromosome*
- ***Telomeric shortening is the molecular clock that triggers senescence***

A model of development and progression of cancer is given in Figure 1.2 (See figure next page)

GENETICS IN GYNECOLOGIC MALIGNANCY

- Familial cancers of the breast, ovary, colon, endometrium and other sites have been observed among the female members of affected families
- Well-defined familial cancer syndromes with **autosomal dominant inheritance** pattern have been described
- **Life-time risk of ovarian cancer in the population as a whole is 1.4%**; Risk is **5% when one first degree** relative is affected and **7% when two or more first degree relatives** are affected
- Familial cancers **account for less than 5% of** all ovarian cancers
- Familial cancers **have an early age of onset**

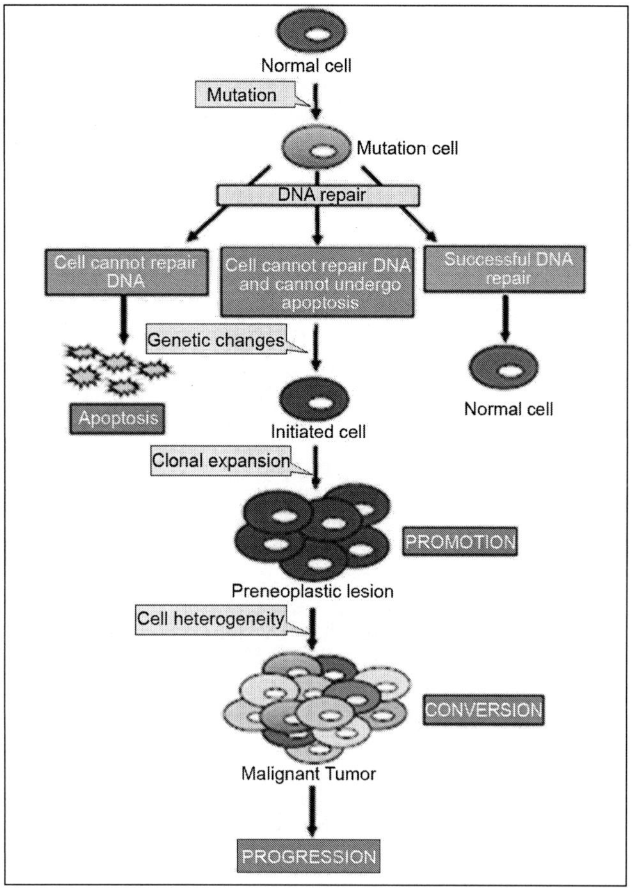

Figure 1.2: Development and progression of cancer

- Oncogenes, tumor suppressor genes and mutator genes are involved with the malignant change of cells
- **Early detection of cancer** may be possible by **detecting mutated copies of gene products (p53, HER-2/neu, K-ras) using polymerase or ligase chain reaction**
- **Common hereditary cancer syndromes that include gynecologic cancers as part of their cancer spectrum include the following (Table 1.3)**
  - **Hereditary Breast and Ovarian Cancer syndrome -caused by germline mutations in *BRCA1* or *BRCA2***
  - **Lynch syndrome-caused by germline mutations in *MLH1, MSH2, MSH6, or PMS2***
- **Other syndromes that include gynecologic cancers include**
  - **Cowden's syndrome (*PTEN* germline mutation)**
  - **Peutz-Jeghers syndrome (*STK11* germline mutation)**
  - **Li-Fraumeni syndrome (*TP53* germline mutation)**
- All of these cancer syndromes are caused **by mutations in tumor-suppressor genes**.
- In order for an individual to develop a cancer associated with one of the hereditary cancer syndromes, both the **maternally and paternally inherited copy of the relevant gene must be inactivated, as described by Knudsen's two hit hypothesis**
- Women with hereditary cancer syndromes have inherited from either their mother or father, a nonworking copy of one of the relevant genes. Therefore, in order for cancer to develop in a susceptible tissue through defects in a specific pathway, only the second working copy of the relevant gene needs to be lost.
  - This explains why the **cancers occur earlier** and **more frequently** in women with hereditary cancer syndromes than in the general population
  - This also explains why **not all individuals with an inherited predisposition develop cancer**, as it is possible that the second working copy of the relevant tumor suppressor gene is never lost in a susceptible tissue

- These syndromes are all caused by **mutations in a single allele of the relevant tumor suppressor gene**, and are **all autosomal dominant disorders** in which **each offspring**[a] **is at 50% risk of inheriting the cancer predisposition**

Table 1.3: Common hereditary syndromes that include gynecologic cancers as part of their cancer spectrum

Syndrome	Gene	Chromosome	Predominant Cancer
Hereditary breast/ovarian cancer	BRCA1	17q21	Breast, ovary
	BRCA2	13q12	
Lynch syndrome	MSH2	2p16	Colon, endometrium, ovary and urinary tract
	MLH1	3q21	
	MSH6	2p16	
	PMS2	7q22	
Cowden syndrome	PTEN	10q23	Breast, thyroid and endometrial
Li-Fraumeni syndrome	TP53	17p13	Breast, sarcomas, leukemias, and brain
Peutz-Jeghers syndrome	STK11	19p13	Colon, breast, gastric, and ovarian sex cord-stromal tumours with annular tubules (SCTAT)

Cancer and Genetic Counselling

- Identifying a woman with hereditary cancer syndrome has tremendous implications for both the patient and her family members
- Recently, increasing emphasis is placed on developing guidelines to assist physicians in recognizing those patients in whom genetic counseling and testing may be helpful

HEREDITARY BREAST AND OVARIAN CANCER SYNDROME

- A diagnosis of hereditary breast and ovarian cancer syndrome (HBOC) is considered, when there are **multiple cases of breast cancer and/or ovarian cancer on the same side of the family**
- It usually **occurs in association with BRCA1 or BRCA2 mutation**
- Mutations are inherited in **autosomal dominant pattern**
- Most hereditary ovarian cancer syndromes are associated with mutations in **BRCA 1 located on chromosome 17**
- **Small proportions** have mutations in **BRCA 2 gene located on chromosome 13**
- The **lifetime risk of ovarian cancer for women with BRCA1 mutations and BRCA2 mutations** has been estimated to be **40% and 20%,** respectively.
- Hereditary ovarian cancers occur **one decade earlier than sporadic cases.** Average age at diagnosis is 50 years. If a malignant ovarian tumor occurs in the premenopausal age group, detailed family history and screening of other family members are to be done
- **Survival** for women with **ovarian cancer related to a BRCA mutation** has been reported to be **longer than for women with a similar stage cancer and no mutation**
- **Risk of ovarian cancer in women with BRCA mutations may be reduced by prophylactic salpingo-oophorectomy, also termed as Risk reduction salpingo- oophorectomy (RRSO)**
- **Criteria for offering risk assessment in HOBC syndrome and Risk reduction recommendations for women with BRCA mutations are given in Tables 1.4 and 1.5**

Table 1.4 : American College of Obstetrician and Gynecologists and Society of Gynecologic Oncologists Criteria for Offering Genetic Risk Assessment for Hereditary Breast and Ovarian Cancer Syndrome
Patients with greater than an approximate 20-25% chance of having an inherited predisposition to breast cancer and ovarian cancer and for whom genetic risk assessment is recommended:
• Women with a personal history of both breast cancer and ovarian cancer[a]
• Women with ovarian cancera and a close relative[a] with ovarian cancer or premenopausal breast cancer
• Women with ovarian cancer[a] who are of Ashkenazi Jewish ancestry

Contd.

Contd.

• Women with breast cancer at age 50 years or younger and a close relative[a] with ovarian cancer[b] or male breast cancer at any age
• Women of Ashkenazi Jewish ancestry in whom breast cancer was diagnosed at age 40 years or younger
• Women with a close relative[b] with a known *BRCA1* or *BRCA2* mutation
Patients with greater than approximate 5%-10% chance of having an inherited predisposition to breast cancer and ovarian cancer and for whom genetic risk assessment may be helpful:
• Women with breast cancer at age 40 years or younger
• Women with ovarian cancer, primary peritoneal cancer, or fallopian tube cancer of high grade, serous histology at any age
• Women with bilateral breast cancer (particularly if the first case of breast cancer was diagnosed at age 50 years or younger)
• Women with breast cancer at age 50 years or younger and a close relative[b] with breast cancer at age 50 years or younger
• Women of Ashkenazi Jewish ancestry with breast cancer at age 50 years or younger
• Women with breast cancer at any age and two or more close relatives[b] with breast cancer at any age (particularly if at least one case of breast cancer was diagnosed at age 50 years or younger)
• Unaffected women with a close relativeb who meets one of the previous criteria
a Cancer of the peritoneum and fallopian tubes should be considered a part of the spectrum of the hereditary breast and ovarian cancer syndrome b Close relative is defined as a first-degree relative (mother, sister, daughter) or second degree relative (grandmother, granddaughter, aunt, niece)

Table 1.5: Risk-Reduction Recommendation for Carriers of *BRCA1* and *BRCA2* Mutations
Breast
• Annual mammography and annual breast MRI starting by age 30
• RRSO to reduce breast cancer risk between age 35 and 40 and when childbearing is complete
• Consider chemoprevention with tamoxifen, raloxifene, or an aromatase inhibitor
• Consider RRM
Ovary/Fallopian Tube
• RRSO to reduce ovarian and fallopian tube cancer risk between age 35 and 40 and when childbearing is complete
• Consider chemoprevention with oral contraceptives
• Consider ovarian cancer screening with every 6 month transvaginal ultrasound and CA-125 from age 30-35 years until definitive risk-reduction with RRSO
RRSO, risk-reducing salpingo-oophorectomy; R.R.M, risk-reducing mastectomy

HEREDITARY NONPOLYPOSIS COLORECTAL CANCER (HNPCC) OR LYNCH SYNDROME

- Hereditary nonpolyposis colorectal cancer (HNPCC) or Lynch syndrome has a high **risk of colon cancer (40-60%) as well as other cancers including endometrial (second most common), ovarian, stomach, small intestine, genitourinary and hepatobiliary tract cancers**
- Lifetime risk of any Lynch syndrome associated cancer is about 75%
- It is an **autosomal dominant** genetic condition
- Women with HNPCC (Lynch II syndrome) have lifetime risk of about **50% for endometrial cancer and 12% for ovarian cancer**
- Average age at diagnosis is **40 years**
- Mutations in **the DNA mismatch repair (MMR) genes MLH1, MSH2, MSH6 or PMS2** account for more than 95% of mutations found in Lynch syndrome
- MSH2 located on chromosome 2p16 and MLH1 locates on chromosome 3p21 are the two most common Lynch syndrome associated mutation
- **Criteria for risk assessment for Lynch syndrome and risk reduction recommendations for women with Lynch syndrome are given in Tables 1.6 and 1.7**

Table 1.6: Society of Gynecologic Oncologists Criteria for Offering Genetic Risk Assessment for Lynch Syndrome
Patients with greater than approximately 20%-25% chance of having Lynch syndrome and for whom genetic risk assessment is recommended:
• Patients with endometrial or colorectal cancer who meet the revised Amsterdam criteria as listed below:
– At least three relatives with a sentinel Lynch associated cancer (colorectal cancer, cancer of the endometrium, small bowel, ureter, or renal pelvis) in one lineage;
– One affected individual should be a first-degree relative of the other two;
– At least 2 successive generations should be affected
– At least 1 Lynch-associated cancer should be diagnosed before age 50
• Patients with synchronous or metachronous endometrial and colorectal cancer with the first cancer diagnosed prior to age 50
• Patients with synchronous or metachronous ovarian and colorectal cancer with the first cancer diagnosed prior to age 50
• Patients with colorectal or endometrial cancer with evidence of a mismatch repair defect (i.e., microsatellite instability (MSI) or immunohistochemical loss of expression of *MLH1, MSH2, MSH6,* or *PMS2*)
• Patients with a first-or second-degree relative with a known mismatch repair gene mutation
Patients with greater than approximately 5%-10% chance of having Lynch syndrome and for whom genetic risk assessment may be helpful:
• Patients with endometrial or colorectal cancer diagnosed prior to age 50
• Patient with endometrial or ovarian cancer with a synchronous or metachronous colon or other Lynch syndrome-associated tumor[a] at any age
• Patients with endometrial or colorectal cancer and a first-degree relative with a Lynch syndrome-associated tumor[a] diagnosed prior to age 50
• Patients with colorectal or endometrial cancer diagnosed at any age with two or more first of second degree-relatives[b] with Lynch syndrome-associated tumors[a], regardless of age
• Patients with a first or second-degree relative[b] that meets the above criteria
a Lynch-associated tumors include colorectal, stomach, ovarian, pancreas, ureter and renal pelvis, biliary tract, and brain (usually glioblastoma as seen in Turcot syndrome) tumors, sebaceous gland adenomas and liceratoacanthomas in Muir-Torre syndrome, and carcinoma of the small bowel
b First and second-degree relatives are parents, sibling, children, aunts, uncles, niece, nephews, grandparents and grandchildren

Table 1.7: Risk-reduction recommendations for Women with Lynch Syndrome
Gastrointestinal
• Colonoscopy every 1-2 years beginning at age 20-25 (or age 30 for women with MSH6 mutations)
• Consider esophagogastroduodenoscopy (EGD) every 2-3 years beginning at age 30-35
• Consider capsule endoscopy every 2-3 years beginning at age 30-35
• Consider chemoprevention with aspirin or NSAIDs
Gynecologic
• Patients should be aware that abnormal vaginal bleeding warrants evaluation
• Consider screening with annual endometrial biopsy and transvaginal ultrasound beginning at age 30
• Consider chemoprevention with oral contraceptives or progestins
• Consider risk-reducing hysterectomy with bilateral salpingo-oophorectomy between age 35 and 40 and when childbearing is complete
Urologic
• Consider annual urinalysis starting at age 25-30

OTHER RARE SYNDROMES: Cowden Syndrome, Li-Fraumeni syndrome and Peutz-Jeghers syndrome are rare autosomal dominant inherited cancer syndromes that include gynecologic cancers as part of their cancer spectrum

A. Cowden Syndrome

- It is caused by germline mutations in the ***PTEN* gene**
- Individuals with Cowden Syndrome are at increased risk for both **benign and malignant** processes that include **gastrointestinal polyps, thyroid disease, benign breast disease, mucocutaneous lesions, as well as breast, thyroid, and endometrial cancer**
- The lifetime risk of **endometrial cancer** in a woman with Cowden syndrome is about be **5-28%**

- Current guidelines recommend **observation for and prompt evaluation of abnormal uterine bleeding in women with Cowden syndrome**
- Screening with endometrial biopsies and/or ultrasound measurement of the endometrial thickness is being evaluated in ongoing research studies

B. Li-Fraumeni Syndrome

- Caused by germline mutations in ***TP53***
- It is characterized by **early-onset breast cancer, soft tissue and bone sarcomas, adrenal cortical tumors and brain tumors**
- Cases of ovarian cancer have been reported in women with **Li-Fraumeni syndrome**
- **Screening breast MRI** is recommended, beginning at age 20 to 25
- There are **no current screening recommendations for gynecologic cancers** in women with Li-Fraumeni syndrome

C. Peutz-Jeghers Syndrome

- It is caused by germline mutations in ***STK11***
- Peutz-Jeghers is generally **characterized by multiple gastro-intestinal polyps and pigmented lesions on the lips and buccal mucosa**
- Women with this syndrome also have a markedly **increased risk for gastrointestinal and breast malignancies**
- Gynecologic cancers associated with this syndrome include **sex cord-stromal tumors with annular tubules (SCTAT) of the ovary and adenoma malignum of the cervix**
  - **SCTAT are typically benign and bilateral**
  - **Adenoma malignum of the cervix** is a rare and aggressive neoplasm, often difficult to diagnose both clinically and histologically. On imaging, the tumor appears as a multicystic endocervical mass. Histologically, the tumor appears well differentiated, but the natural history can be aggressive.
- Due to the rarity of the syndrome and the gynecologic cancers, it is **unclear whether women with Peutz-Jeghers should be screened**
- Yearly **pelvic exam and Pap smear beginning at age 25** have been recommended. However, the role of pelvic imaging is unclear

RECENT UPDATES

CRITERIA TO IDENTIFY FAMILIES LIKELY TO HAVE LYNCH SYNDROME

A. Amsterdam Criteria

- ***Amsterdam criteria*** are a set *of diagnostic criteria used to help identify families, which are likely to have* **Lynch syndrome**, *developed in Amsterdam, in 1990*
- *The initial Amsterdam criteria were a series of clinical criteria known as the "3-2-1" rule, formulated to serve as a common starting point for future research into the genetics underlying the syndrome. The criteria were as follows:*
  1. *At least 3 relatives with histologically confirmed colorectal cancer, 1 of whom is a first degree relative of the other 2; familial adenomatous polyposis should be excluded*
  2. *At least 2 successive generations involved*
  3. *At least 1 of the cancers diagnosed before age 50*

The criteria were expanded in 1998 to include the ***associated non-colorectal cancers****, termed as the* ***Amsterdam II clinical criteria*** *for families with Lynch syndrome*

B. Amsterdam II Criteria

Each of the following criteria must be fulfilled:

- *3* or more relatives with an associated cancer (*colorectal cancer, or cancer of the endometrium, small intestine, ureter or renal pelvis), 1 should be a first-degree relative of the other two*
- *2* or more *successive generations affected*
- *1* or more relatives diagn*osed before the age of 50 years*
- *Familial adenomatous polyposis* (FAP) should be excluded i*n cases of colorectal carcinoma*
- *Tumors should be verified by pathologic examination*

C. Bethesda Guidelines

The National Cancer Institute (NCI) published recommendations in 1997 and revised them in 2004 for identification of individuals who should receive genetic testing for Lynch syndrome related tumors

The Revised Bethesda Guidelines are as follows

- *Colorectal carcinoma (CRC) diagnosed in a patient who is less than 50 years old*
- *Presence of synchronous (at the same time) or metachronous (at another time) CRC or other Lynch syndrome-associated tumors, regardless of age*
- *CRC with high microsatellite instability histology diagnosed in a patient less than 60 years old;*
- *CRC diagnosed in one or more first-degree relatives with a Lynch syndrome-associated tumor, with one of the cancers being diagnosed at less than 50 years of age*
- *CRC diagnosed in two or more first-degree or second-degree relatives with Lynch syndrome-associated tumors, regardless of age*

The Revised Bethesda Guidelines have been reported to be more sensitive than Amsterdam II Criteria in detecting individuals and families at risk of Lynch syndrome

Role of Endometrial Cancer Abnormal MMR Protein in Screening Lynch-Syndrome (LS) Families

- *LS is caused by genetic mutation in one of the DNA mismatch repair (MMR) genes such as MLH1, MSH2, MSH6 or PMS2*
- *MMR gene defect leads to loss of MMR function and results in accumulation of mutations in (coding and non-coding) microsatellites (termed as microsatellite instability; MSI)*
- *The frequency of LS-associated genetic mutations in endometrial cancers is 1.8- 2 %, which is similar to the frequency of LS in colorectal cancer.*
- ***Immunohistochemical staining (IHC) can be used to detect the loss of MMR protein expression and determine the identity of the mutated gene***
- *IHC testing of MMR proteins plays an important role in screening LS and the routine testing of MMR proteins in endometrial cancer can contribute to the screening of LS families (Flow chart 1.1)*

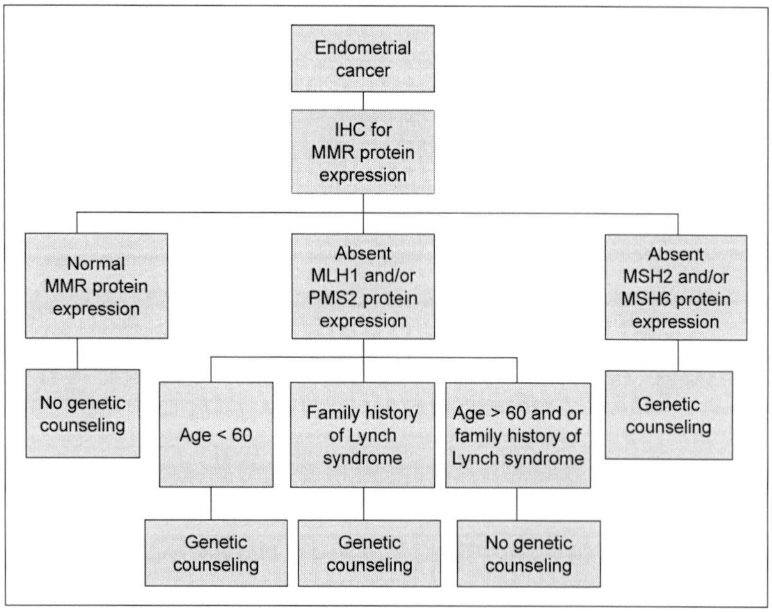

IHC – Immunohistochemistry; MMR-Mismatch repair gene

Flow chart 1.1: Role of endometrial cancer abnormal MMR protein in screening Lynch-syndrome (LS) families

CHAPTER 2

ENDOMETRIAL HYPERPLASIA AND ENDOMETRIAL CANCER

INTRODUCTION

- Carcinoma endometrium is the **most common genital malignancy among females in developed countries. North America and Europe have the highest incidence**
- In **developing countries** like India, **it ranks third amongst genital malignancies next to cervical and ovarian carcinoma**
- **Common reasons for increased prevalence of endometrial carcinoma in developed countries include obesity and increased life expectancy**
- **Differential diagnosis for post menopausal bleeding (PMB) and various uterine causes of post menopausal bleeding are given in table 2.1 and 2.2**

Table 2.1: Differential Diagnosis for Post Menopausal Bleeding

Malignant causes	Benign causes
• Endometrial carcinoma • Endometrial hyperplasia • Cervical carcinoma • Estrogen-producing ovarian tumors • Vaginal and vulvar cancers (rare)	• Atrophic endometritis • Endometrial polyp • Atrophic vaginitis • Local lesions on cervix – cervicitis, cervical polyp, erosion etc.,

Table 2.2: Uterine Causes of Postmenopausal Bleeding

Cause	Percent (%)
Endometrial atrophy	60–80 (**Most common**)
Endometrial hyperplasia	5–10
Endometrial cancer	10
Estrogen replacement therapy	15–25
Endometrial polyps	2–12

Note

- ***Atrophic endometrium** is the **most common uterine cause of PMB***
- ***Endometrial carcinoma** accounts for **10% of uterine cause for PMB***

Endometrial carcinoma progresses through premalignant phase of endometrial hyperplasia (Endometrial intraepithelial neoplasia (EIN)) in a large proportion of cases

Endometrial hyperplasia and endometrial carcinoma are described in subsequent text

ENDOMETRIAL HYPERPLASIA

- It is a **premalignant disease of the endometrium** characterized by **abnormal proliferation of the endometrial glands and stroma**
- **Most common age group : 40 -55 years (perimenopausal) age group**
- **Most common risk factor : prolonged unopposed estrogen exposure** such as in Follicular cysts of ovary, PCOD, Hormone replacement therapy, hormone secreting ovarian tumors (Granulosa cell and theca cell tumors); also associated with glucose intolerance

- **Clinical presentation**
  - **Peri menopausal** women present with **Abnormal uterine bleeding (AUB)**
  - **Post menopausal women** present with **postmenopausal bleeding (PMB)**

  Classification of endometrial hyperplasia (Table 2.3)
- Histopathologically, Endometrial hyperplasia are classified **based on the Architecture and Cellular Atypia** as follows

World Health Organisation 1994 (WHO 94) classification

- Imple hyperplasia
- Complex hyperplasia
- Simple hyperplasia with atypia
- Complex hyperplasia with atypia

In 2014 the WHO published a new, simplified WHO classification of endometrial hyperplasia, which consists of only two categories of hyperplasia: with and without atypia, as opposed to four found in the WHO 94 classification. This reduction to two categories was due to the need to do away with the confusing multitude of terms currently in use.

New WHO 2014 classification of endometrial hyperplasia

- **Non-atypical endometrial hyperplasia (benign hyperplasia)**
- **Atypical endometrial hyperplasia or Endometrial Intraepithelial Neoplasia (EIN)/well differentiated carcinoma**

According to ACOG guidelines (2015), the preferred terminology is "endometrial intraepithelial neoplasia" (rather than "atypical endometrial hyperplasia"). RCOG guidelines (2016) recommend the WHO 2014 classification and present clear algorithms for hyperplasia (with or without atypia) treatment Risk of progression of endometrial hyperplasia to endometrial carcinoma are mentioned Table 2.4

Table 2.3: Histopathology Features in Simple and Complex Hyperplasia

Simple hyperplasia	Complex hyperplasia
Glands are large, cystic with increased glands/stromal ratio (cystoglandular hyperplasia)	Glands number and size increased and glands are thrown into folds (overcrowding of glands)
Scanty mitosis	Numerous mitosis
Stroma is sparsely cellular	Stroma is densely cellular
Simple and complex hyperplasia may be with or without nuclear atypia	
Characteristic Features of nuclear atypia	
• Cell is large in size and irregular • Loss of polarity • Hyperchromatic nucleus and prominent nucleoli • Altered nuclear cytoplasmic ratio	

Table 2.4: Risk of Progression Of Endometrial Hyperplasia to Carcinoma

Type of Hyperplasia	Risk of Progression to Endometrial Carcinoma (%)	Regression (%)
Simple hyperplasia without atypia	1	80
Complex atypia without atypia	3	80
Simple hyperplasia with atypia	8	60
Complex hyperplasia with atypia	29	50

Management of Endometrial Hyperplasia

- Management depends mainly on the **type of endometrial hyperplasia and the age** of the patient
- **High dose progesterone therapy** is found to be effective in reversing hyperplasia with or without atypia.

RCOG 2016 Guidelines on Management of Endometrial Hyperplasia

i. **Management of endometrial hyperplasia without atypia (Table 2.5)**
   - **Hyperplasia without atypia at all ages** can be treated with **progesterone therapy**
   - Both **continuous oral progesterones** [medroxyprogesterone acetate or norethisterone] and **Levonorgestrel – IUD (LNG-IUD) are effective**

Table 2.5: Management of Endometrial Hyperplasia without Atypia

Management in Premenopausal women	Management in Postmenopausal women
LNG-IUD or continuous oral progesterones (Medroxy Progesterone acetate (MPA) or Norethisterone 10–20 mg/day) are prescribed for 6 months	Progesterone therapy can be given as in premenopausal women
Assessment of response to Medical therapy • **Endometrial sampling is repeated after 6 months** to assess response to therapy • Repeat sampling usually shows **histological regression of endometrial hyperplasia in majority of cases**	
• Cases with **persistence of hyperplasia are treated with high-dose progesterones**—MPA 200 mg/day or Megestrol acetate 160 mg/day • In case of **refractoriness to therapy, hysterectomy is done** **Indications for hysterectomy in cases with endometrial hyperplasia without atypia** • Progression to atypical hyperplasia during follow up • No histological regression of hyperplasia despite 12 months of therapy • Persistence of bleeding symptoms • Relapse of endometrial hyperplasia after completing progesterone treatment • Refusal by the woman to undergo endometrial surveillance or comply with medical treatment	

ii. Management of endometrial hyperplasia with atypia (Table 2.6)

Hyperplasia with atypia is **usually a complex hyperplasia. Management of endometrial hyperplasia with atypia is described in Table 2.6**

Table 2.6: Management of Endometrial Hyperplasia with Atypia

Management in Premenopausal women		Management in Postmenopausal women
Women who have completed family	**Younger women desirous of future childbearing**	
Hysterectomy is the treatment of choice for following reasons: • **Associated endometrial carcinoma** may be present in **40%** of women • There is increased risk of progression to endometrial carcinoma	• **LNG-IUD or high-dose continuous progesterone therapy may be prescribed for 9 months** • Patient is counseled about risks of underlying malignancy and subsequent progression to endometrial cancer. **Assessment of response to medical therapy** • Endometrial sampling every 3 months is mandatory to assess response to therapy • **If there is regression of endometrial hyperplasia,** the patient is kept under surveillance with periodic endometrial sampling. Hysterectomy is performed on completion of family • **If there is no regression,** hysterectomy is done.	**Hysterectomy is the treatment of choice**

Extra Edge

Salient points from the RCOG 2016 recommendations on Management of Endometrial hyperplasia (Table 2.7)

Table 2.7: RCOG 2016 Recommendations on Management of Endometrial Hyperplasia

Endometrial hyperplasia without atypia	*Women with atypical endometrial hyperplasia*
• ***LNG-IUD should be the first-line therapy*** *because it has a higher disease regression rate, more favorable bleeding profile, and fewer adverse effects when compared with oral progesterones.* • ***Cyclical progesterones should not be used*** *because they are less effective in inducing regression of endometrial hyperplasia without atypia.* • ***Treatment with oral progesterones or the LNG-IUD should be for a minimum of 6 months*** *in order to induce histological regression of endometrial hyperplasia without atypia.* • ***Endometrial ablation is not recommended for the treatment of endometrial hyperplasia*** *because complete and persistent endometrial destruction cannot be ensured, and intrauterine adhesion formation may preclude future endometrial histological surveillance.* • ***Hysterectomy should not be considered as a first-line treatment for hyperplasia without atypia*** *because progesterone therapy induces histological and symptomatic remission in the majority of women, and avoids the morbidity associated with major surgery.*	• *Women with* ***atypical hyperplasia should undergo a total hysterectomy*** *because of risk of underlying malignancy or progression to cancer* • ***Women desirous of further childbearing,*** *who are treated conservatively and having evidence of histological regression of the disease, should be followed up with endometrial biopsy every 6–12 months, until hysterectomy is performed*

ENDOMETRIAL CARCINOMA

- **Most common gynecological cancer in developed countries**
- Mean age at diagnosis is **60 years (55-70 years)**
- Most **common histological type is endometriod carcinoma**
- Most cases **present in early stages with AUB or PMB**
- Most common **route of spread is direct spread**
- **Risk factors and protective factors for endometrial carcinoma are given in Table 2.8**

Table 2.8: Risk Factors for Endometrial Carcinoma

Characteristic	Relative risk
Nulliparity	2-3
Late menopause (> 52 years)	2-4
Obesity	
• 21-50 lb overweight	3
• >50 lb overweight	10
Diabetes mellitus	2-8
Unopposed estrogen therapy such as (HRT)	4-8
Tamoxifen therapy	2-3
Atypical endometrial hyperplasia	8-29
Hereditary Non Polyposis colorectal cancer (HNPCC) syndrome	20
FACTORS THAT REDUCE THE RISK FOR ENDOMETRIAL CARCINOMA	
• Early age at menopause	
• Multi parity	
• Oral contraceptive pill (OCPs) usage–**OCPs reduce Endometrial cancer risk by 40%;** protection increases with duration of usage and protection lasts even 10 years after discontinuation of OCPs	
• Consumption of a high- fiber diet	
• Physical activity	

Note

- ***Corpus cancer syndrome***– *it refer to* ***combination of DM, obesity, and hypertension*** *in association with carcinoma endometrium*
- *About* ***5% of endometrial cancers are hereditary****. Majority of the hereditary endometrial cancers occur as a* ***part of Lynch II syndrome or Hereditary Non Polyposis colorectal cancer (HNPCC) syndrome*** *(autosomal dominant)*
- *Among women belonging to families with the* ***hereditary HNPCC syndrome, the most common extra-colonic malignancy is endometrial carcinoma***
- *Lifetime risk of endometrial carcinoma in HNPCC is 40- 60%*

Classification of Endometrial Carcinoma

Endometrial cancers can be **Type I or type II.** The pathogenesis and clinical behavior are different in these two types of endometrial cancers (Table 2.9)

Table 2.9: Types of Endometrial Cancers

	Type I Endometrial Carcinoma	Type II Endometrial Carcinoma
Characteristics		
Risk factors	Pre and perimenopausal women with hyperestrogenism, obesity, DM	Elderly postmenopausal women
Role of estrogen	Linked to excess estrogen stimulation	Develops from atrophic endometrium
Incidence	80%	20%
Race	White > Black	White = Black
Differentiation	Well differentiated	Poorly differentiated
Histology	Endometrioid	Non endometrioid (serous, clear cell type)
Stage at diagnosis	Early stages	Late stages
Prognosis	Good	Aggressive and poor prognosis

Contd.

Contd.

Molecular Features		
Ploidy	Diploid	Aneuploid
Associated gene alteration	**pTEN, K-ras**	**p53, p16, HER2/neu** (p53 mutation- shown to play a pivoted role in serous endometrial cancers
Microsatellite instability	**Yes - MLH1/MSH6**	**No**

Histopathological Types

- **Histopathological examination** of endometrium is the **gold standard** for diagnosis of endometrial cancer.
- **Endometrial sampling is obtained** by office **endometrial biopsy, Dilatation and curettage (D and C), fractional curettage or hysteroscopic biopsy**
- **The various histopathological types and grades of endometrial carcinoma are mentioned in Table 2.10**

Table 2.10: Histological Types of Endometrial Carcinoma (WHO classification)

Type	Incidence	Description
Endometrioid carcinoma (adenocarcinoma)	80-85 %	Composed of glands that resemble normal endometrial glands but contain more solid areas, less glandular formation, and more cytologic atypia; well differentiated **(Most common histological type)**
Adenocarcinoma variants		
Endometrial carcinoma with squamous differentiation	15-25%	Tumors with benign-appearing squamous elements (termed adenoacanthomas) and with malignant-looking squamous elements (termed adenosquamous carcinomas); well differentiated
Villoglandular variant	2%	Endometrial cells with characteristics of endometrioid cells, arranged in papillary fibrovascular stalks; well-differentiated
Secretory variant	5%	50% of cells have intracytoplasmic mucin; mostly well-differentiated
Other types		
Papillary Serous adenocarcinoma	3-4 %	Endometrial carcinoma that **resemble serous carcinoma of the ovary and fallopian tube;** very aggressive, poor prognosis **Associated with BRCA1 and BRCA 2 mutations in 5-10%**
Clear cell adenocarcinoma	<5%	Common in older women; very aggressive, poor prognosis Mixed histologic pattern; **Hobnail cells seen**
Squamous	< 1 %	Seen in older women and cervical stenosis; **very poor prognosis** Generally pure cell type, some with glands
Undifferentiated carcinoma	<1%	Poor prognosis
Mixed carcinoma		Carcinoma composed of more than one type, with at least 10% of each component

Apart from the classification of endometrial carcinoma, carcinoma of the endometrium comprising of mixed epithelial and mesenchymal tumors including:

1. Adenomyoma
2. Atypical polypoid adenomyoma
3. Adenofibroma
4. Adenosarcoma
5. Carcinosarcoma: currently carcinosarcomas, in which **both epithelial and mesenchymal components are malignant and aggressive tumors,** are currently considered metaplastic carcinomas, and are treated as aggressive carcinomas

Contd.

Contd.

Histopathological degree of differentiation

Grade	Description
G1	5% or less of nonsquamous or nonmorular solid growth pattern
G2	6% to 50% of nonsquamous or nonmorular solid growth pattern
G3	More than 50% of nonsquamous or nonmorular solid growth pattern
Clear cell and serous adenocarcinomas–***are considered as high grade***	
Adenocarcinoma with squamous differentiation–***grading is allocated according to the nuclear grading of glandular component***	

Note

- ***Endometrioid adenocarcinoma is the most common subtype of endometrial cancer***
- ***Clear cell carcinoma and serous carcinoma are highly malignant***
- ***Serous and clear cell tumors deeply invade the myometrium*** *and there is a* ***propensity for peritoneal spread***
- *Due to the propensity for peritoneal spread,* ***peritoneal biopsy and omental biopsy are taken during surgical staging in Serous and clear cell endometrial tumors***
- ***Serous and clear cell tumors are more likely to have extrauterine spread*** *and* ***preoperative CA-125 and/or imaging is warranted***
- ***If an endometrial carcinoma manifests two or more different cell types****, each representing at least 10% or more of the tumor, it is termed as* ***'mixed cell type'***
- ***Incidence of synchronous endometrial cancer and ovarian cancer is 1.5–3.5%.*** *In most of the cases, both endometrial and ovarian cancers are* ***well-differentiated adenocarcinoma*** *with excellent prognosis.* ***Primary site is assigned to the area having the largest tumor mass and most advanced stage***

Clinical Presentation of Endometrial Carcinoma

- Most common age group 55-70 years
- Abnormal uterine bleeding
- Postmenopausal bleeding
- Brown watery offensive discharge
- Pelvic pain/ discomfort
- Uterus may be bulky or enlarged on palpation
- In older women, cervical stenosis may lead to development of pyometra

Note

- *Endometrial cancer* ***presents in early stages with vaginal bleeding****; therefore, most cases are stage I or II at diagnosis*
- ***Simpson's pain*** *- Unique nature of pain seen in about* ***15% cases with endometrial carcinoma.*** *Pain is mild, appears at the* ***same time every day lasting for 1–2 hours****, in* ***hypogastric region*** *and bilateral iliac fossa. This pain is* ***attributed to expulsive nature of uterine contraction***

Diagnosis

- **Initial evaluation of postmenopausal bleeding is to perform a Transvaginal sonography (TVS)** to assess **endometrial thickness (ET).** TVS can also identify endometrial polyps, pyometra and other pelvic pathology
  - **USG characteristics suspicious of endometrial carcinoma**
    - Endometrial thickness **≥5 mm in a postmenopausal woman** – Postmenopausal ET ≥5 mm is taken as **cut off for endometrial sampling** (TVS is an effective test with **high negative predictive value** when **ET is < 5 mm in PMB**)
    - Non homogenous echo texture of endometrium
    - Irregular and poorly defined margins
    - Polypoidal endometrial growth
    - Fluid collection within the endometrium
- **Endometrial biopsy or endometrial aspiration along with endocervical sampling** is performed as Outpatient procedure using **Vabra aspirator/ Pipelle/ Novak curette.** This procedure requires no cervical dilatation or anesthesia and has high

sensitivity and specificity. **Endocervical and endometrial samples are sent for histopathology** (Endocervical sampling is done to rule out endocervical extension of endometrial cancer or a primary endocervical cancer)

- **TVS + endometrial biopsy has a negative predictive value of 96%**
- **Fractional curettage is done** in women with high index of suspicion, **if the results of endometrial sampling is negative or tissue obtained is inadequate**
  - **Indications for Fractional curettage or Dilatation and curettage (D and C)**
    - Recurrent bleeding with negative endometrial sampling
    - Recurrent bleeding with ET <5 mm
    - Complex atypical hyperplasia in endometrial sampling
- **Pap smear is sensitive only in 50% cases of endometrial carcinoma** (However, Pap smear is indicated in all cases presenting with perimenopausal or postmenopausal bleeding, to rule out carcinoma cervix; if cervix has an obvious growth, cervical biopsy is taken)
- **Role of hysteroscopy**
  - **Fluid distension media** used in hysteroscopy can cause **dissemination of cancer cells intraperitoneal cavity.** Hence, it is **not recommended in suspected endometrial carcinoma**
  - **Hysteroscopy directed biopsy** is done if USG shows **focal endometrial abnormalities or in women with diagnostic uncertainty**

Management of Endometrial Carcinoma

After a histopathological diagnosis of endometrial carcinoma, investigations are done to assess the local extent of tumor, evidence of metastatic disease and perioperative risk

Pretreatment Evaluation

- **Ultrasound abdomen and pelvis** – to look for Myometrial invasion, extension to cervix and Ovarian metastasis, ascites, Liver metastasis and Pelvic and para-aortic lymphadenopathy (USG is less sensitive than CT/ MRI)
- **CT/ MRI** – to assess myometrial invasion, parametrial extension and lymph node metastasis (NOTE- PET-CT is the best imaging method to evaluate lymph nodes and distant metastasis and should be considered in advanced stage diseases)
- **Chest X-ray** – look for pulmonary metastasis
- **Renal and liver function tests**
- **CA 125** – may be elevated in patients with **high grade tumors and in Papillary serous and clear cell endometrial carcinoma;** imaging studies of abdomen, pelvis and chest should be performed if CA 125 is elevated
- **Barium enema and colonoscopy –** done in cases with suspected HNPCC
- **Cystoscopy/ proctoscopy –** if extension to bladder or rectum suspected

Prognostic Tumor Characteristics for High-Risk endometrial carcinoma
Four main histopathologic criteria are recommended to determine high-risk disease: • Tumor grade 3 (poorly differentiated). • Lymphovascular space invasion. • Non endometrioid histology (serous, clear cell, undifferentiated, anaplastic, etc.) • Cervical stromal involvement. **MRI scanning and intraoperative frozen section represent the most accurate means of assessing the depth of myometrial invasion and cervical involvement**

Staging of Carcinoma Endometrium (FIGO, 2009) (Table 2.11 and Fig. 2.1)

Endometrial cancer is **surgically staged.** Clinical staging significantly under stages the disease and is done only in women who are not fit for surgery

Table 2.11: Staging of Carcinoma Endometrium (FIGO, 2009)

Stage I	**Confined to corpus uteri**
1A	No or < less than half of myometrium is involved
1B	Invasion of >= more than or equal to half of myometrium
Stage II	**Involves cervical stroma but does not extend beyond uterus**
Stage III	**Local and / or regional spread of tumor**
IIIA	Involves serosa/adnexa
IIIB	Vaginal/parametrial involvement
IIIC	Metastasis to pelvic and para-aortic nodes
IIIC1	Positive pelvic nodes
IIIC2	Positive para-aortic nodes with/without positive pelvic nodes
Stage IV	**Involves bladder and/or bowel mucosa and/or distant metastasis**
IVA	Involves bladder or bowel mucosa
IV B	Distant metastasis including intra- abdominal metastasis/ inguinal nodes

Note

- ***All stages can be either grade 1, 2 or 3***
- ***Endocervical glandular involvement -Stage I***
- ***Endocervical stromal involvement -Stage II***
- ***Positive peritoneal cytology is reported separately, not included in staging***

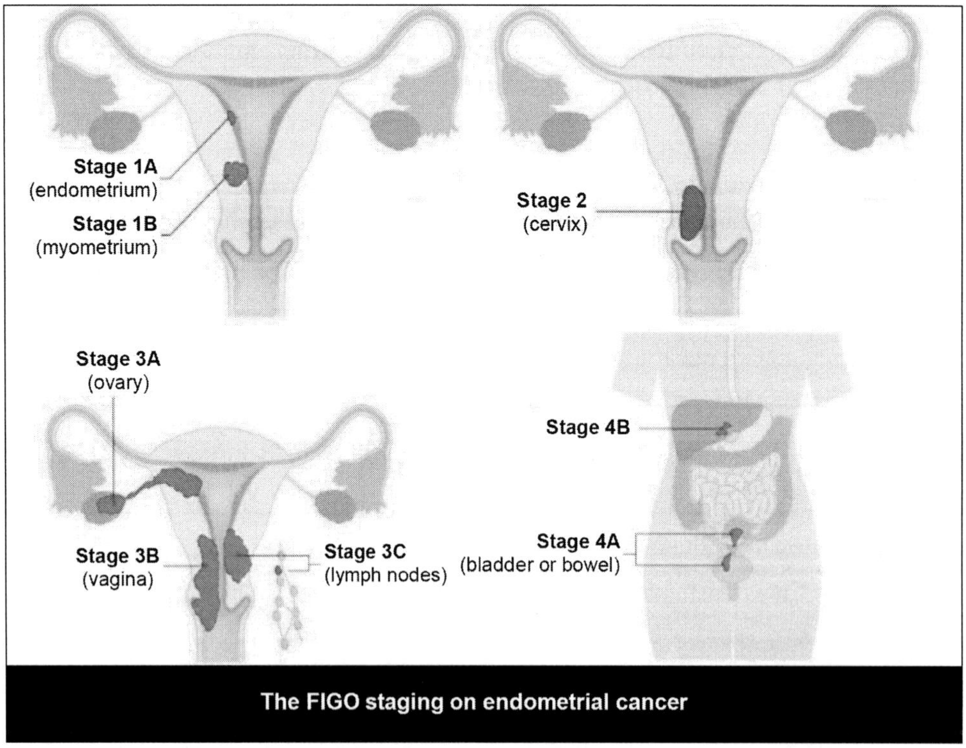

Fig. 2.1: FIGO Staging of Carcinoma Endometrium (FIGO 2009)

Surgical Staging Procedure for Endometrial Carcinoma

Steps of Surgical Staging
• **Midline vertical** incision is given
• Ascitic fluid is collected for cytology. If there is no ascites, **peritoneal wash** with 50–100 mL of normal saline is done and the peritoneal washings are collected **for cytology**

Contd.

Contd.

• **Systematic exploration of the abdomen and pelvis is done**–Paracolic gutters, ascending colon, hepatic flexure, liver, under surface of diaphragm, transverse colon, splenic flexure and spleen, descending colon, omentum, and adnexal surfaces should be inspected and palpated for possible metastasis. This is followed by palpation of any enlarged nodes in pelvic and para aortic region
• **Any suspicious area should be biopsied**
• **Extrafascial hysterectomy and bilateral salpingo-oophorectomy** is performed
• **Uterus specimen should be cut opened to assess tumor size, depth of myometrial invasion, and cervical extension**
• Pelvic and paraaortic lymphadenectomy is recommended in all cases **except in Stage IA (Myometrial involvement < 50%) Grade 1 endometriod carcinoma, with Tumor size of <2 cm**
• **Infracolic omentectomy, peritoneal biopsies** and **diaphragmatic scrapings** should be done **in cases with serous, clear cell and mixed Mullerian tumors** (due to high propensity of intra- abdominal spread and upper abdominal recurrence)

Indications for Pelvic and Para Aortic Lymph Node Sampling

- **Clear cell, serous and squamous tumors**
- **Endometrioid tumors with:**
  - Myometrial invasion >50% (Stage > IA)
  - G2 and G3 histology
  - Tumor size > 2 cm
  - Cervical stromal involvement
  - Extra uterine spread (adnexal or pelvic extension of disease)

Note
• *Pelvic and para-aortic lymphadenectomy is indicated in all cases **except in Stage IA (Myometrial involvement < 50%) Grade 1 endometriod carcinoma with Tumor size of <2 cm***
• *Currently, sentinel lymph node mapping has been introduced into surgical staging of endometrial carcinoma to reduce the morbidity associated with lymphadenectomy and to obtain prognostic information from lymph node status*

Treatment of Endometrial Carcinoma (Table 2.12)

Table 2.12: Treatment of Endometrial Carcinoma

Stage	Treatment
Stage I	**Extrafascial hysterectomy + B/L salpingo- oophorectomy + pelvic and para–aortic lymph node sampling followed by Post operative adjuvant radiotherapy**
Stage II	**Two options are available:** **Initial surgical staging followed by RT (best approach)** • Modified radical hysterectomy + bilateral salpingo-oophorectomy + pelvic and para-aortic lymphadenectomy is performed followed by Post operative radiotherapy **Initial RT followed by surgery** – indicated in patients who are unsuitable for extensive surgery (obese, elderly, medical problems) • The preferred approach is initial radiotherapy followed within 6 weeks by a less extensive surgery (TAH with BSO)
Stage III	Surgery is performed to determine extent of the disease and to remove the tumor bulk, if possible. **Preferred treatment is Surgical debulking of the tumor, pelvic and para-aortic lymphadenectomy, peritoneal biopsy from suspicious areas, and infracolic omentectomy followed by Post-operative adjuvant radiotherapy + chemotherapy** **Extension to pelvic side walls** –indicates inoperable tumor → Primary treatment with RT -> exploratory laparotomy may be considered
Stage IV	Primary aim is to provide **palliative relief** of bleeding and complications involving bladder and rectum Usually involves a **combination of cytoreductive surgery, chemotherapy, radiotherapy and systemic hormonal therapy** • **Patients with extra abdominal metastasis -> chemotherapy or hormonal therapy (if receptor positive)** • **RT provides local control in patients with vaginal bleeding, pain, tumor mass and leg edema due to lymph node involvement**

Adjuvant Therapy

- **A postoperative treatment plan should take into account the following**
  - The prognostic factors determined by the surgical-pathologic staging
  - The available postoperative treatment modalities and their morbidities
- **Patients can be classified into three categories**
  - Cases with high rate of cure without postoperative therapy
  - Cases with low rate of cure without postoperative therapy
  - Cases with reduced rate of surgical cure and may benefit from additional therapy
- **Vaginal brachytherapy and external beam pelvic RT with/without an extended field RT is commonly employed as post operative adjuvant therapy**
- **Chemotherapy is recently supported as an adjuvant treatment for patients with stage III and Stage IV endometrial carcinoma**
- **Serous and clear cell cancers** tend **to spread in a fashion similar to ovarian cancer,** with a high propensity for upper abdominal relapse. **Whole abdomen RT along with systemic chemotherapy is required in these cases**

Post Surgical Radiotherapy Based on Surgical-Pathological Staging (Table 2.13):

- **Radiation therapy remains the standard adjuvant treatment modality** for most patients at risk for recurrence
- **Post operative RT is required in all stages except endometrial Ca. Stage IA, Grades 1 and 2**

Table 2.13: Post surgical Radiotherapy Based on Surgical-Pathological Staging

Surgico- Pathological staging	Post-operative Treatment
Stage I A, G1, 2	*None*
Stage IA, G3 **Stage IB, G1, 2**	*Vaginal cuff radiation only*
Stage IB, G3 **Stage II**	*Pelvic irradiation + vaginal cuff boost*
Positive para-aortic lymph nodes	*Pelvic irradiation + vaginal cuff boost + Extended field radiation*
Adnexal/parametrial involvement	*Whole abdominal radiation and/ or chemotherapy*
Stage IV	*Palliative RT (Combination therapy is currently being considered in advanced stage disease)* • *Pelvic RT for local tumor control* • *Palliative bone, Brain RT in metastatic cases*

Note

- ***Vaginal Vault radiation – reduces vault recurrence** from 15% to 1-2%. Vaginal vault is a common site of recurrence, even in women with tumor confined to the uterus*
- ***External pelvic radiation – reduces pelvic recurrence** in women at high risk such as - grade 3 tumors, deep myometrial invasion and cervical extension*
- ***Extended-field radiation** – indicated in women with **positive para-aortic nodes**. It includes irradiation of pelvic, common iliac and para-aortic nodes*
- ***Whole abdominal radiation (WAR)**– indicated in women with **stage III and IV disease** and **serous and clear cell tumors** Entire abdomen is irradiated **shielding the kidneys. GI and liver toxicities are more with WAR***

Role of Hormonal Therapy in Endometrial Carcinoma
• **No survival benefit for adjuvant progesterone therapy in endometrial cancer**
Indications
• Advanced and metastatic endometrial carcinoma – **Hormonal therapy can provide prolonged remission of metastatic disease in women with receptor positive tumors**

Contd.

Contd.

• Recurrence – **Progesterone's are currently recommended as initial treatment** for **hormone receptor–positive recurrent endometrial cancers** **Agents used** • Oral Medroxy-progesterone acetate (MPA) 200 mg qid • Megestrol acetate 160 mg qid
Role of Chemotherapy in Endometrial Carcinoma
Indications • Chemotherapy is mainly used in management of advanced and metastatic endometrial cancer. Combined RT and chemotherapy is considered **Agents used** • Platinum based chemotherapy is commonly used • Response is **better with combination therapy than single agent chemotherapy** • Carboplatin with Paclitaxel is the standard recommendation for adjuvant therapy of stage III and Stage IV disease. Doxorubicin is another agent that has been used in the combination • Recently, agents targeting specific molecular pathways are under evaluation.
Role of Fertility- Sparing Surgery in Endometrial Carcinoma
• It can be offered only in **women with** endometriod cancer **Stage IA without myometrial invasion, Grade 1** who wish to retain their reproductive potential, after adequate counseling about the risks associated with conservative management • **Megestrol acetate 160 -320 mg/ day or MPA 400-600 mg/day is given for 3 months and then endometrial biopsy is repeated** – Non response or progression of the disease requires surgical management – If there is response, biopsy is repeated every 3 months till two consecutive biopsies are negative. Conception may then be allowed. TAH + BSO is done on completion of family (ovarian preservation for future therapeutic beneficial option may be considered in Grade I intramural endometriod cancers
Role of Vaginal Hysterectomy and Laparoscopy in Endometrial Carcinoma
• Role of Laparoscopic assisted vaginal hysterectomy (LAVH) and laparoscopic hysterectomy (LH) in endometrial carcinoma is debatable • Hysterectomy and BSO by vaginal and laparoscopic surgeries may be preferred in women with **stage IA, grade 1 endometrial carcinoma who are morbidly obese** • These procedures are associated with less postoperative morbidity, early ambulation and better wound healing **Disadvantages** – Complete Staging may not be possible. – Approach to upper abdomen and para-aortic lymph nodes is compromised. – Laparoscopy can lead to port site metastasis.
Role of Hormone Replacement Therapy Following Surgery in Endometrial Carcinoma
• Estrogens are withheld for initial few years (1–3 years) following treatment of endometrial carcinoma which is the most common time period for cancer recurrence • Alternatively, **topical estrogens can be used to treat vaginal symptoms** • Symptomatic relief of **hot flushes can be achieved with progestin's** only therapy and non-hormonal agents like such as **clonidine** • Selective estrogen receptor modulators (SERMS) such as raloxifene and weight–bearing exercises can help to reduce bone loss
Role of Tumor Markers in Endometrial Carcinoma
• CA- 125 is useful in **predicting extrauterine spread and in follow-up of patients with advanced and recurrent cancer** • **Serous and clear cell tumors are more likely to have extrauterine spread and preoperative CA-125 and/or imaging is warranted** • Surveillance with CA-125 levels is reserved for patients with an elevated value at initial diagnosis

SPECIAL CONSIDERATIONS

Post hysterectomy Diagnosis of Endometrial carcinoma

- Several therapeutic management problems have been reported to arise from post hysterectomy diagnosis, especially where the adnexae have not been removed

- Recommendations for further postoperative therapy are based on known risk factors for extrauterine disease related to the histologic grade and depth of myometrial invasion
- Individuals with grade 3 lesions, deep myometrial invasion, or LVSI require additional surgery to remove the adnexae, or adjuvant RT
- Patients with a grade 1 or 2 lesion with minimal myometrial invasion and no LVSI involvement require no further therapy

Medically Inoperable Patients

- Common reasons for medically inoperable endometrial carcinoma are morbid obesity and severe cardiopulmonary disease
- In such cases, uterine brachytherapy plus EBRT is advised
- For patients with contraindications to general anesthesia, and who are unsuitable for radiotherapy high-dose progestin's may be used
- Trials using intrauterine hormone releasing devices instead of oral progestin's are underway

Follow-Up of Patients Treated for Endometrial Carcinoma

- ACOG recommends follow-up of patients every 3-4 months for 2-3 years, and then every 6 months. After 5 years, patients can have routine annual follow-up
- Patients with tumor recurrence often present with symptoms

Routine Post-Treatment Surveillance is as Follows

- Patient education is given regarding symptoms of recurrence such as vaginal bleeding and pelvic pain
- During each visit, history and clinical examination including pelvic examination should be done
- Pap smears routinely at each follow-up visit – not found to be beneficial
- Annual chest X-ray – not cost effective
- USG, CT scan, MRI, and IVP are done only if clinically indicated
- CA- 125 is helpful in follow up of patients with advanced disease, uterine serous and clear cell carcinoma and those with previously elevated levels
- Factors Affecting Survival In Endometrial Carcinoma and 5 year survival rates are mentioned in Table 2.14 and 2.15

Table 2.15: Factors Affecting Survival in Endometrial Carcinoma

Factor	Prognosis
Lymph node metastasis	Most important prognostic factor ; positive nodes – poor prognosis
Age at diagnosis	Older women – poor prognosis
Stage of the disease	Advanced stage at presentation - poor prognosis
Histological type	Endometriod carcinoma –good prognosis; papillary serous and clear cell – poor prognosis
Histological grade	Grade 3 – poor Prognosis
Myometrial invasion	Increased depth of myometrial invasion associated with risk of extrauterine spread and recurrence
Tumor size	Tumor size >=2 cm associated with more lymph node involvement
Cervical extension	Associated with risk of extrauterine spread, lymph node metastasis and recurrence
Hormone receptor status	positive receptor status has good prognosis
Ploidy status	DNA aneuploidy – poor prognosis
Peritoneal cytology	Role of positive Peritoneal cytology is controversial

Table 2.16: Five Year Survival Rate in Endometrial Carcinoma

Stage I	80-90%
Stage II	60-80%
Stage III	50%
Stage IV	20%

Recurrence of Endometrial Carcinoma

- **25% of the patients treated for endometrial carcinoma develop recurrent disease**
- Majority of recurrence occurs **within 3 years** of initial treatment
- Most recurrences tend to be **vaginal or pelvic**
- **Vaginal bleeding** is the **most common symptom with vault recurrence**
- Pelvic pain is often present with pelvic recurrence

Management of recurrence:

- **Treatment choice depends on primary therapy that was administered. Treatment may be with surgery/ RT or both. Cases not amenable to surgery or RT are treated with chemotherapy**

Local recurrence:

- Local recurrences are treated with surgery/ radiotherapy or both
- Pelvic or vaginal recurrence in patients who have not received prior pelvic irradiation - treated with **external pelvic RT and vaginal brachytherapy**
- **Role of surgery in recurrent disease**
  - Surgical resection of a metastatic vaginal nodule >2 cm prior to radiation may improve local control.
  - In patients with isolated central pelvic recurrence who had prior RT, exploratory laparotomy and pelvic exenteration may be done (Performing surgery in irradiated field increases morbidity such as pain, fistula formation)
  - Patients with intraperitoneal recurrence may need **surgery to relieve intestinal obstruction**

Distant metastasis:

- **Hormone receptor positive ->** Progesterone therapy -> if progesterone treatment fails -> palliative chemotherapy. Maximum response is observed only after 3 or more months of treatment
- **Hormone receptor negative -> palliative Chemotherapy**

Role of Screening for Endometrial Carcinoma
Routine screening for endometrial cancer is not recommended for the following reasons:
• More than **95% of patients are symptomatic and present with vaginal bleeding at an early stage** and hence screening for endometrial carcinoma is not warranted.
• There is Lack of an appropriate, cost-effective and acceptable screening test that reduces mortality
• **PAP smear cannot be used as a screening test as only 50% of endometrial cancers have malignant cells in Pap smear**
• **CA 125- has no role in screening (not cost effective)**
• **Screening by TVS and endometrial sampling is recommended for only high-risk women, such as those with a family history of Lynch II syndrome or HNPCC syndrome with a wish to preserve fertility**
• **TVS + endometrial biopsy performed annually from 35 years onwards until hysterectomy is performed. Prophylactic surgery (TAH + BSO) is recommended at 40 years in women with Lynch II mutation carriers to prevent endometrial and ovarian cancers**

RECENT UPDATES

Tailored surveillance programs for gynecologic cancer related with Lynch syndrome (LS)

- *LS or hereditary non-polyposis colorectal cancer (HNPCC), is an autosomal dominant genetic condition caused by germ-line mutations in the mismatch repair (MMR; MSH2, MLH1, MSH6, PMS2) genes*
- *The mutations in these onco-protective genes eventually lead to neoplastic changes and tumorigenesis, hence carriers of germ-line mutations in the mismatch repair are at high-risk of colorectal cancer and other cancers including endometrial cancer (second most common), ovary, stomach, and small intestine.*
- *The international collaborative group on HNPCC defined the Amsterdam I and II criteria that are widely used to identify candidates for genetic testing which can make a diagnosis of LS (Refer recent updates in Chapter 1).*
- Families meeting Amsterdam criteria should be counseled on colorectal and endometrial cancer risk, and those with certain genetic mutations could be offered tailored cancer surveillance programs (JAMA Oncology in 2017). Based on the published results, the recommendations were as follows:
  - *The most commonly identified mutation was **MSH2*** in study population

- *Gynecological surveillance should be focused from:*
  - *Age 30 years for those with MSH2* mutations
  - *Age 35 years for those with non-truncating MLH1* mutations
  - *Age 40 years for those with MSH6* and truncating *MLH1* mutations
- *Routine pathologic screening of mismatch repair deficiencies in the endometrial cancer specimen, similar to colorectal cancer is increasingly being introduced in practice*
- *In most women with mismatch repair deficiency this is caused by **MLH1 promoter hypermethylation** and testing of this is recommended.*
- *Survivors of endometrial cancer have increased risk of second cancer when compared with a matched population, mainly related to lifestyle factors and genetic susceptibility. These women should hence be counseled on exercise and weight loss programs*

Sentinel Lymph Node (SLN) Mapping Acceptable in Endometrial Cancer

- *SLN mapping has been developed for several solid malignancies to identify lymph node metastases, that reduced the surgical morbidity from performing a complete lymphadenectomy*
- *SLN mapping is established as one of the standard staging procedures in breast cancer and melanoma*
- *SLN use in endometrial cancer is unsatisfactory until now. However, it has been revealed recently that SLN mapping have a high diagnostic accuracy in detecting nodal metastases and can safety replace complete lymphadenectomy in endometrial cancer staging*
- *Fluorescence Imaging for Robotic Endometrial Sentinel lymph node biopsy (FIRES) trial in 2017 was designed with primary objective to estimate the sensitivity and negative predictive value of SLN mapping using indocyanine green (ICG) dye in detecting nodal metastases in patients with endometrial cancer. FIRES trial reported 97% sensitivity to detect nodal metastases and a negative predictive value of 99.6%*
- *SLN mapping can accurately stage endometrial cancer, thereby the morbidity of complete lymphadenectomy*
- *A systematic review and meta-analysis investigating the utility of SLN mapping for endometrial cancer staging was reported in American Journal of Obstetrics and Gynecology (2017). It was reported that SLN mapping successfully identified nodal metastases in endometrial cancer with pooled sensitivity at 96%*
- *Although the evidences from SLN mapping studies in endometrial cancer seems to be promising, there are still many controversies. Among them, consensus for the appropriate patient selection and optimal treatment algorithm to differentially manage high- and low- risk patients are important*
- *Society of Gynecologic Oncologists (SGO) has recommended that SLN mapping can appropriately stage endometrial cancer of low-risk histology and can safely replace lymphadenectomy in staging of endometrial cancers*

Genomic and Immunohistochemistry Studies

- *The Cancer Genome Atlas studies have identified molecular subgroups with distinct prognosis - POLE mutation, mismatch repair deficiency, TP53 mutation*
- *IHC marker studied to differentiate low and high risk endometrial cancer is L1 cell adhesion molecule (L1CAM) -> promising marker for identifying patients with poor outcomes*
- *Markers of the p53 pathway, hormone receptor expression and microsatellite instability are several of the other relevant biomarkers to predict prognosis of endometrial cancer*
- *Currently ongoing trials*
  - *STATEC trial – role of lymphadenectomy to direct adjuvant therapy for high risk endometrial cancers*
  - *PORTEC -4a trial – investigates use of IHC markers to determine use of adjuvant RT*

CHAPTER 3

MESENCHYMAL TUMORS OF THE UTERUS

INTRODUCTION

- **Mesenchymal uterine tumors or uterine sarcomas are rare uterine malignancies; account for 7-8% of all uterine cancers and 1% of all genital malignancies**
- Uterine sarcomas arise from **smooth muscle and connective tissue of the uterus**
- **Uterine sarcomas are aggressive and have poor prognosis** when compared to endometrial adenocarcinomas
- **Leiomyosarcomas are the most common subtype (excluding carcinosarcomas, which are currently classified as metaplastic carcinomas)**
- Majority of **leiomyosarcomas are high-grade tumors** associated with poor prognosis even when apparently confined to the uterus.
- **Low-grade endometrial stromal sarcomas** are indolent tumors associated with long-term survival. **High-grade endometrial stromal sarcomas** and **undifferentiated endometrial sarcomas** behave more aggressively
- **Adenosarcomas** have a favorable prognosis except for tumors showing myometrial invasion or sarcomatous overgrowth
- Carcinosarcomas usually have worse prognosis than grade 3 endometrial carcinomas
- **Tumor stage is the single most important prognostic factor for uterine sarcomas**

MESENCHYMAL UTERINE TUMORS

- **WHO classification** of mesenchymal uterine tumors is given in Table 3.1

Table 3.1: WHO (2014) Classification of Mesenchymal Uterine Tumors
Smooth muscle Tumors • Leiomyoma • Smooth muscle tumor of uncertain malignant potential (STUMP) • Leiomyosarcoma • Unusual smooth muscle mimics of Leiomyosarcoma • Epitheloid smooth muscle tumors – benign/malignant • Myxoid smooth muscle tumors – benign/malignant
Endometrial stromal sarcoma (ESS) • Endometrial stromal nodules • Low grade Endometrial stromal sarcoma • High grade Endometrial stromal sarcoma • Undifferentiated uterine sarcoma
Miscellaneous mesenchymal tumors • Rhabdomyosarcoma • Perivascular epitheloid cell tumor • Uterine tumor resembling ovarian sex cord tumor
Other • Rare uterine tumors

Note
***Carcinosarcoma** –It belongs to **Malignant mixed mesodermal tumor, also termed as malignant mixed müllerian tumors (a mixed epithelial-nonepithelial tumor)**. It was earlier classified under uterine sarcomas, but now reclassified as a metaplastic form of carcinoma of endometrium rather than a sarcoma*

Epidemiology

- **Leiomyosarcomas are the most common uterine mesenchymal tumors** (when excluding carcinosarcomas)
- Leiomyosarcomas account for **2/3rd cases of true uterine sarcomas; Endometrial stromal sarcomas account for 25% of true uterine sarcomas**
- **Carcinosarcomas and leiomyosarcomas account for 4% and 1.5% of all uterine malignancies** respectively
- More common in **African-American women**
- Mostly occur in older **post menopausal age group women (carcinosarcomas and adenosarcomas occur in more older women compared to leiomyosarcomas and ESS)**

Risk Factors (Table 3.2)

Table 3.2: Risk Factors For Carcinosarcomas and Uterine Sarcomas

Risk factors for carcinosarcomas (Risk factors are similar to endometrial adenocarcinomas)	Risk factors for uterine sarcomas
• Obesity • Diabetes • Anovulation • Nulliparity • Prior radiation exposure	• **Prior radiation exposure** • **Prolonged Tamoxifen use** • Hereditary predisposition – **HNPCC and hereditary Retinoblastoma**

NOTE- Sarcomas in previously irradiated patients present in advanced stages (RT associated cervical stenosis obscures uterine bleeding)

Histopathological Classification

Malignant mesenchymal tumors can be classified into pure (single cell type) and mixed (more than one cell type) as follows (Table 3.3a and b):

Table 3.3a: Gynecologic Oncology Group (GOG) Classification of uterine sarcomas

Pure Mesenchymal Tumors	Mixed Epithelial-Mesenchymal Tumors
A. Leiomyosarcoma B. Endometrial stromal sarcoma C. Undifferentiated endometrial sarcoma D. Smooth muscle tumor of uncertain malignant potential (STUMP) E. Mixed endometrial stromal and smooth muscle tumor F. Other soft tissue tumors	A. Adenosarcoma – • Homologous • Heterologous B. Carcinosarcoma (malignant mixed mesodermal tumor or malignant mixed müllerian tumor) • Homologous • Heterologous

Table 3.3b: Homologous and heterologous types of uterine sarcomas

Homologous Types	Heterologous Types
Pure sarcoma	
• Leiomyosarcoma–**Most common** • Endometrial stromal sarcoma (ESS)	• **Rhabdomyosarcoma**–Most common • Chondrosarcoma • Osteosarcoma • Liposarcoma

Contd.

Contd.

Mixed type – Carcinosarcoma	
Carcinoma + homologous sarcoma	Carcinoma + heterologous sarcoma

Note

- ***Homologous*** *is defined as tumor with native tissue elements (smooth muscle).*
- ***Heterologous*** *is defined as tumor with tissue elements that are not native (cartilage, striated muscle, bones).* ***This is due to the totipotential nature of endometrial stromal cells***

Clinical Presentation

- Most often occurs in **post menopausal women**
- **Vaginal bleeding** is the most common presenting symptom – **post menopausal bleeding**
- **Carcinosarcoma** may present with **vaginal bleeding and fleshy protruberant mass through cervix**
- Uterine enlargement with **presumptive diagnosis of leiomyoma may often be present in cases with leiomyosarcoma**; often diagnosed only after hysterectomy
- **Distant spread usually involves the lungs,** so preoperative assessment should include thoracic imaging
- **Most common histological cell type is spindle cell type**
- **FIGO staging of uterine sarcomas is given in Table 3.4**

Table 3.4: Figo Staging of Uterine Sarcomas (2009)

	Stage	Definition
Leiomyosarcomas and endometrial stromal sarcomas		
I		Tumor limited to uterus
	IA	Less than 5 cm
	IB	More than 5 cm
II		Tumor extends beyond the uterus, within the pelvis
	IIA	Adnexal involvement
	IIB	Involvement of other pelvic tissues
III		Tumor invades abdominal tissues (not just protruding into the abdomen)
	IIA	One site
	IIIB	More than one site
	IIIC	Metastasis to pelvic and/or para-aortic lymph nodes
IV	IVA	Tumor invades bladder and/or rectum
	IVB	Distant metastasis
Adenosarcomas		
I		Tumor limited to uterus
	IA	Tumor limited to endometrium/endocervix with no myometrial invasion
	IB	Less than or equal to half myometrial invasion
	IC	More than half myometrial invasion
II		Tumor extends to the pelvis
	IIA	Adnexal involvement
	IIIB	Tumor extends to extrauterine pelvic tissue
III		Tumor invades abdominal tissue (not just protruding into the abdomen)
	IIIA	One site
	IIIB	More than one site
	IIIC	Metastasis to pelvic and/or para-aortic lymph nodes
IV	IVA	Tumor invades bladder and/or rectum
	IVB	Distant metastasis

NOTE – Uterine carcinosarcomas are staged using the two endometrial adenocarcinoma staging system

Leiomyosarcomas

- **Leiomyosarcomas are the most common uterine sarcomas (excluding carcinosarcomas)**
- **More common in African Americans**
- Median age at diagnosis is early 50s **(occurs in younger age group compared to other uterine sarcomas)**
- **Presents with vaginal bleeding**
- Can arise **de novo (more common)** or **from leiomyoma**
- **Sarcomatous change of fibroid**
  - Occurs in about **<0.5 % cases**
  - **Suspected sarcomatous change in a fibroid is indicated by the following:**
    - Rapid enlargement of fibroid
    - Enlargement of fibroid in post menopausal women who is not on any hormone replacement therapy (HRT)
  - The fibroid becomes soft while undergoing malignant change
- Two thirds of leiomyosarcomas are **intramural and are typically voluminous tumors with diameter of 10 cm or more**
- Leiomyosarcomas are **poorly circumscribed** and cannot be shelled out from surrounding myometrium - **capsule is absent**
- Cut section shows loss of **whorled appearance, soft, bulging, fleshy, necrotic, hemorrhagic mass**
- Test Characteristics Using **Dynamic MRI and Serum Lactate Dehydrogenase** may help in differentiating Uterine Leiomyosarcomas from Degenerating Leiomyomas
- **85% of women diagnosed with a leiomyosarcoma have clinical stage I or II disease**
- Vascular invasion and extrauterine tumor spread are associated with poor prognosis
- Histopathological diagnosis of leiomyosarcomas is made **when any 2 of the following 3 criteria are present:**
  - Coagulative Tumor cell necrosis
  - Diffuse moderate to severe cytological atypia
  - 10 or more mitotic figures per 10 HPF

Table 3.5: Management of Leiomyosarcomas

Stage I and II	• Total abdominal hysterectomy/ debulking of the tumor (if present outside the uterus) is performed • Lymph node involvement and ovarian metastasis are rare and the **role of lymphadenectomy and removal of ovaries is controversial** • **In young women** with leiomyosarcoma confined to the uterus, ovaries can be conserved Adjuvant therapy in Stage I and II • **Adjuvant chemo/RT considered in patients with high risk features** • Role of adjuvant chemo/RT is uncertain in completely resected, uterus confined disease
Stage III and IV (advanced disease)	• Treated with **combination chemotherapy or targeted RT** • Combination chemotherapy usually used are doxorubicin, ifosfomide, docetaxel and gemcitabine

Note

- ***Leiomyosarcomas do not respond well to radiotherapy***
- *High rates of* ***local recurrence and distant metastasis***
- ***Most common site of metastasis is lungs***
- ***Poor prognosis even when confined to uterus***

Smooth Muscle Tumors of Uncertain Malignant Potential (STUMP)

- Uterine smooth muscle tumors that show some worrisome histologic features (i.e. necrosis, nuclear atypia, or mitoses), but do not meet all diagnostic criteria for leiomyosarcoma, fall into the category of atypical smooth muscle tumors (STUMP) i.e., Smooth muscle tumors with **histological features not conclusive of sarcomas are termed as STUMP**

- They have higher degree of cytologic atypia and higher mitotic index than benign leiomyomas
- Most tumors classified as STUMP have been associated with favorable prognosis and only follow-up of the patients is recommended

Smooth Muscle Tumors of Uncertain Malignant Potential [STUMP]
Tumor cell necrosis in a typical leiomyoma
Necrosis of uncertain type with ≥10 MF/10 HPFs, or marked diffuse atypia
Marked diffuse or focal atypia with borderline mitotic counts
Necrosis difficult to classify

Extra Edge

Uterine Smooth Muscle Proliferations with Unusual Growth Patterns (Table 3.6)

This includes:

- Disseminated peritoneal leiomyomatosis
- Benign metastasizing leiomyoma
- Intravenous leiomyomatosis

Table 3.6: Smooth Muscle Proliferations with Unusual Growth Patterns

Terminology	Description
Leiomyomatosis peritonealis disseminata	• *Benign smooth muscle tumor that* ***grows over peritoneal surfaces*** • *Arises from* ***metaplasia of subperitoneal mesenchymal stem cells*** *under influence of estrogen and progesterone to form smooth muscle, fibroblasts, myofibroblasts* • *TAH, BSO, omentectomy and excision of gross disease should be done* • *May be* ***associated with pregnancy and COC pills. Regression usually occurs after termination of pregnancy***
Intravenous leiomyomatosis	• *Benign smooth muscle tumor that* ***grows into venous channels within broad ligaments, uterine and iliac veins*** • ***Prognosis*** *following surgery is* ***excellent*** • ***Regression occurs after menopause***
Benign metastasizing leiomyoma	• *Benign smooth muscle tumor that* ***originates in the uterus and spreads elsewhere, usually to the lungs*** • ***Surgical resection and hormonal therapy*** *are generally recommended*

Leiomyoma Variants that May Mimic Malignancy

- Mitotically active leiomyoma
- Cellular leiomyoma
- Hemorrhagic leiomyoma and hormone-induced changes
- Leiomyoma with bizarre nuclei (atypical leiomyoma)
- Myxoid leiomyoma
- Epithelioid leiomyoma
- Leiomyoma with massive lymphoid infiltration

Endometrial Stromal Tumors

- Arise from endometrial stromal cells, predominantly intramural tumors
- **Classification of Endometrial stromal tumors based on the type of tumor margin**
  - **Benign (well circumscribed tumors)** – Endometrial stromal nodule (ESN)
  - **Malignant (exhibit myometrial invasion and permeation of lymphovascular space)**
    - Endometrial stromal sarcoma (ESS) (low grade)
    - Endometrial stromal sarcoma (high grade)
    - Undifferentiated Endometrial stromal sarcoma

Endometrial Stromal Nodules

- **Benign tumors,** often distinguished from endometrial stromal sarcomas only after hysterectomy
- **Features differentiating ESN from ESS include:**
  - Absence of Infiltrating margins
  - Absence of myometrial invasion and lymphovascular space involvement

Endometrial Stromal Sarcomas (Low Grade ESS)

- **Least aggressive of all sarcomas – has a favorable prognosis**
- Peak incidence in **fifth decade of life** – **premenopausal and post menopausal age group**
- Clinical features–Patients commonly present with abnormal uterine bleeding, pelvic pain, and dysmenorrhea
- **HPE- endometrial stromal sarcomas consist of well-differentiated endometrial stromal cells with only mild nuclear atypia and characteristically invade the lymphovascular spaces of the myometrium. Tumor cell necrosis is rarely seen**
- 60% of low-grade endometrial stromal tumors have **cytogenetic abnormalities such as rearrangements of chromosomes 6, 7 and 17**
- The **most characteristic translocation of these tumors, t(T7;17) (Tp15;q21),** generates a fusion of the **JAZF1 and JJAZ1 genes both of which encode zinc finger proteins** that can be detected by fluorescence in situ hybridization (FISH) as well as by reverse transcriptase–polymerase chain reaction (rt-PCR).

Treatment

- **Standard treatment includes TAH and BSO**
- **Role of lymphadenectomy is not clear.** Performed in cases with extrauterine spread
- These tumors **often express estrogen and progesterone receptors–so adjuvant treatment with Progestins, GnRH analogs, or Aromatase inhibitors** are given
- Tends to have local recurrence and frequently spreads to lungs
- Late recurrences can occur even in patients with Stage I disease; thus, long-term follow- up is required
- Recurrences most commonly in the **pelvis and abdomen,** and less frequently in the lungs and vagina
- Low-grade endometrial stromal sarcomas have favorable prognosis
- **Stage of the tumor is the most significant prognostic factor**
- **Five-year** survival for patients with Stages I and II tumors is 90% compared with 50% for Stages III and IV

Endometrial Stromal Sarcoma (High-Grade)

- Tumors with features that are intermediate between low-grade ESS and undifferentiated sarcomas
- Occurs in age group – 30-60 years
- Clinical presentation – abnormal vaginal bleeding and enlarged uterus
- The tumors may appear as intracavitary polypoid masses and the cut surface is fleshy with extensive areas of necrosis and hemorrhage
- Microscopically, they consist predominantly of high-grade round-cells. Mitotic activity is typically greater than 10 per 10 HPF. Necrosis is usually present
- Often show extrauterine extension at the time of diagnosis
- High-grade ESS typically harbors the YWHAE-FAM22 genetic fusion as a result of t(10;17) (q22;p13)
- Prognosis is intermediate, between low-grade ESS and undifferentiated uterine sarcomas
- Patients with high-grade ESS have earlier and more frequent recurrences (often <1 year)
- Advanced or recurrent tumors should be treated aggressively with a combination of radiation and chemotherapy

Undifferentiated Endometrial Sarcoma

- Rare tumor, highly aggressive tumors
- Occurs in postmenopausal age group (mean age is 60 years)
- Present with postmenopausal bleeding or signs/symptoms secondary to extrauterine spread
- Tumors exhibit myometrial invasion, severe nuclear pleomorphism, high mitotic activity and/or tumor cell necrosis, and **lack smooth muscle or endometrial stromal differentiation**
- Undifferentiated endometrial sarcomas are associated with a **very poor prognosis**
- Patients should be treated by **hysterectomy and bilateral salpingo-oophorectomy and adjuvant radiation and/or chemotherapy**

Adenosarcoma

- Mixed mullerian tumors with a **benign epithelial component and malignant stromal component**
- Occurs mainly in post menopausal women
- They appear as polypoidal tumors that fill and distend the uterine cavity
- **Low malignant potential and better prognosis** than carcinosarcoma
- The **stromal component is usually a low grade sarcoma, usually of endometrial stromal type**
- **Microscopically, the stroma typically concentrates around the glands forming hypercellular periglandular cuffs. The presence of hypercellular periglandular cuffs distinguishes adenosarcoma from its benign counterpart, the adenofibroma**
- **Other features on microscopy include the following**
  - 2 or more mitosic figures/10 HPF
  - Marked stromal hypercellularity
  - Stromal cell atypia
- **Sarcomatous overgrowth** – This term is used when **> 25% of tumor is composed of high grade sarcomas**
- Stromal overgrowth and myometrial invasion are associated with poor prognosis
- **Treatment – TAH + BSO**
- Majority express **Estrogen receptor** in sarcomatous component
- **Heterologous mesenchymal elements, usually rhabdomyosarcoma, are found in 10 -15% of cases**
- **Vaginal or pelvic recurrence are common**

Uterine Carcinosarcoma/Malignant Mixed Müllerian Tumors (MMMT)

- Uterine carcinosarcomas are also **referred to as malignant mixed mullerian tumors**
- It is composed of distinctive but admixed, malignant-appearing epithelial and mesenchymal elements. The sarcomatous component may be **homologous or heterologous**
- Common in seventh decade, but can occur from 4th to 9th decades–biphasic pattern
- **Most common symptom** is vaginal bleeding. Another typical presentation is in the form of polypoid mass that protrudes through the cervical os
- Carcinosarcomas in **previously irradiated patients present in advanced stage** because radiotherapy associated cervical stenosis obscures vaginal bleeding
- 90% of carcinosarcomas harbor **TP53 mutations**
- **The behaviour of carcinosarcoma is predicted by the carcinomatous component**
- Metastasis occurs through lymphatics similar to endometrial carcinoma

- Most **metastasis and recurrences are composed of pure carcinomas**
- **Adverse prognostic factors** include the presence of **heterologous elements and high percentage of sarcomatous component** in the main tumor
- **Treatment includes TAH + BSO, pelvic lymphadenectomy followed by adjuvant therapy with RT or chemotherapy**
- **Ifosfamide** is found to be very active in these cases
- Carcinosarcomas have a **high risk of recurrence** up to 60%. Even stage I tumors have 50% risk of recurrence
- Poor prognosis

Note
Mullerian carcinosarcoma *-malignant tumor with both stromal and epithelial components malignant*
Mullerian adenosarcoma *- epithelial component is benign and stromal component is malignant (Vice versa is very rare)*
Mullerian adenofibroma *- benign tumor with both stromal and epithelial components benign*

Salient Points in Management of Uterine Sarcomas (Table 3.7)

- **Surgery is the cornerstone in the treatment of uterine sarcomas**
- **TAH is performed in majority of malignant mesenchymal tumors of uterus, including leiomyosarcoma, undifferentiated endometrial stromal sarcoma and carcinosarcoma**

Table 3.7: Salient Points in Management of Uterine Sarcomas

	Leiomyosarcoma	**ESS**	**Carcinosarcoma**
Role of Oophorectomy	Risk of ovarian metastasis is low and hence oophorectomy is not indicated in premenopausal women	Indicated	Indicated
Role of lymphadenectomy	Not indicated in leiomyosarcoma confined to uterus	Not indicated in ESS confined to uterus	Indicated
Role of RT	Role of RT remains undefined	Role of RT remains undefined	• RT in carcinosarcoma provides good local control of tumor
Role of chemotherapy • Active agents are different for carcinosarcoma and leiomyosarcoma • Combination chemotherapy is better than single agents	• Used in advanced and recurrent cancers • Active agents used – doxorubicin, ifosfamide, gemcitabine and docetaxel	• Used in advanced and recurrent cancers • Hormonal therapy with progestins, GnRH analogs and aromatase inhibitors have role in treatment of ESS	• Combined sequential treatment with chemotherapy and RT might be beneficial • Active agents used – ifosfamide, cisplatin/ carboplatin and paclitaxel • Ifosfamide is the most active single agent studied
Role of uterine preservation	Option in young women diagnosed with STUMP carcinoma who want to preserve fertility.	-	-

Flowchart 1: Management of Leiomyosarcoma

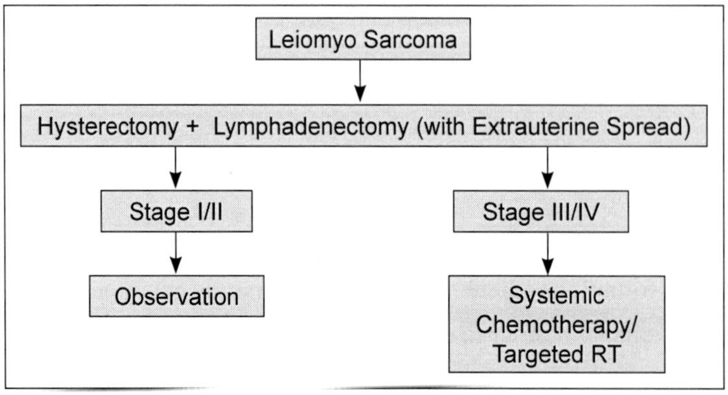

Flowchart 2: Management of Endometrial stromal sarcoma

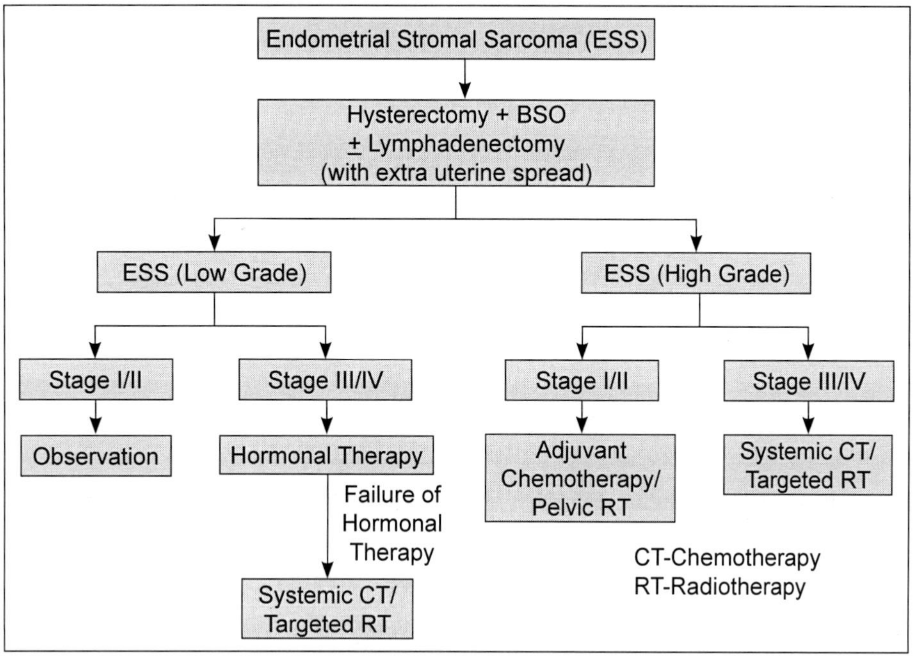

Flowchart 3: Management of carcinocarcoma

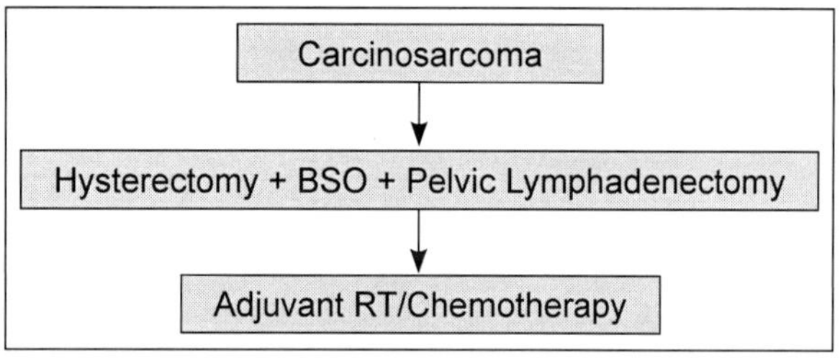

Follow-Up of Sarcomas

- Follow-up should be determined by the risk of recurrence
- As metastasis to the lungs is common, efforts must be made to rule this out
- Low-grade sarcoma patients can be followed for local relapse every 4–6 months for the first 3–5 years, then annually
- High-grade tumors can be followed-up every 3–4 months for the first 2–3 years, twice a year for the next 2–3 years, and then annually

Prognosis

- **Uterine sarcomas have high rate of distant metastasis** even in the absence of intraperitoneal or lymph node metastasis. **This is due to the hematogenous spread of tumor**
- **Even stage I disease had 50% risk of recurrence in carcinosarcoma**
- **Leiomyosarcoma (worst prognosis) > carcinosarcoma > ESS (favorable prognosis)**
- **Patients with ESS** tend to present with **low grade and early stage disease** and have **better prognosis** when compared to leiomyosarcoma and carcinosarcoma

MISCELLANEOUS TUMORS

Sarcoma Botryoides (Embryonal Rhabdomyosarcoma)

- **Special type of mixed mesodermal tumor (rhabdomyosarcoma) commonly arises from cervix and sometimes from vagina or uterus**

- **Age group–common at <8 years of age–Young girls**
- **High grade aggressive tumor**
- Spreads to **lungs and by direct extension to surrounding organs**

Clinical Features

- Blood stained watery vaginal discharge
- Anemia and cachexia
- Vaginal examination reveals **pinkish, grape-like polypoidal soft growth arising from the cervix, often fills up whole vagina**

Diagnosis

- Diagnosis is confirmed by **histology**
- **Histopathology** reveals **loose myxomatous stroma, pleomorphic malignant cells with striated rhabdomyoblasts**

Treatment

- Intravenous administration of **VAC chemotherapy** (vincristine, actinomycin-D, cyclophosphamide) followed by surgery is found to be effective
- Drugs should be **administered every 3 weeks over a period of 6 months**
- **Chemotherapy with local resection of the disease gives better result**
- Radiation therapy may be needed
- The results of multimodality approach are better

Prognosis

- Local recurrence and distant metastases are common
- Prognosis is poor

Perivascular Epithelioid Cell Tumors (Pecomas)

- These are rare mesenchymal tumors **derived from perivascular epithelioid cells that coexpress melanocytic and smooth muscle markers**
- Other tumors that belong to the same family include angiomyolipoma, lymphangioleiomyomatosis, and myelomelanocytic tumor of ligamentum teres/falciform ligament
- About **8% of PEComas occur in patients with tuberous sclerosis complex**

Other Rare Uterine Tumors

HEMANGIOPERICYTOMA

- Tumor is of **both benign and malignant form**
- **Arises from pericytes**
- Consists of **masses of blood vessels, each surrounded by one or more layers of round, oval, or spindle cells**
- Symptoms are similar to that of **adenomyosis or endometrial carcinoma depending on whether benign or malignant nature**
- Uterus is often palpably enlarged, so clinical diagnosis is usually leiomyoma or adenomyosis.
- True nature of the lesion is **only revealed by histological examination** of the specimen following hysterectomy

LYMPHOMAS

- Lymphomas were formerly rare, but now occurrs with increasing frequency
- **Most common sites in genital tract–Ovaries and tubes**
- Growth can infiltrate the uterine wall, broad ligaments and other tissues to produce physical signs similar to advanced carcinoma cervix

- Development of **ascites** is often the lead to lymphomatous tissue in the adnexa
- **Treatment is as for the primary cancer**

RECENT UPDATES

MED12 and uterine smooth muscle oncogenesis

- *The relationship between benign uterine leiomyomas and their malignant counterparts, i.e. leiomyosarcomas and smooth muscle tumors of uncertain malignant potential (STUMP), is still poorly understood*
- *Recently **MED12 mutations** have been reported in uterine leiomyomas. MED12 is a subunit of the multiprotein complex Mediator, a regulator of transcription*
- *Oncogenic mutations in MED12 occur in nearly 70% of uterine leiomyomas, and together with overexpression of **High mobility group (HMGA2) genes**, represent the most common genetic anomalies in leiomyoma*
- *MED12 mutations are restricted to benign smooth muscle tumors (leiomyomas) of the uterus but decreased protein expression has also been observed in uterine leiomyosarcomas independently of mutational status, that suggests a possible epigenetic mechanism*

Immunohistochemistry and molecular biology in uterine sarcomas

- *Leiomyosarcomas usually express smooth muscle markers such as desmin, H-caldesmon, smooth muscle actin, and histone deacetylase 8 (HDCA8). Epithelioid and myxoid leiomyosarcomas may show lesser degrees of immunoreaction for these markers*
- *Leiomyosarcomas are often immunoreactive for CD 10 (mainly considered a marker of endometrial stromal differentiation) and epithelial markers including keratin and EMA*
- *Leiomyosarcomas express estrogen, progesterone and androgen receptors in 30- 40% of cases*
- *Uterine leiomyosarcomas have higher levels of Ki67 compared with benign smooth muscle tumors*
- *Uterine leiomyosarcomas have overexpression of p16 and may prove to be a useful adjunct immunomarker for distinguishing between benign and malignant uterine smooth muscle tumors*
- *The vast majority of uterine leiomyosarcomas are sporadic. Patients with germline mutations in fumarate hydratase are believed to be at increased risk for developing uterine leiomyosarcomas as well as uterine leiomyomas*
- *Ancillary parameters including p53, p16, Ki 67, and Bcl-2 have been used in leiomyosarcomas to try to predict outcome. Combination of tumor size, mitotic index, Ki67, and Bcl-2 protein expression allows two groups of leiomyosarcomas to be distinguished, with different survival as follows:*

Leiomyosarcomas-Worse prognosis	Leiomyosarcomas-Better prognosis
• *Tumors greater than or equal to 10 cm in diameter*	• *Smaller leiomyosarcomas*
• *Greater than or equal to 20 MF/10 HPF*	• *Less than or equal to 20 MF/10 HPF*
• *Greater than or equal to 10% immune reactive nuclei for Ki67*	• *Less than 10% immuno reactive nuclei for Ki67*
• *Negative for Bcl-2*	• *Positive or negative for Bcl-2*

- *Targeted therapies such as **trabectedin and olaratumab** have been investigated as treatment in advanced stage or metastatic leiomyosarcoma with some appreciable disease control*

Immunohistochemistry and Molecular Biology in ESS

Low grade ESS

- *The tumor cells are strongly immunoreactive for CD10*
- *ESS is positive for smooth-muscle actin and less frequently for desmin and Negative for H-caldesmon and HDAC8*
- *Estrogen, progesterone and androgen receptors and WT-1 are typically positive*
- *Nuclear beta-catenin expression has been shown in up to 40% of low-grade endometrial stromal sarcomas*

- *The most common cytogenetic abnormality of low-grade endometrial stromal sarcomas is a recurrent translocation involving chromosomes 7 and 17 t(7;17) (p15;q21)], which results in a fusion between JAZF1 and SUZ12 (formerly designated as JJAZ1)*

High-grade ESS

- *High grade ESS are CD10, estrogen receptor, and progesterone receptor negative*
- *Shows strong diffuse cyclin D1 immunoreactivity (>70% nuclei)*
- *They are also typically c-Kit positive but DOG1 negative*
- *High-grade ESS typically harbors the YWHAE-FAM22 genetic fusion as a result of t(10;17) (q22;p13)*

Adenosarcomas

- *Immunoreactions for cell proliferation markers (Ki-67 and P53) are stronger in adenosarcomas with sarcomatous overgrowth than in typical adenosarcomas*
- *The expression of markers of cell differentiation (CD10 and PR) is higher in typical adenosarcomas than in adenosarcomas with sarcomatous overgrowth*

CHAPTER 4

PREMALIGNANT AND MALIGNANT LESIONS OF THE CERVIX

INTRODUCTION

- Carcinoma cervix is the **most common female genital malignancy in developing countries like India**
- **Majority of new cases and deaths occur in low and middle income countries**
- It often presents with **abnormal uterine bleeding or postmenopausal bleeding**
- **Ca. cervix occurs at an average age of 35-65 years**
- Cancer cervix goes through **preinvasive stages for several years (10-15 years)** before turning cancerous.
- HPV vaccine against infection by high risk HPV groups. HPV is the major etiological agent in Cancer cervix. Effective **screening tests and treatment modalities** are available to diagnose and treat preinvasive lesions of cervix; hence, **cancer cervix is a preventable disease**
- **Pap smear has reduced the incidence of cervical cancer by nearly 80% and death due to Ca. cervix by 70%**
- **WHO has called for elimination of cancer cervix and HPV vaccine is now included in national programs in > 80 countries**

Causes of Post Menopausal Bleeding

- **Cervical causes**–Carcinoma cervix; Benign lesions of cervix such as erosion, polyp, cervicitis, decubitus ulcer
- **Endometrial causes**–Endometrial hyperplasia and carcinoma; Benign conditions of endometrium such as senile endometritis, atrophic endometritis
- **Vaginal causes**–vaginal carcinoma; senile vaginitis, atrophic vaginitis, forgotten vaginal pessary
- **Ovarian**–Hormone secreting ovarian tumors such as Granulosa cell tumor, Theca cell tumor
- Hormone replacement therapy

Differential Diagnosis for Cervical Lesion

- Carcinoma of cervix
- Tubercular ulcer of cervix
- Syphilitic ulcer
- Cervical polyp
- Cervical fibroid
- Cervical papilloma or warts
- Retained products of conception in the cervical canal

Note: Lymphatic Drainage of Cervix
• *Lymphatics from Parametrial and paracervical nodes → obturator nodes → external iliac nodes → common iliac and internal iliac nodes*
• *Lymphatics from posterior part of cervix → Uterosacral and rectal lymph nodes*

CERVIX PREMALIGNANT LESIONS/CERVICAL INTRAEPITHELIAL NEOPLASIA (CIN)

- **Premalignant Lesions of Cervix or Cervical Intraepithelial Neoplasia (CIN)** is a premalignant condition involving the cervix, where the **stratified squamous epithelium is replaced by cells showing varying degree of dysplasia, without invasion of basement membrane**
- **Dysplasia** refers to the **abnormal maturation of the cells of stratified squamous epithelium** of cervix. There is alteration in cell morphology and disorderly arrangement of the cells of stratified squamous epithelium of cervix
- Dysplasia is described as **mild, moderate, and severe dysplasia** and carcinoma in situ based on the involvement of lower 1/3rd, 2/3rd cells or full thickness of the epithelium respectively
- **Dysplasias of all grades can progress to invasive cancer, and hence the terminology (mild, moderate and severe dysplasia) has been replaced by the term CIN in histological grade**
- CIN which involves squamous epithelium is termed as squamous intraepithelial lesion (SIL) which is a spectrum of intraepithelial changes that begins with minimal atypia and progresses through stages of greater intraepithelial abnormalities to invasive squamous cell carcinoma
- The terms CIN, dysplasia and squamous intraepithelial lesion (SIL) are commonly used interchangeably

Characteristics of Cells Showing Dysplasia

- There is loss of stratification and polarity
- The cells vary in size and shape
- The nuclei stain deeply with presence of frequent mitosis and abnormal chromatin pattern
- The nuclei are larger and hyperchromatic with scanty cytoplasm
- The basement membrane remains intact

Pathogenesis of CIN (Fig 4.1 a-d and Fig 4.2)

- The ectocervix and the vagina are lined by squamous epithelium and the endocervix by columnar epithelium. The junction between the two is known as the **squamocolumnar junction (SCJ).**
- **SCJ of cervix is a dynamic point** that keeps moving up and down in relation to different phases of life (see figure below)
- **At birth,** SCJ is located on the ectocervix and is termed as the original SCJ (Figure 4.1a)
- **At puberty and pregnancy, under the influence of estrogen,** the endocervix everts to expose the columnar epithelium (Figure 4.1b). Under the influence of estrogen, the columnar epithelium becomes filled with glycogen and lactobacilli colonize the epithelium ->Lactobacillus acts on the glycogen to produce lactic acid, thereby reducing the vaginal pH ->Reduced vaginal pH stimulates the columnar epithelium to undergo metaplasia and converts it into immature squamous and later mature squamous epithelium ->Metaplasia advances cephalad from original SCJ toward external os. This process establishes an area called **transformation zone (TZ),** which **extends from the original SCJ to the new SCJ** (new SCJ is the junction between the metaplastic squamous epithelium and the columnar epithelium) (Figure 4.1c)
- **The entire TZ with early metaplastic cells is susceptible to oncogenic effects leading to CIN and HPV infection is the most common etiological agent. Most cervical malignancies occur in the region of TZ**
- **CIN is more likely to begin following menarche or pregnancy** when metaplasia is most active.
- **In postmenopausal women,** the new SCJ moves further cephalad and lies within the endocervical canal (Figure 4.1d)

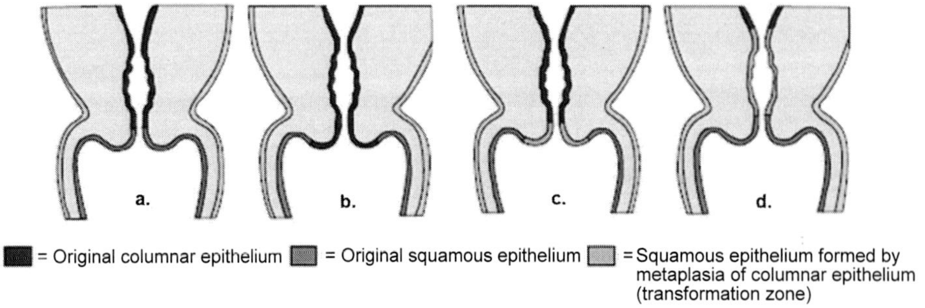

Figure Dynamic squamocolumnar junction of the cervix. **a.** Before puberty, the ectocervix is covered with squamous epithelium. **b.** Increased estrogenic activity during puberty exposes the columnar epithelium onto the ectocervix. **c.** Replacement of columnar epithelium by squamous epithelium to form the transformation zone (TZ). Junction is situated at or slightly outside the external os during reproductive period. **d.** Indrawing of the squamocolumnar New squamocolumnar junction and the TZ into the cervical canal following menopause

Fig 4.1: (a-d) Dynamic squamocolumnar junction of cervix

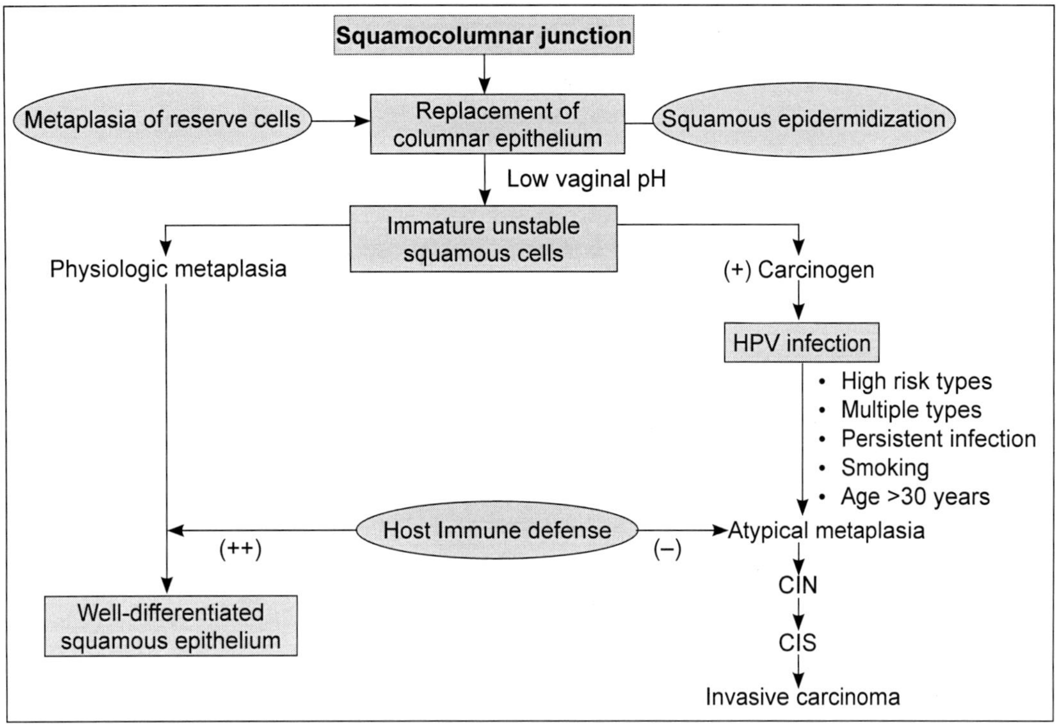

Fig 4.2: Pathogenesis of CIN and Invasive carcinoma

HUMAN PAPILLOMA VIRUS (HPV) INFECTION

- **Persistent HPV infection is the major etiological agent for to preinvasive lesions of cervix and carcinoma cervix**
- HPV infection is **detected in > 95% of preinvasive and invasive carcinoma cervix.** It is also detected in 50% of vaginal cancers and its precancers, > 50% of vulvar cancers and its precancers, 50% of penile cancers and >70% of anal cancers
- **HPV belongs to the Papova** family of DNA viruses
- More than 100 serotypes of HPV are identified, of which about 40 types cause genital tract infection
- Depending on the risk for causing cervical cancer, **HPV are grouped as Low, intermediate risk and high risk HPV (Table 4.1)**

Table 4.1: HPV Groups and their Oncogenic Potential

HPV Type	Oncogenic Potential	Comment
6, 11	Low	• Anogenital warts
31, 33, 35,51, 52	Intermediate	• CIN 1, 2, 3
16, 18, 45, 56	High	• CIN 2, 3 • Invasive CA

Pathogenesis of HPV Infection (Fig. 4.3)

- **E6 and E7 oncoproteins** in the **high-risk HPV group** play an important role in the molecular pathogenesis of cervical cancer
- Proteins encoded by E6 and E7 genes of HPV 16 respectively bind and inactivate p53 and Rb proteins respectively, thereby invalidating their tumor suppressor functions
- HPV types 16 and 18 are found in 70% of invasive cancers
- **HPV-16 is most common HPV seen in invasive cancer cervix and CIN 2-3** (50% cases)
- **HPV-16 is not very specific** as it is also the most common HPV type in women with normal cytology
- **HPV-18 is more specific than HPV-16 for invasive tumors**

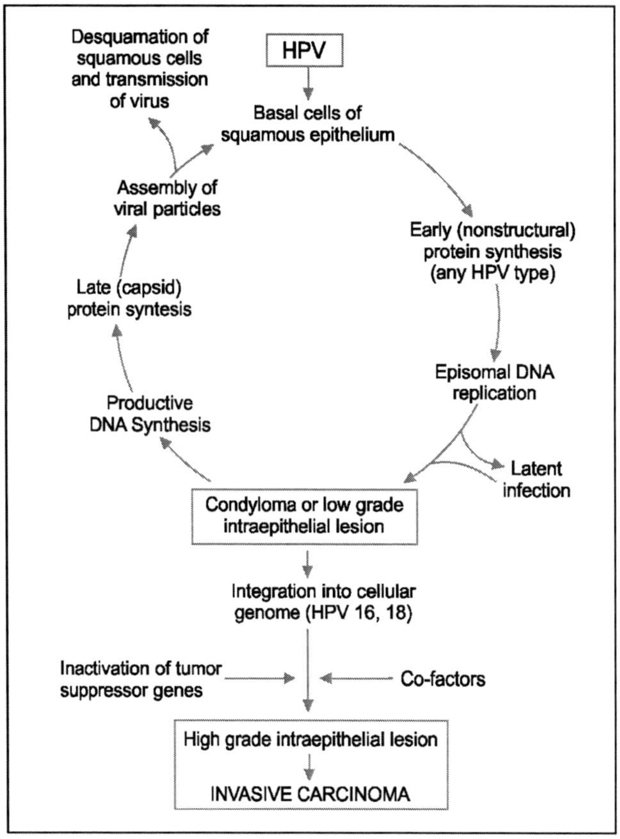

Fig. 4.3: Role of HPV in pathogenesis of cervical cancer

CIN CLASSIFICATION

CIN is classified into three histological grades - CIN 1, 2, 3 based on the involvement of thickness of epithelium (Fig 4.4)

The grades of CIN and comparison with other classification system is given in Table 4.2

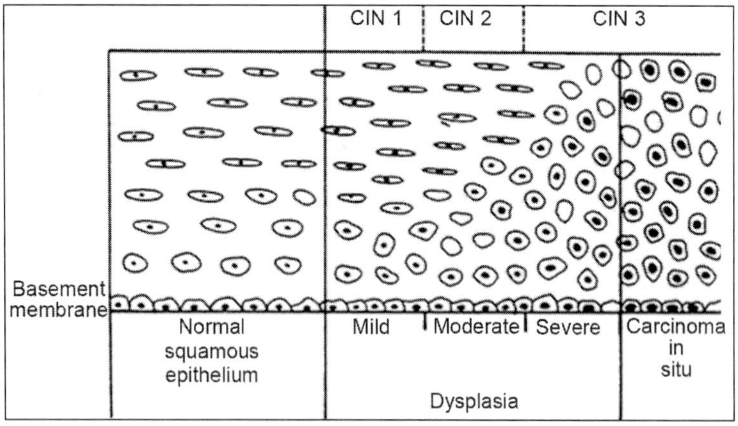

Fig 4.4: Grades of CIN

Table 4.2 Grades of CIN and Comparison with Other Classification Systems

CIN classification				Bethesda system
Histological grade	**Corresponding dysplasia**	**Description**	**Cause and progression**	**Corresponding terminology**
CIN 1	Mild dysplasia	Atypical changes are limited to lower one-third of epithelium	• CIN 1 represents low-grade lesion	Low-grade squamous intraepithelial lesion (LSIL) for CIN 1

Contd.

Contd.

			• CIN 1 lesion are caused by HPV during the infectious phase • Most CIN 1 lesions regress spontaneously	
CIN 2	Moderate dysplasia	Atypical changes extend to middle one-third of epithelium	• CIN 2 and 3 lesion represent high-grade lesions • They are caused by persistent HPV infection	High-grade squamous intraepithelial lesion (HSIL) for CIN 2 and 3
CIN 3	Severe dysplasia and carcinoma in situ	Atypical changes are severe and extend through the entire thickness of epithelium. Basement membrance is intact	• They are not necessarily preceded by CIN I • Progression to invasive cancer occurs more often (5% and 20% in CIN II and CIN III respectively)	

CIN, cervical intraepithelial neoplasia

CIN Progression

- CIN has the potential to develop invasive carcinoma over time. However, there is a long latent period between CIN and invasive carcinoma, which can be detected by screening **(Table 4.3 and Fig 4.5)**

Table 4.3: Progression of CIN

Scheme 2: Life cycle of unstable cervical epithelium

Cervical epithelium	**CIN I**	**CIN II**	**CIN III/CIS**
Regression to normal (%)	60	40	30
Persistence (%)	30	35	50
Progression to CIN III/CIS (%)	5-10	15-20	–
Progression to invasion (%)	< 1	5	20

	Normal	**CIN I, II**	**CIN III/CIS**	**Invasion**
Duration of disease progression (years)	0	5	10	20
Age of the patient (years)		25-30	30-35	40-45

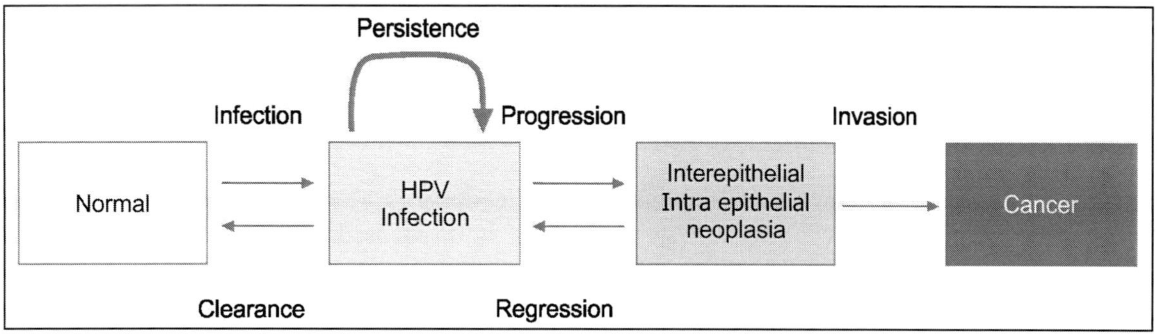

Fig 4.5: Progression of CIN

SCREENING TESTS FOR EARLY DETECTION OF PREINVASIVE LESIONS OF CERVIX

- Screening is public health intervention done to identify individuals with a high probability of having or developing a disease
- Screening for cervical cancer has reduced its incidence by early detection and treatment of precursor lesions namely CIN 1, 2, 3 and adenocarcinoma
- Screening for cervical cancer is easy to perform for the following reasons:
  - The cervix can be easily visualized and tests can be performed

- Cervical cancer goes through premalignant changes and there is a long latent period of 10–20 years before the disease progresses from a premalignant to malignant lesion
- Several screening modalities are available, but **Pap smear (exfoliative cytology) is a time-tested method of screening for cervical cancer and is most widely used**

Screening methods include the following:

- Pap smear
- Thin Prep–liquid-based cytology (LBC)
- HPV DNA testing
- Visual inspection after acetic acid (VIA)
- Visual inspection after Lugol's iodine (VILI)

Screening Guidelines (Table 4.4)

Table 4.4: The American College of Obstetrics and Gynecology (ACOG) and US Preventive Services Task Force (USPSTF) recommendations for cervical cancer screening (2012)

Question	Recommendation
When to start screening?	Screening should begin by 21 years of age or within 3 years of being sexually active, whichever is earlier
How frequently should screening be done and by which method?	At < 30 years, screen every 3 years with pap smear–HPV testing should not be used. At > 30 years, conventional cytology or liquid based cytology can be used • Screen every 5 years with Pap smear and HPV cotesting • Screen every 3 years with Pap smear alone • Women at high risk for cervical cancer must be screened more frequently
How long should screening continue?	Stop screening at 65 years, if previous smears are negative
Should screening be continued after total hysterectomy?	• Screening is not required after hysterectomy, except if done for CIN 2 and 3 • Continue the screening for women treated for CIN 2/3
CIN–cervical intraepithelial neoplasia	

Note

WHO has recommended at least one Pap smear in a woman's lifetime at 35 years for low resource settings where recommended screening cannot be done. If multiple smears can be performed, screening intervals can be increased to 10 years. The incidence of cervical cancer can be reduced remarkably even with such infrequent testing

SCREENING PROCEDURES

PAP Smear

Principle: It is a conventional cytological technique based on exfoliative cytology. The abnormal cells of the cervix exfoliate, that can be collected, smeared and stained. Ayre's wooden spatula and Cytobrush are used for the procedure

Prerequisites for taking a PAP smear: 48 hours prior to taking a Pap smear, ensure that the patient:

- Should not use vaginal cream
- Should not do vaginal douching
- Should not have sexual intercourse

Procedure (Fig 4.6)

- The cervix is visualized by placing a Sims' or Cuscos' speculum.
- Sample should be taken prior to use of lubricants and bimanual examination to prevent dislodgement of exfoliative cells
- The ectocervix is scraped using an Ayre's spatula by rotating the spatula 360° at external os and endocervix scraped with a Cytobrush

- The cells are smeared on a glass slide and fixed with liquid fixative or fixative spray. Fixation is done immediately to avoid air drying that can lead to artifacts
- The slides are stained using Papanicolaou stain which consists of Hematoxylin, Eosin and Orange G and then examined under microscope
- **Fixatives used** are the following:
  - Ethyl alcohol 95% (1:1 mixture of 95% ethanol and ether)
  - Isopropyl alcohol 85%
  - Methanol
  - Surgical spirit

Efficacy of Pap smear: Pap smear has a high specificity (98%) but low sensitivity (60%) and high false-negative rate (50%)

False-negative values occur due to the following:

- Sampling error
- Fixation error
- Interpretation error

Advantages of Pap smear as a screening test:

- Easy to perform on an OPD basis
- Reasonable sensitivity and specificity
- Not very expensive

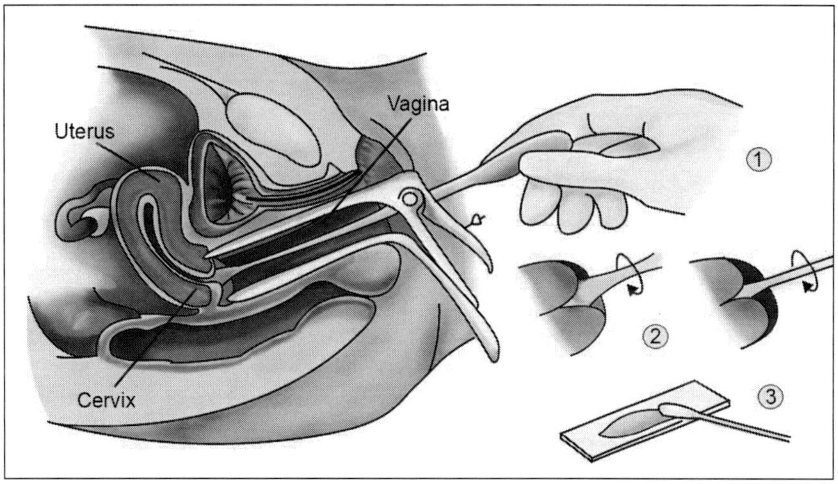

1. Cuscos speculum introduced, Ayre's spatula introduced
2. Ectocervical sample collected by rotating Ayre's spatula 360 deg. at cervical os; endocervical sampling done with a Cytobrush
3. Sample is smeared on a glass slide

Fig 4.6: Pap Smear Procedure

Extra edge

Uses of Ayre's spatula

- To take a PAP smear
- Surface biopsy in Carcinoma cervix
- Hormonal cytology–smear from lateral vaginal wall
- To take a vault smear–Follow up after surgery/RT for recurrence
- To take a buccal smear

Thinprep—Liquid-Based Cytology

Principle: A liquid based medium is used to collect the sample, then filtered and and a monolayer of cells is prepared.

Procedure (Fig. 4.7)

- Sample from cervix is collected in the usual way using a spatula and endocervical brush or by using a special broom sampling device
- Sample is rinsed in a vial containing liquid-based medium–80–90% cells are transferred to the liquid medium and transported to the laboratory
- Cells are separated by passing the liquid through a filter that traps large epithelial cells
- Thin monolayer of cells is prepared, fixed and is interpreted by a cytologist

Advantages

- Decreases sampling and preparation errors
- Eliminates artifacts due to air drying
- Removes blood and other cells that interfere with interpretation
- High specificity and Low false-negative rates
- Fewer unsatisfactory smears
- Can use the residual sample for HPV testing

Disadvantages

- It is expensive.
- Laboratory staff need special training to do the procedure

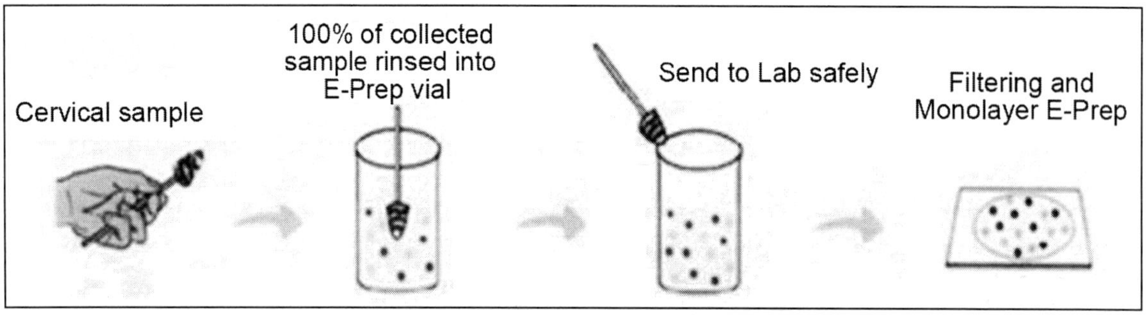

Fig 4.7 Liquid based cytology procedure

HPV – DNA Testing

- Tests for detection of high-risk HPV DNA are commonly used
- **In women <30 years,** prevalence of HPV infection is high and transient. Hence, **HPV- DNA testing has poor sensitivity in this age group**
- **In women >30 years, HPV testing may be used along with cytology (HPV cotesting). The screening interval can be increased to 5 years, if HPV testing is negative**

Visual Inspection After Acetic Acid (VIA)

Principle: Abnormal cells have increased chromatin density and are rich in protein that get coagulated with acetic acid and hence turn white, while normal cells containing glycogen remain normal

- Areas of HPV-related changes, CIN and neoplasia turn acetowhite with acetic acid application

Procedure - Acetic acid 5% is applied to the cervix ->abnormal areas turn acetowhite ->Biopsy taken from acetowhite areas

Advantages

- Health workers can be trained to identify abnormal areas after application of acetic acid on cervix. If VIA is positive, the patient has to be referred to a higher institution for colposcopic evaluation
- This method has been extensively studied in developing countries including India and is currently recommended as the primary screening test for cancer cervix in developing countries

Disadvantages

- Specificity of the test is less (80%) and the false-positive rate is high, resulting in large number of referrals for further evaluation

Visual Inspection After Lugol's Iodine

Principle: When Lugol's iodine or Schiller's iodine is applied on the cervix, normal cervical epithelium, which is rich in glycogen, stains mahogany brown (Schiller test).The abnormal areas rich in protein do not take up the iodine and appear mustard yellow

- Lugol's iodine consists of **10% potassium iodide with 5% iodine**

Advantages and disadvantages are similar to those of VIA

REPORTING OF CERVICAL CYTOLOGY (Table 4.5 and 4.6)

Table 4.5: The Bethesda System Classification of Epithelial Cell Abnormalities

Squamous cell abnormalities	Glandular cell abnormalities
• Atypical squamous cells of undetermined significance (ASCUS)	• Atypical endocervical cells
• Atypical Squamous cells high grade (ASC-HG)	• Atypical endometrial cells
• Low-grade squamous intraepithelial lesion (L-SIL)	• Atypical glandular cells (AGC)
• High-grade squamous intraepithelial lesion (H-SIL)	• Endocervical adenocarcinoma in situ
• Squamous cell carcinoma	• Adenocarcinoma

Table 4.6: Comparison of Various Classification Systems for Reporting Cervical Cytology

Pap Class System (1954)	Scheme I Reagan (1956) (WHO)	Scheme II Richart (2001)	Scheme III Bethesda (1988)
Class 1	Negative for malignant cells	Negative	Within normal limits
Class 2	• Inflammation • Squamous atypia • Koilocytes		Reactive and reparative changes (ASCUS)
Class 3	Mild dysplasia	• CIN-I (HPV)	• LSIL (HPV)
Class 4	• Moderate dysplasia • Severe dysplasia • Carcinoma in situ	• CIN-II • CIN-III	• HSIL • HSIL
Class 5	Invasive cancer	Invasive cancer	Invasive cancer

EVALUATION AND MANAGEMENT FOLLOWING CERVICAL CYTOLOGY REPORT (Table 4.7)

Bethesda system assures uniformity of reporting and provides clear guidelines for further evaluation and management

Table 4.7: Evaluation Following Cytology Report

Cervical cytology	Further evaluation/management
Normal	Continue screening as usual
Atypical squamous cells of undermined significance (ASCUS)	HPV testing (or) repeat cytology after 1 year
Atypical squamous cells-high grade (ASC-HG)	Colposcopy
LSIL	Colposcopy
HSIL	Colposcopy
AGC	Colposcopy, ECC
Adenocarcinoma in situ	Colposcopy, ECC and endometrial sampling, if > 35 years

AGC, atypical glandular cells; HSIL, high-grade squamous intraepithelial lesion; LSIL, low-grade squamous intraepithelial lesion; ECC, endocervical curettage

Approach to women undergoing screening with cervical cytology–adapted from American Society For Colposcopy and Cervical Pathology (ASCCP) Guidelines-2012 for Management of Abnormal Cervical Cytology (Flowcharts)

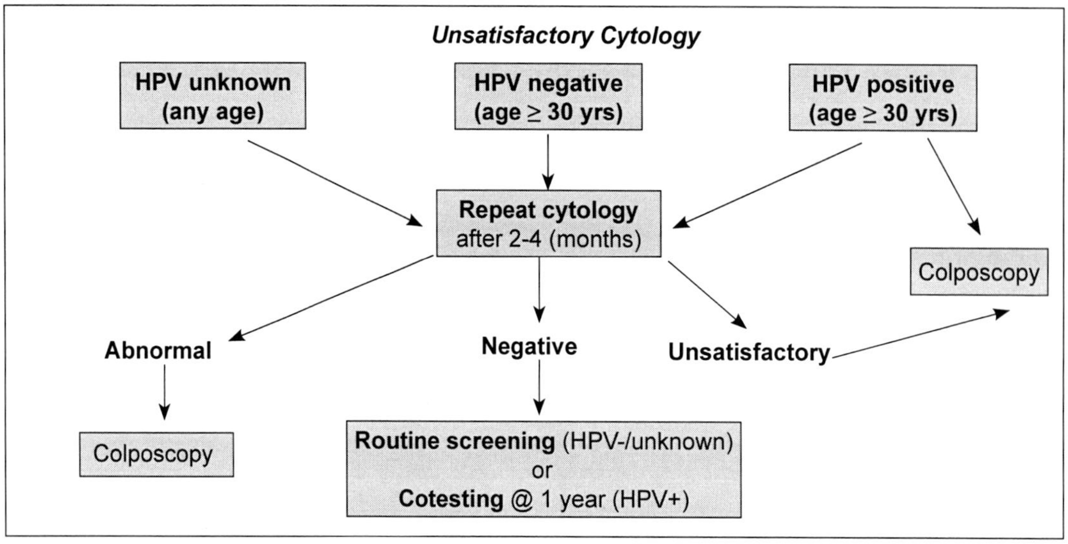

Flowchart 1: Management of Unsatisfactory Cytology

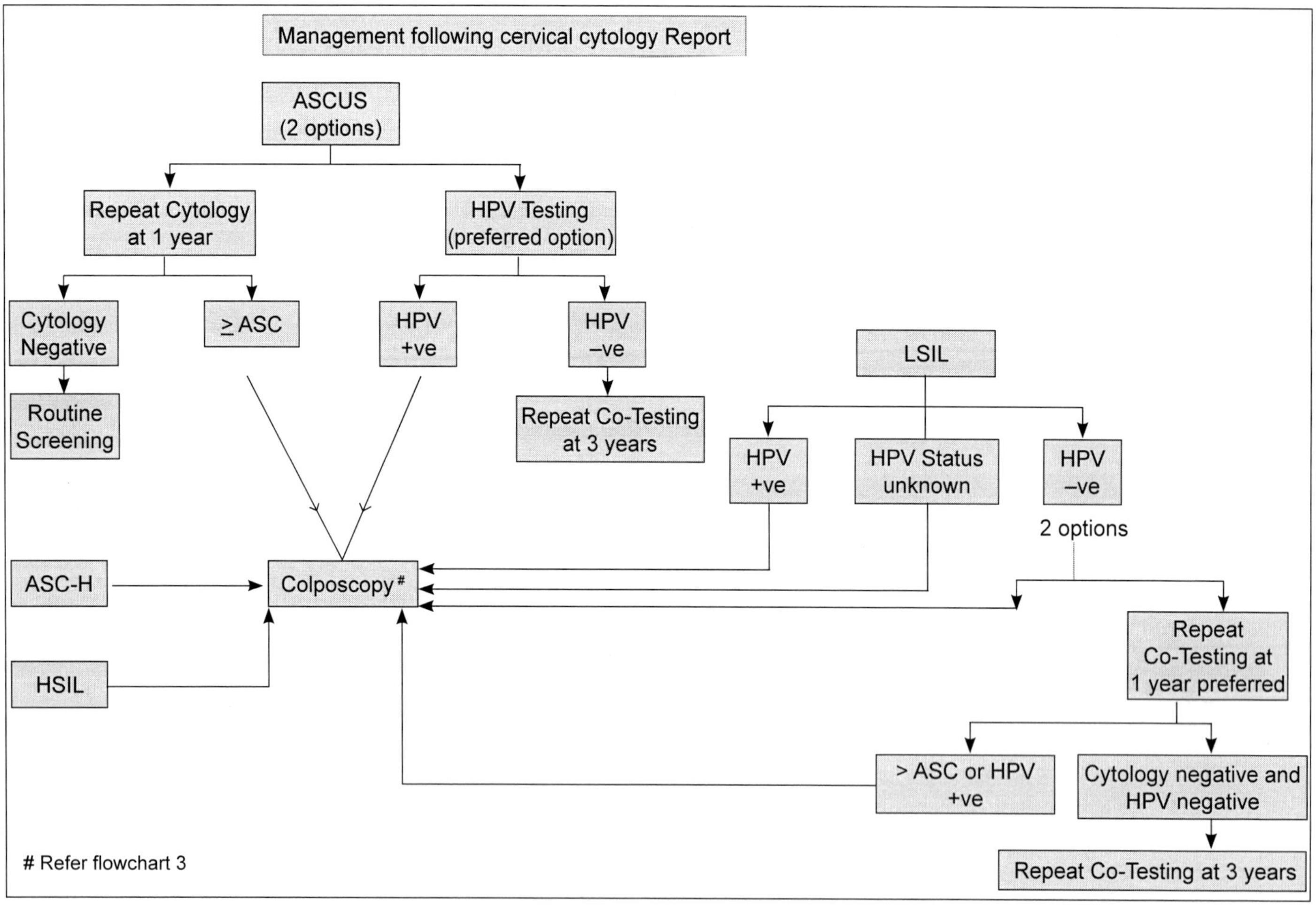

Flowchart 2: Management of Abnormal Cervical Cytology

COLPOSCOPY

- Colposcopy is **visualization of the cervix, vagina and vulva under a low-magnification microscope** to detect premalignant and malignant lesions. It helps to localize abnormal areas from where biopsy has to be taken
- **Acetic acid 5%** can be applied and biopsies are taken when indicated
- It is **complementary and not a substitute for cytology**

Satisfactory colposcopy is indicated by visualization of the squamo-columnar junction (SCJ), transformation zone, and the columnar epithelium

Indications

- Abnormal Pap smear
- Cervix looks suspicious but Pap is normal
- Lesion is not clinically detected–to locate abnormal areas and to study the extent of lesion
- To plan colposcopic guided conservative procedures
- To follow-up of patients who are conservatively managed

Abnormal Colposcopic Findings

Atypical transformation zone
Keratosis
Aceto-white epithelium
Punctation
Mosaicism
Atypical vessels
Suspect frank invasive carcinoma
Unsatisfactory colposcopic findings

Reid's Colposcopic Index (RCI)

- RCT is a Systematic objective method of colposcopic grading of severity of premalignant cervical lesions
- It is a well-known scoring system designed to standardize colposcopic assessment and assist in the prediction of histological diagnosis (Table 4.8)
- The index **considers four colposcopic signs: lesion margin, color of acetowhitening, blood vessels, and iodine staining**
- By evaluating 4 colposcopic features, **maximum score of 8 can be obtained; the score achieved is reported to be 97% accurate at predicting the grade of cervical intraepithelial neoplasia**

Table 4.8: Scoring system for Reid's Colposcopic Index (RCI)

	Score		
Colposcopic Sign	**Zero Points**	**One Point**	**Two Points**
Margin	Exophytic condylomas; areas showing a micropapillary contour Lesions with distinct edges Feathered, scalloped edges Lesions with an angular, jagged shape "Satellite" areas and acetowhitening distal to the original squamocolumnar junction	Lesions with a regular (circular or semicircular) shape, showing smooth, straight edges	Rolled, peeling edges Any internal demarcation between areas of differing colposcopic appearance
Color	Shiny, snow-white color Areas of faint (semitransparent) whitening	Intermediate shape (shiny, but gray-white)	Dull reflectance with oyster-white color
Vessels	Fine-caliber vessels, poorly formed patterns	No surface vessels	Definite, coarse punctation or mosaic pattern
Iodine	Any lesion staining mahogany brown; mustard-yellow staining by a minor lesion (by the first three criteria)	Partial iodine staining (mottled pattern)	Mustard-yellow staining of a significant lesion (an acetowhite area scoring 3 or more points by the first three criteria)

Swede's Colposcopic Index (SCI)

- The Swede score is a **new scoring system devised by Strander et al.**
- **This includes lesion size as a variable to be scored in addition to the 4 variables found in the Reid colposcopic index, along with modifications to definitions of the scores for the remaining variables** (Table 4.9)
- This scoring index showed that the **specificity for a total score of 8 or higher was 90% and that no lesion of CIN 2 or higher resulted in a score of less than 5**

Table 4.9: Scoring system for Swede's Colposcopic Index (SCI)

Swede Score	0	1	2
Aceto uptake	Zero or transparent	Shady, milky Neither transparent nor opaque	Distinct Opaque White
Margins/surface	Diffuse	Sharp but irregular, jagged, geographic satellites	Sharp, even difference in surface level, includes cuffing
Vessels	Fine, regular	Absent	Coarse of Atypical
Lesion size	< 5 mm	5-15 mm or Two quadrants	> 15 mm or Three to four quadrants or undefined endocervically
Iodine staining	Brown	Faintly or patchy yellow	Distinct yellow

DIAGNOSTIC CONIZATION/CONE BIOPSY

- It refers to **excision of a cone-shaped tissue from the cervix,** with base of cone at ectocervix and apex in the endocervical canal, close to the internal os. Procedure is done under anesthesia

Indications for conization

- Unsatisfactory colposcopy–entire limits of the lesion or the transformation zone not visible in colposcopy
- Large lesions extending into the endocervical canal
- Cytology–colposcopy discordance (cytology shows more severe grade lesion)
- Suspected microinvasive cancer
- CIN reported in endocervical curettage
- Histological diagnosis of adenocarcinoma in situ
- It serves as therapeutic purpose in CIN II,III lesions

Methods for Cone Biopsy

- Cold knife cone biopsy
- Large loop excision of transformation zone (LLETZ)
- Loop electrosurgical excision procedure (LEEP)
- Needle excision of transformation zone (NETZ)

TREATMENT OF PRE INVASIVE LESIONS OF CERVIX ON HISTOLOGY

Management of CIN 1 histology (Table 4.10)

- Most cases of CIN 1 regress spontaneously overtime
- Risk of progression to invasive cancer is <1%

Table 4.10: Management of CIN 1 Histology

Management in women <25 years of age	Management in women >25 years of age
Repeat cytology at 12 and 24 months. If cytology shows persistent LSIL,then colposcopy and biopsy are indicated	Management options include the following:

Contd.

Contd.

	• **Follow-up** with cytology/HPV co-testing at 12 and 24 months – If cytology is positive or HPV testing is positive, colposcopy and biopsy are indicated. – If cytology is negative and HPV testing is negative -> age appropriate retesting can be done 3 years later • **If patient cannot be followed** up -Treat with excision/ablative procedure

Management of CIN 2 and 3 histology (Table 4.11)

- Risk of progression of CIN 2 to invasive cancer is 5% and of CIN 3 to invasive cancer is 12%. Therefore, colposcopy and prompt treatment is mandatory

Table 4.11: Management of CIN 2 and 3 Histology

Management in young women desirous of future reproductive function	Management in women who have completed family
• **If colposcopy is satisfactory, options are as follows:** – Follow up with cytology and colposcopy every 6 months and HPV co-testing after 1 year. If HSIL persists, repeat biopsy – Treat with excision procedure	• **If colposcopy is satisfactory,** excision or ablation procedure is recommended; excision procedure is preferred
• **If colposcopy is unsatisfactory,** excision procedure is recommended	• **If colposcopy is unsatisfactory,** excision procedure is recommended

LAST PROJECT (Lower Anogenital Squamous Terminology Standardization Project for HPV-Associated Lesions-2012)

LAST PROJECT RECOMMENDATIONS

- **A two-tiered nomenclature LSIL and HSIL, was recommended for noninvasive HPV associated squamous proliferations of Lower anogenital tract, which may be further qualified with appropriate _IN terminology**
- **CIN1 is equivalent to histopathological LSIL and CIN 2, 3 is equivalent to histopathological HSIL (see flowchart below)**

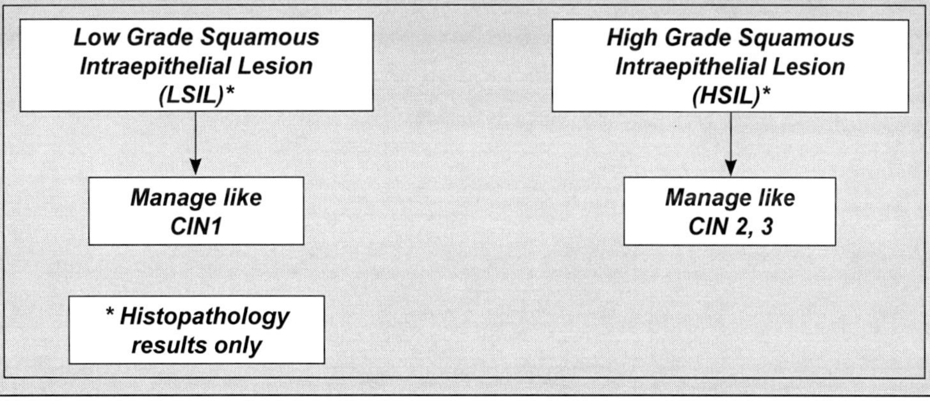

Note

- ***Histopathological CIN1 is equivalent to histopathological LSIL***
- ***Histopathological CIN 2-3 is equivalent to histopathological HSIL***
- *But, histopathological CIN1 and CIN2,3 are not equivalent to cytological LSIL and HSIL* ***(Bethesda system)***

MANAGEMENT OF CIN HISTOLOGY–American Society for Colposcopy and Cervical Pathology (ASCCP) Guidelines-2012

- **For managing cervical pre cancer, the histopathological classification is two-tiered (LAST recommendation), applying the terms CIN1 to low-grade lesions (LGIL) and CIN 2, 3 to high-grade lesions (HGIL) –Flowchart 3**

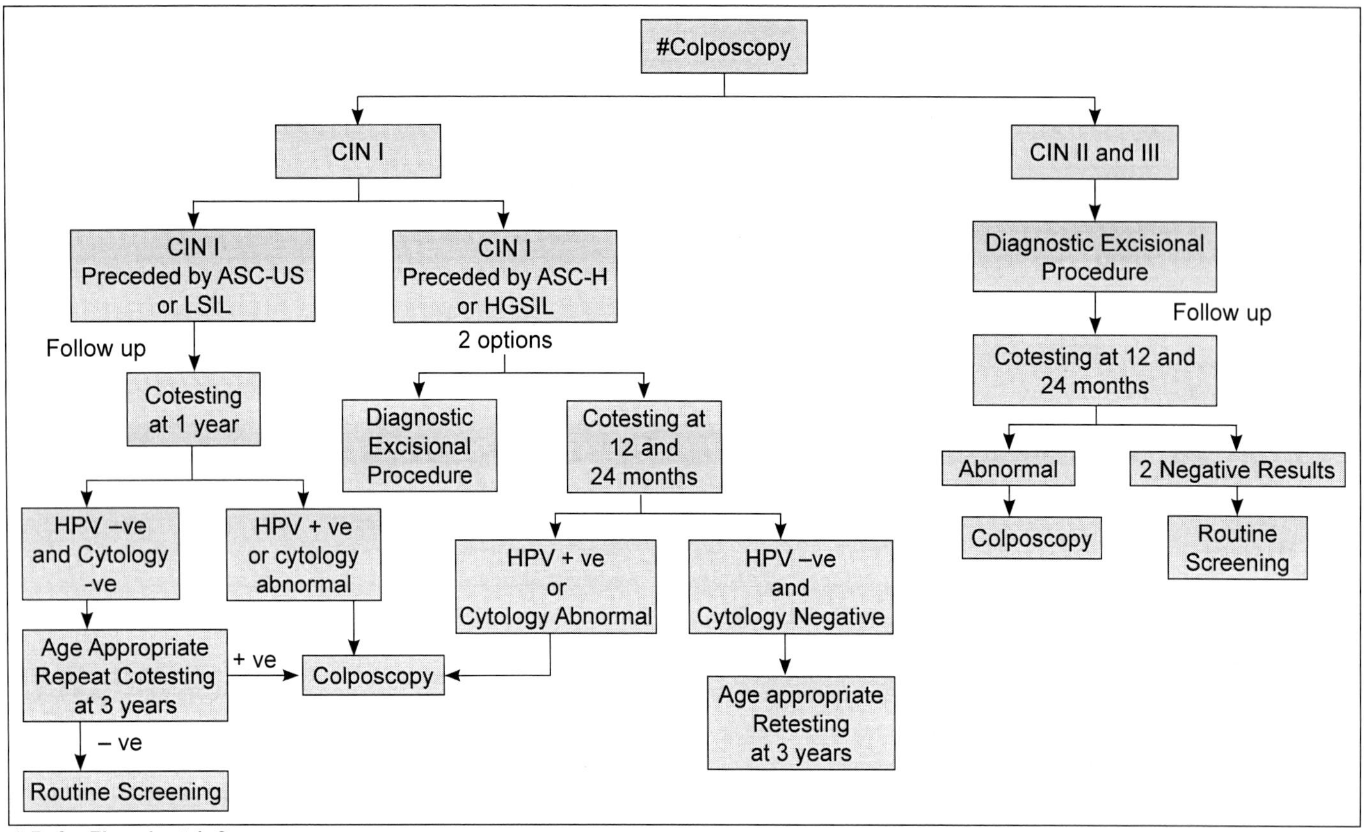

Refer Flowchart 1, 2

Flowchart 3- Management of CIN Lesions on Colposcopy

Treatment Modalities Available for Pre Invasive Lesions of Cervix (Table 4.12)

Table 4.12: Procedures available for treatment of pre invasive lesions of cervix

	Ablative procedures	Excision procedures
Procedures	• Cauterization (thermoablation) • Cryotherapy (Figure) • Laser ablation	• Cold knife conization • Laser conization with CO_2 laser • Large loop excision of transformation zone (LLETZ) • Loop electrosurgical excision procedure (LEEP)
Advantages	• Easy to perform • No risk of excessive bleeding • Useful in low-resource settings	• Specimen obtained for histopathological examination • Can identify occult microinvasive lesion or adenocarcinoma of endocervix (tissue biopsy obtained)
Disadvantages	• These procedures cause local destruction of tissue and hence no tissue is obtained for histopathology • Cryotherapy can cause profuse watery discharge for 2-4 weeks	• Cold knife conization can be associated with immediate complications such as hemorrhage and infection and late complications such as cervical stenosis, cervical incompetence, recurrent pregnancy loss, and preterm labor • Laser conization equipment is expensive and expertise is required for performing the procedure

CARCINOMA CERVIX

Risk Factors for Cancer Cervix

- Coitus at an early age (<16 years)
- Child birth at early age < 20 years
- Multi parity
- Multiple sexual partners
- Pills - OCPs (OCPs usage for >5 years doubles the risk of endocervical carcinoma)
- Papilloma virus (HPV -16, 18) – ***major etiological agent in cervical cancer***
- Infections
  - HIV, STDs *(Ca. cervix is an AIDS defining cancer)*
  - HSV-2, Chlamydia trachomatis – act as co factors
- Immunosuppression
- Socioeconomic group–low SES
- Smoking cigarette *(smoking for 20 years doubles the risk for Ca. cervix)*
- Smegma from uncircumscribed male partners *(increased incidence of Ca. cervix in African Americans and decreased risk in Jews and Muslims who undergo circumcision)*

Clinical Features

Symptoms

- Carcinoma cervix usually occurs in multiparous women between the age group of 35 and 65 years
- It may be asymptomatic in early stages
- **Common presentation include the following:**
  - PMB
  - Metrorrhagia/heavy menstrual bleeding (HMB)
  - Postcoital bleeding
  - Intermenstrual bleeding
- Vaginal discharge
  - Blood-stained discharge
  - Foul-smelling purulent discharge (due to infection of necrotic tissue in the growth)
- Back pain: It is a late symptom due to infiltration of sacral nerves
- Cachexia and weight loss may be present in advanced stages
- Invasion of surrounding structures can present with following symptoms
  - *Hematuria:* Bladder involvement
  - *Tenesmus and bleeding per rectum:* Rectal involvement
  - *Renal failure and uremia:* Compression of ureters (uremia is the most common cause of death in carcinoma cervix)
  - *Pain radiating to legs:* Sciatic nerve involvement
  - *Edema of lower limbs:* Lymphatic and venous compression

Signs

- Cancer cervix will have the following features on speculum examination:
  - The cervical lesion may be exophytic (cauliflower like proliferative growth), endophytic (hard, barrel-shaped cervix), or ulcerative.
  - The lesion will have the following **characteristic features–friability, bleeding on touch, induration and fixity**
- Rectal and rectovaginal examinations should be done in all cases of suspected carcinoma cervix, to check for involvement of parametrium, pelvic side walls, rectal mucosa and recto vaginal septum

Confirmation of Diagnosis

- **Cervical punch Biopsy should be taken from the margin of the growth** and sent for histopathology
- Biopsy should not be taken from the center because it would contain only necrotic tissue due to reduced blood supply

Varieties on macroscopic or naked eye appearance of cervical cancer

- **Exophytic** – proliferative, cauliflower like growth arising from anterior or posterior lip of cervix with rough granular bleeding surface
- **Infiltrative or endophytic**–Infiltrates the cervical stroma without any obvious growth. **Arises mostly from endocervical canal. Barrel shaped cervix in P/R examination**
- **Ulcerative** – lesion excavates the cervix like an irregular crater

Histological Types of Cervical Cancer

- **Squamous cell carcinoma**–Carcinoma arises from squamous epithelium of cervix – **most common type (80 -90%). It is of** 3 subtypes
  - Large cell keratinizing-shows foci of keratinization with keratin pearls
  - Large cell non keratinizing–no keratin pearls
  - Small cell carcinoma–poorly differentiated carcinoma
- **Adenocarcinoma**–arises from columnar cells lining the endocervical canal
  - 10-20 % cases
  - Prognosis is poor when compared to squamous cell carcinoma

Mode of Spread of Carcinoma Cervix

- Direct spread–to uterus, vagina, bladder, rectum, parametrium
- Lymphatic spread to parametrial, obturator, external iliac, common iliac, internal iliac, para aortic lymph nodes
- Hematogenous spread to distant organs
- Intra peritoneal spread

Risk of Ovarian metastases

Squamous cell carcinoma of the cervix	0.5 %
Adenocarcinoma of cervix	1.7%

Causes of Death In Cancer Cervix

- **Uremia**–This is due to ureteric obstruction following parametrial involvement by the tumor leading to hydroureter and hydronephrosis. Infection sets in, thereby compromising kidney functions further, leading to uremia
- **Hemorrhage**–The vaginal bleeding from the growth may be brisk or continuous leading to anemia
- **Sepsis**–Pelvic or generalized peritonitis may occur which may be fatal.
- **Cancer Cachexia**–The cancerous tissues have got depressant action on general metabolism leading to cachexia

Extra Edge

Causes of nodularity of utero sacral ligament

- *Endometriosis*
- *Carcinoma cervix*

Causes of Pouch of Douglas (POD) deposits

- *Endometriosis*
- *Secondary deposits from ovarian tumor*

STAGING OF CARCINOMA CERVIX

Once histological diagnosis of cervical cancer is made, next step is to stage the disease to formulate the most effective therapy. **Cervical cancer is clinically staged (Table 4.13 and Fig 4.8)**

Table 4.13: Staging of Carcinoma Cervix (FIGO 2009)

Stage	Description
Stage I:	Cancer is confined to cervix
IA:	Microinvasive cancer (diagnosed only on microscopy)
1B:	Clinically visible lesion
IA1:	Depth of stromal invasion ≤3 mm and horizontal extension of ≤7 mm
IA2:	Depth of stromal invasion >3 and ≤5 mm, horizontal extension of ≤7 mm
IB1:	Clinically visible lesion of ≤4 cm
IB2:	Clinically visible lesion of >4 cm
Stage II:	Cancer spreads beyond cervix, but not to pelvic side walls or lower one-third of vagina.
IIA:	Involves upper two-third of vagina without parametrial involvement
IIA1	Lesion of ≤4 cm
IIA2	lesion of >4 cm
IIB:	Parametrium involved but not up to pelvic side walls
Stage III:	Cancer extends to pelvic side walls and/or involves lower one-third of vagina and/or causes hydronephrosis or nonfunctioning kidney
IIIA:	Involves lower one-third of vagina but not the pelvic side walls
IIIB:	Extends to pelvic side walls and/or hydronephrosis or nonfunctioning kidney
Stage IV:	Cancer extends beyond true pelvis or involves mucosa of bladder or rectum.
IVA:	Involves mucosa of adjacent organs–bladder and rectum
IVB:	Distant metastasis

NOTE

- *Parametrium involvement up to pelvic sidewalls means that on rectal examination, there is no cancer-free space between the tumor and the pelvic sidewalls*
- *All cases of Carcinoma cervix with hydronephrosis or nonfunctioning kidney are included under Stage 3B, unless they are known to be due to other causes*
- *Bullous edema of bladder as such does not permit the case to be allotted to stage IV. Mucosal involvement of bladder or rectum is considered as Stage IV*
- *Involvement of vascular or lymphatic spaces does not change the stage allotment*

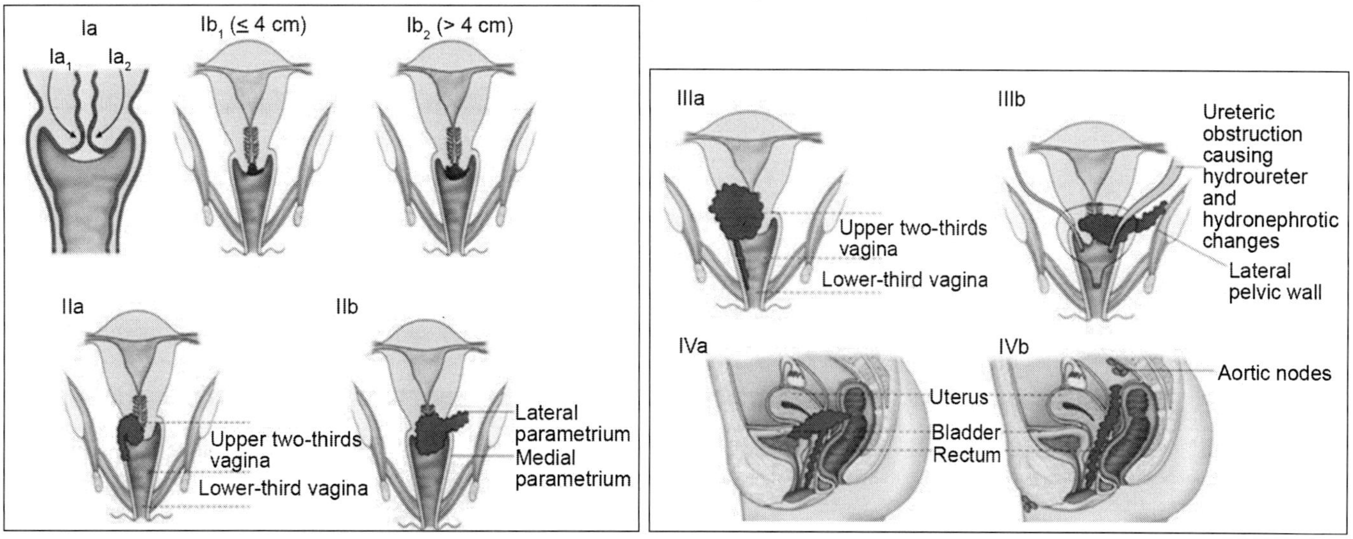

Fig 4.8: FIGO 2009 Staging of carcinoma cervix

Standard staging procedures accepted by International Federation of Gynecology and Obstetrics (FIGO)

- Per speculum examination, bimanual pelvic examination and rectal examination to assess tumor size, vaginal extension, and parametrial invasion
- Cervical biopsy, endocervical curettage, or conization to confirm diagnosis
- Colposcopy in early stage disease
- Cystoscopy and proctoscopy in women with advanced disease to look for bladder and rectal involvement
- Hysteroscopy in endocervical lesions and to detect extension to uterus
- Intravenous pyelography (IVP) to detect hydroureteronephrosis
- Chest X-ray to detect lung metastasis

Other Modalities for Staging

- **Ultrasonography:** To assess tumor volume, hydroureteronephrosis, liver metastasis, and associated gynecological pathology
- **CT scan:** To assess lymph nodes, regional extension and distant metastasis
- **MRI:** To assess parametrial infiltration and regional extension, lymph nodes, tumor volume, hydroureteronephrosis, and distant metastasis **(MRI is better than CT for assessment of local invasion and parametrial involvement)**
- **Positron emission tomography (PET) scan:** To assess lymph nodes and distant metastasis (best method)
- **Sigmoidoscopy:** To assess large bowel involvement
- **Sentinel node biopsy:** To assess lymph node involvement

Note

- *Routine supplementary investigations include chest X-ray, iIVP, cystoscopy, and proctoscopy*
- *In cases of suspected pelvic inflammation, a course of antibiotic should be given prior to clinical staging*
- *If any doubt exists as to which stage to be assigned, the lower stage should be chosen*
- *The results of other modalities for staging can change the proposed treatment but do not alter the FIGO staging*
- *Once assigned, the stage remains the same. Staging cannot be changed once therapy has begun*

Disadvantages of Clinical staging

- Difficult to assess the **lymph node involvement** on clinical examination which is **a main factor determining prognosis**
- Difficulty in differentiating inflammatory and malignant induration of the parametrium

Extra Edge

RECENT ADVANCES IN INVESTIGATION OF CERVICAL CANCER

Fluoro-2-deoxy-glucose (FDG) PET scan*: This test is based on the fact that malignant cells exhibit glycolysis more than normal cells and FDG accumulates in malignant cells.* ***FDG PET scan is a gold standard investigation for carcinoma cervix but very expensive***

Tumor marker for Cancer cervix

Squamous cell carcinoma (SCC) *antigen is a serum marker for carcinoma cervix. Although the antigen is not specific, it has been found to be useful to monitor treatment response and to predict tumor recurrence*

Sentinel lymph node sampling

- ***Sentinel lymph node (SLN) is the first node that drains a primary tumor*** *that can be detected by* ***intraoperative lymphatic mapping****. This is done by* ***injecting methylene blue dye*** *into the tumor or by lymphoscintigraphy using* ***technetium-99***
- *It has been studied in Ca. breast, Ca. vulva, Ca. cervix and Ca. penis*

Microinvasive Cancer Cervix

- Diagnosis of Stage IA1 and IA2 made on microscopic examination of a tissue/specimen obtained by doing a LEEP (loop electrosurgical excision procedure) or cone biopsy specimen or trachelectomy or hysterectomy is termed as microinvasive lesion

Contd.

Contd.

- Lymphovascular space involvement is very less at this depth of invasion and hence called as microinvasive lesion
- Lesion with ≤ 3mm depth of invasion – lymph node metastasis is rare
- Lesion with >3 to ≤ 5 mm depth of invasion – 5% involvement of lymph nodes
- The term **"early stage cervical cancer"** is used for stages **IA, IB, and IIA**
- The term **"locally advanced cervical cancer"** is used **for stages IIB–IVA**
- **Carcinoma in situ is not included in FIGO staging**

Revised FIGO Staging of Carcinoma of the Cervix (2018)

- **Until 2018, the FIGO staging was based on clinical examination with the addition of certain procedures that were allowed by FIGO to change the staging**
- **In 2018, this has been revised by the FIGO Gynecologic Oncology Committee to allow imaging and pathological findings, where available, to assign the stage**
- **The revised staging is shown in Table 4.14 (presented at the FIGO XXII World Congress of Gynecology and Obstetrics)**

Table 4.14: Revised FIGO Staging of Cervical Cancer - 2018

Stage	Description
I	The carcinoma is strictly confined to the cervix (extension to the uterine corpus should be disregarded)
IA	Invasive carcinoma that can be diagnosed only by microscopy, with maximum depth of invasion < 5 mm[a]
IA1	Measured stromal invasion ≤ 3 mm in depth
IA2	Measured stromal invasion > 3 mm and ≤ 5 mm in depth
IB	Invasive carcinoma with measured deepest invasion > 5 mm (greater than Stage IA), lesion limited to the cervix uteri"[b]
IB1	Invasive carcinoma > 5 mm depth of stromal invasion and ≤ 2 cm in greatest dimension
IB2	Invasive carcinoma > 2 cm and ≤ 4 cm in greatest dimension
IB3	Invasive carcinoma > 4 cm in greatest dimension
II	The carcinoma invades beyond the uterus, but has not extended onto the lower third of the vagina or to the pelvic wall
IIA	Involvement limited to the upper two-third of the vagina without parametrial involvement
IIA1	Invasive carcinoma ≤ 4 cm in greatest dimension
IIA2	Invasive carcinoma > 4 cm in greatest dimension
IIB	With parametrial involvement but not up to the pelvic wall
III	The carcinoma involves the lower third of the vagina and/or extends to the pelvic wall and/or causes hydronephrosis or non-functioning kidney and/or involves pelvic and/or para-aortic lymph nodes[c]
IIIA	The carcinoma involves the lower third of the vagina, with no extension to the pelvic wall
IIIB	Extension to the pelvic wall and/or hydronephrosis or non-functioning kidney (unless known to be due to another cause)
IIIC	Involvement of pelvic and/or para-aortic lymph nodes, irrespective of tumor size and extent (with r and p notations)[c]
IIIC1	Pelvic lymph node metastasis only
IIIC2	Para-aortic lymph node metastasis
IV	The carcinoma has extended beyond the true pelvis or has involved (biopsy proven) the mucosa of the bladder or rectum. (A bullous edema, as such, does not permit a case to be allotted to Stage IV)
IVA	Spread to adjacent pelvic organs
IVB	Spread to distant organs

When in doubt, the lower staging should be assigned

a. Imaging and pathology can be used, where available, to supplement clinical findings with respect to tumor size and extent, in all stages

b. The involvement of vascular/lymphatic spaces does not change the staging. The lateral extent of the lesion is no longer considered

c. Adding notation of r (imaging) and (pathology) to indicate the findings that are used to allocate the case to Stage IIIC. Example: If imaging indicates pelvic lymph node metastasis, the stage allocation would be Stage IIIC1r, and if confirmed by pathology findings, it would be Stage IIIC1p. The type of imaging modality or pathology technique used should always be documented

Key Amendments to Staging of Cancer of the Cervix Uteri
The following amendments to the staging classification of carcinoma of the cervix uteri were made by the FIGO Committee for Gynecologic Oncology in 2019:
1. Allowing the use of any imaging modality and/or pathological findings for allocating the stage
2. In stage I, amendments to microscopic pathological findings and to size designation, allowing the use of imaging and/or pathological assessment of the size of the cervical tumor
3. In stage II, allowing the use of imaging and/or pathological assessment of size and extent of the cervical tumor
4. In stages I through III, allowing assessment of retroperitoneal lymph nodes by imaging and/or pathological findings and, if deemed metastatic the case is designated as stage IIIC (with notation of method used for stage allocation)
5. No recommendations for routine investigations, which are to be decided on the basis of clinical findings and standard of care

General Recommendations
1. The revised staging system does not mandate the use of a specific imaging technique, lymph node biopsy, or surgical assessment of the extent of tumor. In low-resourced conditions, clinicians can continue to assess the patient clinically as before
a. The size of the primary tumor can be assessed by clinical evaluation, (pre- or intraoperative) imaging, and/or pathological measurement
b. Identification of lymph node metastasis to be accomplished using imaging technique(s) and/or pathological assessment methods available to the provider, and the choice of technique depends on its availability
2. It is recommended that the method used for imaging (e.g., ultra-sound, computed tomography (CT), magnetic resonance imaging (MRI), position emission tomography [PET], PET-CT. MRI-PET, etc.) and /or the pathological technique used (e.g., evaluation of the operative specimen, lymph node biopsy, or find needle aspiration cytology), and the results there of, should be recorded, so that subsequent data analysis can be performed. The imaging method can be used for the following:
a. For measurement of the primary tumor size
b. For assessment of extension into the surrounding tissues and adjacent organs
c. For assessment of location and characteristics of the retroperitoneal lymph nodes:
3. It is recognized that there will be limitations for imaging findings in low-and lower-middle-income countries as a result of paucity, non-availability, or inadequate access to extensive imaging services
4. As in the previous staging, when in doubt, the lower staging should be assigned

TREATMENT OF CANCER CERVIX

Two main modalities of treatment are surgery and radiotherapy (RT); chemotherapy is a valuable adjunct therapy. Treatment depends on following:

- Stage of the cancer
- Age of the patient
- Associated comorbidities
- Associated gynecological problems (fibroid, ovarian tumor)
- Facilities and expertise available
- Patient's choice

Pretreatment evaluation

- Complete hemogram (to detect and correct anemia before surgery or chemo radiation)
- Blood grouping and typing, reservation
- Urine albumin, sugar, and microscopy examination (to detect RBCs in urine)
- Renal function test (to detect renal failure; to obtain a baseline value prior to starting therapy)
- Liver function test (may be abnormal in advanced malignancy with metastasis; to obtain a baseline value prior to starting therapy)
- Tests for HIV and HBsAg

Pretreatment preparation

- General health of the patient must be improved prior to therapy by correcting anemia and malnutrition for the following reasons:
  - To make the patient sufficiently fit to withstand surgery
  - To improve tissue oxygenation for effective ionizing effect of RT

Treatment options include the following:

- **Surgery:** Surgical treatment is reserved only till stage IIA
- **RT:** Stages IIB to IVB, primary chemoradiation is the treatment of choice. However, RT can be given in all stages

Table 4.15: Treatment Options for Various Stages of Carcinoma Cervix

Stage	Options	Procedure
IA1 without LVSI	Surgery/RT	• If fertility is desired, therapeutic conization can be done. Further management is based on histopathology – If margins are positive: Radical trachelectomy – If patient has completed her family, type I hysterectomy is done • If patient has completed her family, type I hysterectomy is done
IA 1 with LVSI	Surgery/RT	• If fertility is desired, radical trachelectomy with PLND is done • If patient has completed family, type II hysterectomy with PLND is done
IA2	Surgery/RT	• If fertility is desired, radical trachelectomy with PLND is done • If patient has completed family, type II hysterectomy with PLND is done • Patients may require postoperative chemoradiation
IB1	Surgery/RT	• Type III hysterectomy with PLND • Most patients require postoperative adjuvant chemoradiation • If fertility is desired, radical trachelectomy can be done, provided the lesion is less than 2 cm
IB2 and IIA	Surgery/RT	• Type III hysterectomy with PLND and para-aortic LND with postoperative adjuvant chemoradiation or • Primary chemoradiation (better option)
IIB, IIIA, IIIB	RT	• Chemoradiation is the treatment of choice
IVA	RT	• Chemoradiation is the treatment of choice
IV B	Palliative chemotherapy RT	• Symptomatic treatment with least morbidity is the main concern in these patients

LVSI, lymphovascular space involvement; PLND, pelvic lymph node dissection; RT, radiotherapy

Note

Surgery as initial treatment is not encouraged in Stage IB3 (FIGO 2018 staging) and IIA2 disease since 80% of them require Post operative RT or concurrent chemo radiation (CCRT). Addition of adjuvant radiotherapy to surgery increases morbidity and compromises quality of life. Additionally, combined modality treatment will overburden the surgical and radiation facilities, which are already inadequate in low-resource countries

Therefore, CCRT is the standard of care for Stage IB3 and IIA2 disease. CCRT includes external radiation and intracavitary brachytherapy (Tumor size of more than 4 cm was incorporated in the FIGO staging system 2009 as Stage IB2 and now in the 2018 FIGO staging revised as Stage IB3)

ROLE OF SURGERY IN CANCER CERVIX

Indications–Surgery is limited to stage I up to stage IIA lesions

***Surgical options for Ca. cervix* include the following**

- Cone biopsy
- Radical trachelectomy

- Extrafascial or Type I hysterectomy
- Radical hysterectomy–Modified radical hysterectomy(MRH), Radical hysterectomy (RH) and extended RH
- Recent advances–nerve-sparing surgery and laparoscopic radical hysterectomy

Advantages of Surgery

- Ovaries are preserved
- A more pliable vagina is retained for sexual intercourse
- Bladder and bowel complications associated with RT are avoided
- Pelvic lymph nodes can be removed
- There is the psychological benefit of the disease being removed
- Quality of life and patient satisfaction are better with surgery
- Specimen is obtained for histopathological examination

Disadvantages of Surgery

- Not applicable to all stages
- Anesthetic complications
- Complications due to surgery (Table 4.16)

Table 4.16: Complication of Surgery

Intra operative complications	Post operative complications
• Hemorrhage • Injury to surrounding structures like bowel, bladder, ureter etc.,	• **Immediate/ acute complications**–Hemorrhage, intestinal obstruction, sepsis, febrile morbidity, pulmonary embolism, Vescico vaginal fistula • **Late / chronic complications**–Bladder atony/hypotony, lymphocyst formation

Specific indications for surgery in Carcinoma cervix
- Associated PID
- Associated fibroid, ovarian tumor, prolapse uterus, endocervical carcinoma
- Stump carcinoma
- Radioresistant adenocarcinoma of cervix
- Young patient
- Recurrence after radiation therapy

Surgical Procedures for Cancer Cervix

CONE BIOPSY

- It is a conservative treatment option for women who desire preservation of uterus and fertility for **Stage IA1 without lymphovascular space involvement**
  - **If margins are negative -> follow up**
  - **If margins are positive -> trachelectomy has to be performed**

RADICAL TRACHELECTOMY

- It is a conservative treatment option for women who desire preservation of uterus and fertility
- **It can be done in**
  - **Stage I A1 with margins positive**
  - **Stage I A2 and I B1**

- It can be done via abdominal/vaginal route
- PLND and cervical encerclage are done along with the procedure
- Long term outcome is uncertain as experience with this procedure is limited
- Limited data on pregnancy outcome- increased risk of abortions, preterm labor, PROM
- If recurrence occurs – definitive treatment with surgery/ RT is necessary

Schauta Mitra's operation

- Radical vaginal hysterectomy with extraperitoneal pelvic lymphadenectomy

Various Types of Hysterectomy -Table 4.17

Table 4.17: Types of Hysterectomy–Piver Classification

Type	Description
Type I	**Extra fascial hysterectomy** • Cervical fascia–completely removed • Bladder–partially mobilized • Rectum–recto vaginal septum partially mobilized • Ureters–not mobilized • Cardinal ligaments resected medial to ureters • Uterosacrals resected at level of cervix • Vaginal cuff–small rim removed
Type II	**Modified radical hysterectomy or Wertheim's hysterectomy** • Cervical fascia–completely removed • Bladder–completely mobilized • Rectum–recto vaginal septum partially mobilized • **Uterine artery** is ligated at the level of ureter preserving the ureteric branch to ureter • **Ureter** is not dissected from vesico uterine ligament (unroofed in ureteric tunnel) • **Parametrium**–Medial half of parametrium is removed (cardinal ligaments resected at level of ureter and uterosacrals partially resected)) • **Vagina**–Small margin of vagina (1-2 cm) removed
Type III	**Radical hysterectomy or Meig's hysterectomy** • Cervical fascia–completely removed • Bladder–completely mobilized • Rectum–recto vaginal septum completely mobilized • **Uterine artery** is ligated at its origin • **Ureter** is dissected from vesico uterine ligament (completely dissected to bladder entry) • **Parametrium**–Entire parametrium is removed (cardinal ligaments resected at pelvic side walls and uterosacrals at post pelvic insertion)) • **Vagina**–Upper 1/3rd of vagina is removed
Type IV	**Extended radical hysterectomy–Structures removed in addition to type III hysterectomy are** • Periureteric tissue • Superior vesical artery • Vagina–3/4th of vagina removed
Type V	**Pelvic exenteration surgery** • Distal ureter and segment of bladder and rectum are removed

ROLE OF RADIOTHERAPY IN CANCER CERVIX

Indications

- It is a primary treatment modality that can be used for all stages (curative role)
  - CCRT is the standard treatment for patient with FIGO stage IIB – IV A
  - Although surgery is preferred for early stage disease (FIGO stage IA, IB, IIA) in cases with contraindications for surgery or anesthesia, radiotherapy provides equally good results in terms of local control and survival
- Postoperative RT (adjuvant therapy) following surgery is indicated in high- and intermediate risk cases as follows:
  - Positive margins
  - Positive lymph nodes
  - Microscopic parametrial involvement
  - Large tumor size
  - Lymphovascular space involvement (LVSI)
  - Cervical stromal invasion
- Palliative therapy for alleviating distressing symptoms in patients with advanced incurable disease
- In case of recurrence following surgery, RT can be given
- Hemostatic RT can be given to control brisk hemorrhage

Factors Considered for Decision on Adjuvant Radiotherapy/ Chemoradiation Following Surgical Treatment

- Patients with high- and intermediate-risk factors are associated with an increased risk of recurrence and hence require adjuvant radiotherapy/ CCRT (Table 4.18)

Table 4.18: Various prognostic factors to decide on post operative adjuvant RT

High-risk factors(Peter's criteria)	Intermediate-risk factors (Sedlis criteria)
• Positive lymph nodes	• Large tumor size (> 4cm)
• Positive surgical margins	• Lymphovascular space involvement (LVSI)
• Microscopic parametrial involvement	• Deep cervical stromal invasion
• 40% risk of recurrence within 3 years	• 30% risk of recurrence within 3 years
• Offered Concurrent chemoradiation	• Require Post operative RT without chemotherapy

- **Most important variable associated with survival is the status of lymph node involvement**

Advantages

- It can be given in all stages of cancer cervix
- It can be given as an OPD procedure
- Patients with comorbid conditions who are unfit for surgery can be treated by RT
- Complications due to surgery are avoided
- Survival rates are similar to those for surgery

Disadvantages

- Urinary fistulas and strictures can develop following RT
- Radiation fibrosis of bowel and bladder can occur
- RT causes stricture and shortening of vagina, leading to dyspareunia
- It leads to ovarian destruction

- It can lead to avascular necrosis of femur head
- There is a possibility of secondary sarcomas because of destruction of the surrounding normal structures
- Patient satisfaction is less (tumor lesion is not removed)
- Quality of life is poor with RT

METHODS OF ADMINISTRATION OF RT

Technique of RT

- Radiation dose is expressed in rad (radiation absorbed dose) or Gray
- 1 Gray = 100 rad; hence, 1 rad = 1 cGy (centigray)
- Radiation obeys the "inverse square law," that is, the dose of radiation at a given point is inversely proportional to the square of distance of that point from the radiation source
- **RT is of the following types (Table 4.19):**
  - **External beam RT (EBRT; teletherapy)**
  - **Intracavitary RT (ICRT; brachytherapy)**
- **In early stages:** Brachytherapy is given first followed by EBRT
- **In advanced stages:** EBRT is given first to shrink the primary tumor and make the insertion of intracavitary source feasible, followed by brachytherapy

Teletherapy

- Radiation is given from a distance targeting the **tumor bed and the draining lymph nodes**
- **The aim** is to deliver the maximum tolerated dose to the tumor, while avoiding damage to the surrounding normal tissues
- EBRT is given by a **linear accelerator,** which can deliver a high dose of radiation to deeper tissues with relative sparing of superficial structures suchas skin
- **A dose of 45–50 Gy is usually prescribed**
- Treatment of carcinoma cervix requires delivery of adequate doses of irradiation to the pelvic lymph nodes. Ideally, three-dimensional imaging with CT, MRI, or both will be used to ensure adequate coverage
- **Intensity modulated radiation therapy (IMRT) is an advanced and refined** newer **technique of irradiation explored in the postoperative setting to reduce the toxicity**

Intensity-Modulated Radiation Therapy

- IMRT refers to the delivery of radiation beams with varying intensity patterns that create a dose distribution,which **covers the target with the prescribed dose while limiting doses to normal surrounding structures**
- Treatment planning is done **based on three-dimensional imaging utilizing CT.** MRI and PET images can be fused with planning CT scans to delineate the treatment volume more accurately

Potential benefits of IMRT

- It can preferentially limit the dose of radiation to normal tissues
- It can safely deliver higher tumor doses
- Enables the treatment and retreatment of tumors that are not otherwise treatable

Extended Field Radiation Therapy

- Extended field radiation therapy (EFRT) can be used either prophylactically or therapeutically to treat the lymph nodes located in **the paraaortic chain**
- **The paraaortic chain is surrounded by organs of limited radiation tolerance (spinal cord, kidneys and small intestine) and thus its use is related to increased acute and late toxicities**

Brachytherapy

- The tumor and surrounding areas are treated by direct contact with high-energy sources placed in the vagina or cervix
- Radioactive sources commonly used are cesium-137 and iridium-192
- Intracavitary radiation is delivered by using a tandem inserted into the uterus and ovoids inserted into the vagina

Brachytherapy Procedure

- After cervical dilatation, a hollowtube (tandem) is inserted into the cervical canal
- Two ovoids (hollow, round applicators) are put, one in each lateral fornix. Roller gauze is packed between them and both vaginal walls. Cesium or iridium is then transferred to the applicators by “Afterloading” remote technique
- **“Afterloading technique” is performed to avoid radiation hazard to hospital staff**

Calculation of Radiation Dose

The radiation dose is calculated according to the amount of radiation received at two arbitrary points A and B (Fig 4.9)

- **Point A**
  - It is 2 cm above and lateral to externalos
  - Corresponds to the point of crossing of uterine artery with ureter in the parametrial tissue
- **Point B**
  - It is 3 cm lateral to point A
  - Corresponds to obturator nodes on lateral pelvic wall
- Standard dose to the whole pelvis **with EBRT** is **45-50 Gy** delivered by four-field box or IMRT technique
- Standard ICRT is usually performed using a tandem and two ovoids. Any of the dose rate systems, namely low-dose-rate (LDR), high-dose-rate (HDR), or pulsed-dose-rate (PDR) may be practiced as all three yield comparable survival rates
- With **LDR,** a dose of 30–40 Gy is prescribed in one or two sessions
- With **HDR,** a dose of 5.5–8 Gy is delivered by 3–5 weekly fractions
- PDR is rarely used, however the overall treatment time and dose remains the same as in LDR, except that the treatment is given in multiple hourly pulses, each lasting for a few minutes
- The total combined dose with EBRT and ICRT should be in the range of 80–90 Gy (The **total dose of 80 -90 Gy at point A and 50–65 Gy at point B** limits the bladder and rectal dose to less than 60Gy)

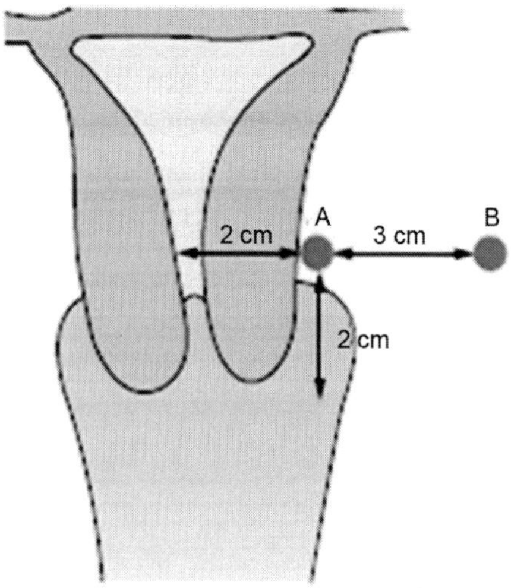

Points A and B used in radiotherapy. Point A is 2 cm above and lateral to the external os. Point B is 3 cm lateral to point A.

Fig 4.9: Points A and B used in radiotherapy for cancer cervix

Table 4.19: EBRT and brachytherapy administered for treatment of carcinoma cervix	
External beam radiotherapy	**Intracavitary RT**
Delivers uniform dose of radiation to the tumor and entire pelvis	Delivers maximum dose to the tumor, parametrium, and paravaginal tissue, and the radiation diminishes toward the lateral pelvic wall
It is administered using linear accelerator	Uterine tandems and vaginal ovoids are used as applicator
It is administered in fraction, 5 days/week for 5 weeks (25 fractions)	The does is delivered as follows: • Low-dose rates over 36-48 hours using cesium-137 (or) • High-dose rates–once a week for 2-3 weeks using iridium-192

Complications of Radiotherapy –Table 4.20

Table 4.20: Complications of RT	
Early complications	**Late complications**
• Uterine perforation at the time of insertion of applicators in brachytherapy • In teletherapy, nausea, vomiting, diarrhea, and abdominal cramps • Skin rashes and bone marrow depression	• Vaginal stenosis • Vesicovaginal fistula and rectovaginal fistula • Cystitis • Proctitis leading to diarrhea, tenesmus, and rectal bleeding • Small bowel obstruction and strictures • Premature menopause due to ovarian failure

Note:

Late toxicity following RT is due to gradually increasing ischemia and fibrosis, owing to progressive obliterative endarteritis caused by chronic effects of radiation on tissues

Role of Chemotherapy in Carcinoma Cervix

- It is used for **adjuvant therapy and palliative therapy**
- Drugs commonly used include cisplatin, bleomycin, 5-flurouracil (5-FU), vincristin, mitomycin and adriamycin.
- **Chemoradiation**
  - It is the concomitant administration of chemotherapy along with RT
  - Chemotherapy acts as a radiosensitizer and the synergistic action of the two therapies gives better results
  - The **drug commonly used is cisplatin 40 mg/m2 with appropriate hydration, administered as once weekly infusion for 6 weeks in combination with RT (usually during EBRT)**
  - **Chemoradiation is the treatment of choice for cervical cancer stages IIB to IVA**

Prognostic Factors in Cancer Cervix

- Stage of the disease
- Lymph node metastasis (most important factor)
- Parametrial involvement
- Tumor volume
- Histological type
- Tumor differentiation (grade)

5–Year Survival Rate (Table 4.21)

Table 4.21: Lymph node involvement and 5- year survival rate in carcinoma cervix			
Stage	**Pelvic lymph nodes (%)**	**Para-aortic lymph nodes (%)**	**5-year survival (%)**
IA1	0.5-1	0	95-100
IA 2	5	<1	

Contd.

Contd.

IB	15	8	80-90
IIA	25	10	65-70
IIB	35	20	40-45
III	45	30	20-40
IV	55	40	15-20

Follow-Up of Treated Cases

- The patient is followed up every 3 months for the first 2 years and then annually for the rest of the life
- During follow-up visits, H/o symptoms such as bleeding P/V, discharge P/V and pelvic pain are noted
- **Examination includes the following:**
  - Speculum examination of the vaginal vault
  - Bimanual and rectal examination to palpate for any recurrence of disease
- **Investigations**
  - Pap smear of the vault during every visit (Patients should return to annual population-based screening after 5 years of disease-free survival)
  - Chest X-ray is done every year
  - Other investigations are done depending on the clinical findings and resources available

Note
DISEASE PERSISTENCE–*Persistent cervical cancer refers to the one that has not completely regressed after 3 months of radiotherapy*
DISEASE RECURRENCE–*Recurrence refers to new lesion that develops after completion of primary therapy*

RECURRENT DISEASE

- Recurrences may occur locally in the pelvic or para-aortic nodes or may develop distant metastases
- The risk of both pelvic and distant metastasis increases in proportion to tumor volume
- Most recurrences are seen within 3 years and the prognosis is poor
- Uremia is the most common terminal event

Treatment of Recurrence

- The treatment plan depends on the **site and extent of recurrence and/or metastases,** and **prior treatment received**
- Pelvic or regional **recurrences after definitive surgery** alone are **managed with RT** or chemoradiation
- Salvage options for central **recurrence after definitive or adjuvant RT** are limited **to exenteration surgeries.** In selected patients, reirradiation using interstitial radiation implants or EBRT/ IMRT is done
- If there is only limited metastatic disease, a trial of platinum based chemotherapy is justified
- If there is extensive local or distant metastatic disease, the patient is assigned to palliative therapy with chemotherapy and/ or RT

Palliative Radiotherapy

- Common symptoms in patients with advanced incurable disease include **vaginal bleeding, pelvic pain, malodorous discharge, and symptoms related to metastatic disease**
- Short course radiotherapy is very effective in palliation of such symptoms
- There is no standard dose fraction schedule; A dose of 20 Gy in 5 fractions over 1 week or 30 Gy in 10 fractions over 2 weeks is commonly practiced
- Control of bleeding is usually achieved after 12–48 hours of radiotherapy

- In patients with pain arising from enlarged para-aortic or supraclavicular nodes, skeletal metastases and symptoms associated with cerebral metastases, palliative radiotherapy is given as larger fractions over shorter periods of time

PREVENTION OF CANCER CERVIX

- Persistent HPV infection denotes the presence of the same type-specific HPV DNA on repeated sampling after 6-12 months
- Only one-tenth of all infections become persistent, and these women could develop cervical precancerous lesions

Approaches for control of cervical cancer include the following:

- **Primary prevention**
  - Prevention of HPV infection by HPV vaccination
  - Use of condom, increasing the age of marriage and of first child birth, limitation of family, maintenance of local hygiene and treatment of STIs are steps in prevention
  - Removal of cervix during hysterectomy done for benign conditions helps prevention of stump carcinoma (Incidence is 1%)
- **Secondary prevention**
  - Screening for cervical precancerous lesions

Primary prevention of cervical cancer with HPV vaccination

- Cervical cancer accounts for >90% of all HPV related cancers
- Age-specific cross-sectional HPV prevalence peaks in **women aged < 25 years,** suggesting that the infection is predominantly transmitted through sexual route
- Prophylactic HPV vaccination as a preventive strategy should target women before initiation of sexual activity, focusing on **girls aged 10–14 years**
- **HPV vaccines prevent HPV infection** and therefore cervical cancer. It also prevents other HPV related cancers such as **anal, vaginal, vulvar and oropharyngeal cancers**
- Three HPV vaccines are currently available for use in females and males from 9 years of age, for the prevention of premalignant lesions and cancers affecting the cervix, vulva, vagina, and anus caused by high-risk HPV types:
  - A bivalent vaccine targeting HPV16 and 18–**Cervarix (Table 4.22)**
  - A quadrivalent vaccine targeting HPV 6 and 11 in addition to HPV16 and 18–**Gardasil**
  - A nanovalent vaccine targeting HPV types 31, 33, 45, 52, and 58 in addition to HPV 6, 11, 16, and 18
  - The quadrivalent and nanovalent vaccines target anogenital warts caused by HPV 6 and 11 in addition to the malignant and premalignant lesions
- All the vaccines are recombinant vaccines composed of virus-like particles (VLPs) and are not infectious since they do not contain viral DNA
- For girls and boys aged 9–14 years, a two-dose schedule (0. 5 mL IM at 0 and 6-12 months) is recommended
- For girls aged 15 years and above, and for immune compromised patients, the recommendation is for three doses (0.5 mL at 0, 1, 6 months)
- HPV vaccine can be given in women who already had sexual exposure. It will prevent acquisition of new infections, though it cannot act against infections that are already established
- WHO has stated that there is no safety concern regarding HPV vaccines
- There is evidence for the effectiveness of vaccination in terms of reduced prevalence of high-risk HPV types, anogenital warts and high-grade cervical abnormalities
- The vaccine covers only some high-risk types of HPV; hence **continued cervical cancer screening is recommended even after the vaccination** to detect cytological abnormalities caused by other types of HPV

Table 4.22: Vaccines for Prevention of Cancer Cervix

	Gardasil	Cervarix
HPV types	6, 11, 16, 18	16, 18
Dose schedule	0.5 mL IM 0, 2, 6 months	0.5 mL IM 0, 1–2, 6 months
Indications	Cervical cancer, CIN, Vulvar cancer, VIN, Vaginal cancer, VAIN, Anogenital warts	Cervical cancer, CIN
Population approved	Males and females aged 9–26 years	Females aged 9–25 years
Advisory Committee on Practices (ACIP) recommendations	Females aged 11 and 12 years with catch-up vaccination for females aged 13-26 years. Permissive for boys aged 9–26 years	

CIN -cervical intraepithelial neoplasia, VIN - vulvar intraepithelial neoplasia, VAIN - vaginal intraepithelial neoplasia

Down Staging for Cervical Cancer (WHO)

- It is defined as **"detection of the disease at an earlier stage when it is still curable. Detection is done by nurses and other paramedical health workers using a simple speculum for visual inspection of the cervix"**
- The "down staging screening" is an alternative to regular cytologic screening in developing countries, where effective mass screening cannot be extended and majority of carcinoma cervix cases are diagnosed at an advanced stage
- This method is **suboptimal when compared to cytological screening.** However, in places where prevalence of cancer is high and cytological screening is not available, "down staging screening" is useful
- This strategy can minimize the cervical cancer death through early detection

Downstaging procedure

- A female primary health care worker is trained for 2–3 weeks to perform speculum examination and to distinguish a normal cervix from an abnormal cervix
- Characteristics of a normal cervix- Pink in color, smooth surface and does not bleed on touch
- Characteristics of an abnormal cervix - Reddish, patchy red or white areas, growth or ulcer on the surface and bleeds on touch.
- Once any abnormality is suspected, the case is referred to a center where diagnosis and treatment of premalignant and malignant lesions are done.

RECENT UPDATES

IMMUNOCYTOCHEMICAL MARKERS FOR DYSPLASTIC CELLS:

Various immunocytochemical markers have been evaluated in staining dysplastic cells either in biopsies or in cytological smears

- *Colposcopy is usually done on women with abnormal smears and/or positive HPV test. A newer concept of triage using biomarkers p16INK4a and Ki-67 dual immunostaining has been advocated to avoid over referral for colposcopy*
- *Diffuse immunostaining with p16INK4a and dual staining with Ki-67 is the hallmark of HSIL (CIN2 and CIN3), regardless of HPV status*

Diagnosis/Entry	*p16*	*Ki-67*
HSIL	Strong and diffuse block positive staining	Cluster of at least two strongly stained epithelial nuclei above the upper two-thirds of epithelium
LSIL	Negative or weak band-like staining	Cluster of at least two strongly stained epithelial nuclei above the lower third of the epithelium
Benign/reactive atypia	Negative or weak band-like staining	Parabasal location and/or throughout epithelium in inflammatory cells
Atrophy and immature squamous metaplasia	Negative or weak band-like staining	Limited to parabasal cells
Tangentially cut epithelium through basal-layer	Negative or weak band-like staining	Diffuse positivity

HSIL: High-grade squamous intraepithelial lesion, LSIL: Low-grade squamous intraepithelial lesion

Update on Human Papillomavirus (HPV) Vaccination

- *HPV vaccines, including the bivalent HPV 16 and 18 vaccine and the quadrivalent HPV 6, 11, 16, and 18 vaccine, are effective in preventing up to 70% of cervical and other HPV-related cancers*
- *In addition to HPV subtypes 6, 11, 16, and 18, a 9-valent HPV vaccine would also protect against HPV subtypes 31, 33, 45, 52, and 58, and could prevent around 90% of cervical cancers*
- *Huh et al reported in Lancet (2017), that prophylactic administration of the 9vHPV vaccine is highly efficacious in preventing HPV infection, cervical cytological abnormalities and high-grade cervical intraepithelial neoplasia (CIN) histology*
- *The Centers for Disease Control and Prevention's Advisory (CDC) Committee on Immunization Practices (ACIP) recommends routine HPV vaccination at age 11 or 12 years, and it can be given starting at age 9 years. In 2016, the ACIP recommended reducing the number of HPV vaccine shots from 3 to 2 for girls and boys between the ages of 9 and 14. Based on the available immunogenicity evidence, a 2-dose schedule (0, 6–12 months) will have similar efficacy to a 3-dose schedule (0, 1–2, 6 months), if the HPV vaccination schedule is started before the 15 years*

Pembrolizumab in Advanced Cervical Cancer

- *Pembrolizumab is a highly selective humanized monoclonal antibody that blocks the interaction between programmed death (PD)-1 receptor and its ligands, PD-L1 and PD-L2, and allows the immune system to destroy cancer cells*
- *US Food and Drug Administration (FDA) has approved pembrolizumab for advanced melanoma, non-small cell lung cancer, head and neck squamous cell carcinoma, classical Hodgkin lymphoma, urothelial carcinoma, and gastric cancer till now*
- *The recent identification of a higher PD-L1 expression in HPV-inducing cervical cancers suggests that PD-1 also may be an attractive therapeutic target for patients with advanced cervical cancer and several trials are going on to assess the safety and efficacy of pembrolizumab in PD-L1-positive advanced cervical cancer*

CHAPTER 5

EPITHELIAL OVARIAN TUMORS

INTRODUCTION

- Ovarian malignancy constitutes about **15–20% of genital malignancy**
- It is more prevalent in USA and Scandinavian countries and less in Latin American and Asian countries including Japan and India
- Highest incidence is recorded in the industrialized countries (USA, UK and Sweden)
- Ovarian malignancy accounts for 5% of all gynecological cancers in India

Ovarian tumors are classified as follows:

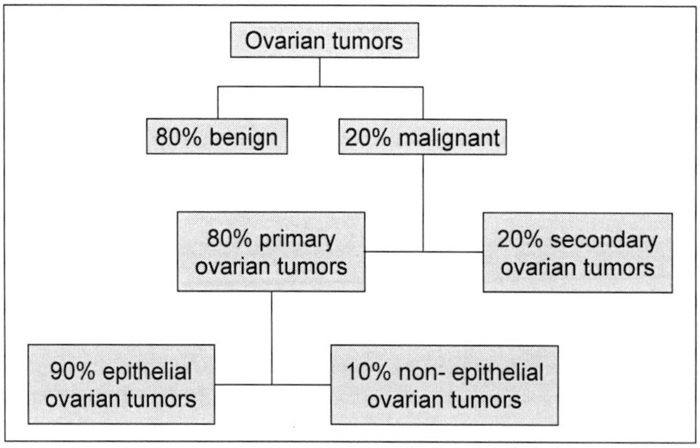

Etiology

- **'Incessant ovulation' theory** (Fathalla, 1971) suggests repeated ovulatory trauma to the ovarian epithelial lining is a promoting factor for carcinogenesis
- **Risk factors and protective factors for ovarian cancers are given in Table 5.1**

Table 5.1: Risk Factors and Protective Factors for Ovarian Cancers

Risk Factors for Ovarian Cancer	Protective Factors for Ovarian cancer
• Advancing age – common in age group 50–70 yrs • Obesity • Nulliparity (due to prolonged repetitive ovulation) • Early menarche • Late menopause • Family history of ovarian, breast, endometrial and colorectal malignancy • Carriers of BRCA 1 or 2 mutation • Hormone replacement therapy (estrogen only HRTs)	• Multiparity • Breast feeding • Oral contraceptive pills (OCP use for 5 years–50% risk reduction) • Salpingectomy/tubal ligation • Hysterectomy has been associated with reduction in the risk • Physical activity

Note

- *There is **no consistent relationship reported of specific dietary components** to ovarian cancer risk*
- *There is **weak or no association between infertility treatment and development of ovarian cancer***

Significance of Age in Ovarian Tumor

- More than **80% of epithelial ovarian cancers occur in postmenopausal women,** usually between 50 and 70 years of age
- **30% of ovarian tumors in postmenopausal age group are malignant,** whereas only 7% in premenopausal age group are malignant
- 70% of ovarian tumors that occur in women **<20 years of age are germ cell tumors**

Genetics in Ovarian Malignancy

Hereditary ovarian cancer occurs in two forms:

Hereditary nonpolyposis colorectal cancer (HNPCC) or Lynch II syndrome:

- Hereditary nonpolyposis colorectal cancer (HNPCC) or Lynch syndrome has a **high risk of colon cancer as well as other cancers including endometrial (second most common), ovarian, stomach, small intestine, genitourinary and hepatobiliary tract cancers**
- It is an **autosomal dominant** genetic condition
- Women with HNPCC (Lynch II syndrome) have lifetime risk of about **50% for endometrial cancer and 12% for ovarian cancer**
- Average age at diagnosis is **40 years**
- Mutations in the three DNA mismatch repair genes **MLH1, MSH2 and MSH6** account for > 95% of mutations found in Lynch syndrome

Hereditary Breast and ovarian cancer syndrome:

- A diagnosis of hereditary breast and ovarian cancer syndrome (HBOC) is considered when there are multiple cases of breast cancer and/or ovarian cancer on the same side of the family
- It usually occurs in association with BRCA1 or BRCA2 mutation
- Mutations are inherited in **autosomal dominant pattern**
- Most hereditary ovarian cancer syndromes are associated with mutations in **BRCA 1 located on chromosome 17**
- Small proportions have mutations in **BRCA 2 gene located on chromosome 13**
- The lifetime risk of ovarian cancer for women with **BRCA1 mutations and BRCA2 mutations** has been estimated to be **40% and 20%,** respectively
- Hereditary ovarian cancers **occur one decade earlier than sporadic cases.** Average age at diagnosis is **50 years.** If a malignant ovarian tumor occurs in the premenopausal age group, detailed family history and screening of other family members are to be done
- Survival for women with ovarian cancer related to a BRCA mutation has been reported to be longer than for women with a similar stage cancer and no mutation
- Risk may be reduced by **prophylactic salpingo-oophorectomy**

WHO Classification of Ovarian Tumors (Nine Major Groups)

- The World Health Organization Histological Classification for ovarian tumors separates ovarian neoplasms according to the most probable tissue of origin: surface epithelial (65%), germ cell (15%), sex cord-stromal (10%), metastases (5%), miscellaneous
- Surface epithelial tumors are further classified by cell type (serous, mucinous, endometrioid, etc) and atypia (benign, borderline [atypical proliferation, low malignant potential] or malignant; malignant may be invasive or non-invasive)
- Most malignant tumors are surface epithelial (90%)

- **Surface Epithelial tumors (may be benign, borderline malignant, or malignant) – arises from coelomic epithelium**
  - Serous tumors
  - Mucinous tumors
  - Transitional cell tumor
  - Clear cell tumor
  - Endometrioid tumors
  - Mixed epithelial tumor
  - Undifferentiated carcinoma
  - Unclassified
- **Sex cord stromal tumors – arises from gonadal stroma**
  - Granulosa cell tumors and theca cell tumors
  - Androblastomas
  - Gynandroblastomas
  - Unclassified
- **Germ cell tumors – arises from germ cells**
  - Dysgerminoma
  - Endodermal sinus tumor
  - Embryonal cell carcinoma
  - Polyembryoma
  - Choriocarcinoma
  - Teratoma
  - Mixed forms
- **Gonadoblastoma—pure/mixed with germ cells**
- **Lipid cell tumors**
- **Soft-tissue tumors**
- **Secondary (metastatic) tumors**
- **Unclassified**

EPITHELIAL OVARIAN TUMORS

- These may arise de novo as malignant or may result from malignant changes of benign tumors
- **Serous tumors** are believed to arise de novo from the surface epithelium of the ovary or from the mucosa of fallopian tube, and progress rapidly. This makes screening and early detection difficult and hence **majority of fatal ovarian cancers are high-grade serous carcinomas**
- **Recent advance**–It is believed that **most serous tumors originate from a precursor lesion 'STIC' (Serous tubal intraepithelial carcinoma) in the distal fallopian tube. Low grade serous carcinoma** is a recently described small subset of ovarian serous tumors that appears to follow a **slow to invasive carcinoma**

- **Mucinous carcinomas mostly transit through a mucinous cystadenoma- borderline tumor–carcinoma sequence**
- **Clear cell carcinomas** and majority of **endometrioid carcinomas arise in endometriosis**

Histological Classification of Epithelial Ovarian Tumors - Table 5.2 and 5.3

Table 5.2: Histology of Epithelial Ovarian Tumors

Epithelial ovarian tumors	**Histological resemblance**
Serous tumors	Lining of fallopian tube
Mucinous tumors	Endocervical-like and intestinal type
Endometriod umors	Endometrial lining
Clear cell tumors	Resembles clear cell-renal cell carcinoma (ccRCC)- both feature clear cytoplasm
Transitional cell tumors (Brenner's tumor)	Urinary bladder

Table 5.3: Histological Classification of Epithelial Ovarian Tumors

Surface Epithelial - Stromal Tumors
Serous tumors: Benign (cystadenoma) Borderline tumors (serous borderline tumor) Malignant (serous adenocarcinoma)
Mucinous tumors, endocervical-like and intestinal type: Benign (cystadenoma) Borderline tumors (mucinous borderline tumor) Malignant (mucinous adenocarcinoma
Endometrioid tumors: Benign (cystadenoma) Borderline tumors (endometrioid borderline tumor) Malignant (endometrioid adenocarcinoma)
Clear cell tumors: Benign Borderline tumors Malignant (clear cell adenocarcinoma)
Transitional cell tumors: Brenner tumor Brenner tumor of borderline malignancy Malignant Brenner tumor Transitional cell carcinoma (non-Brenner type)
Epithelial-stromal: Adenosarcoma Carcinosarcoma (formerly mixed Müllerian tumors)

SEROUS TUMORS

- It arises from the totipotent surface epithelium of the ovary
- It accounts for **40% of ovarian tumors (most common ovarian tumors)**
- **Bilaterality– 40%**
- **Risk of malignancy–40%**
- **Serous tumors can be benign, borderline or malignant (Table 5.4)**

Table 5.4: Incidence and age at diagnosis of serous tumors

Serous Tumor Type	Incidence	Age at Diagnosis years
Benign	78%	40-50
Borderline tumors	2%	45-50
Malignant	20%	50-60

Serous cystadenomas

- Serous cystadenomas are not very large unlike mucinous cystadenoma
- **Gross appearance**
  - The cyst wall is smooth, shiny and greyish white. At times, there are papillary projection
  - The content fluid is clear, rich in serum proteins–albumin and globulin
  - May be uniloculated or multiloculated on cut section
- **Microscopic examination**
  - Lined by a single layer of cuboidal epithelium. There may be presence of ciliated, secretory and peg cells **resembling tubal epithelium**
  - The papillary projections consist of dense fibrous stroma covered by single or multiple layersof columnar epithelium
  - May contain **Psammoma Bodies**–tiny, spherical, laminated calcified structures often found in areas of cellular degeneration

Borderline serous tumors

- Often **confined to the ovary** and associated with a **survival of almost 100%**
- **Micropapillary serous tumors** are a subtype of borderline tumor, likely to be associated with invasive implants and hence have a worse prognosis
- Microinvasion is present in 10% of borderline tumors. The presence of microinvasion does not appear to affect the prognosis of these tumors
- May spread to lymph nodes, but this does not worsen the overall good prognosis of these tumors

Serous adenocarcinomas

- **Gross appearance:** Present as solid masses bounded by a capsule, containing areas of necrosis and hemorrhage; size ranges from small (2 to 3 cm) to quite large
- **Microscopy**–Large sheets of **polygonal cells** growing without stromal support accompanied by a desmoplastic response. The nuclei are large, pleomorphic, with variably sized nucleoli and numerous mitotic figures
- The ovary from which the neoplasm has arisen is usually not apparent in gross or microscopic examination
- Graded as **high-grade** (5-year survival rate 25%) **and low-grade** serous carcinomas (5-year survival rate 85%). Refer figure 5.1
- **90% of advanced-stage serous carcinomas belong to the high-grade group**
- **Low-grade neoplasms** are characterized by cells with mild to moderate nuclear atypia, evenly distributed chromatin, variable nucleoli, and **less than 10 mitoses/10 hpf**
- **CA 125 level is often elevated**
- **Immunohistochemical analysis-Carcino embryonic antigen (CEA) negative; stain positive for WT1, cytokeratin (CK)** 7, and **negative for CK20 and calretinin.** These tests are employed to evaluate a carcinoma whose primary site is uncertain
  - **Pancreatic and breast carcinomas have the same CK7/ CK 20 profile,** and thus other markers are needed for differentiation. **GCDFP-15 (gross cystic disease fluid protein) is positive in breast carcinoma and often negative in ovarian carcinoma**

MUCINOUS TUMORS

- It arises from the **totipotent surface epithelium of the ovary**
- It accounts for **20–25% of all ovarian tumors**
- **Bilateral in 10% cases**
- **Risk of malignancy is 10%**
- Primary ovarian mucinous tumors include three types as given in table 5.5

Table 5.5: Incidence and mean age at diagnosis of Mucinous tumors

Type	Incidence	Mean age
Benign Cystadenomas	82%	40-50 years
Borderline tumors	13%	45-50 years
Primary ovarianmucinous carcinomas	5%	50-60 years

Mucinous cystadenoma

- It may enlarge to a huge size and is the **largest benign ovarian tumor**
- **Gross appearance**
  - The cyst wall is lobulated with a bluish white hue
  - The cyst is usually **multiloculated** and cut section shows **honeycomb pattern**
  - The content of the **cyst is thick and viscid mucin,** a glycoprotein with high content of neutral polysaccharides
- **Microscopic examination:** The cyst is lined by a single layer of tall columnar epithelium with dark staining basal nucleus without any cilia. The epithelial characteristics are like those of endocervix. There are 2 types of mucinous tumors: the **gastrointestinal (more common) and endocervical type.**

Borderline mucinous tumors

- Borderline mucinous tumors are **often stage I** at diagnosis with **almost 100% survival**
- The presence of microinvasion does not appear to affect the benign prognosis of these tumors

Primary Ovarian Mucinous Carcinoma

- Primary ovarian mucinous carcinomas are multicystic masses filled with thick tenacious mucinous material. They may contain solid areas, areas of necrosis and can rupture with surface involvement
- **Most present as stage I cancers**
- Mucinous carcinomas with **secondary spread to ovaries are more common than primary ovarian mucinous carcinomas**
- **Metastatic mucinous carcinomas** are usually recognized when the ovarian tumors exhibit any or all of the following features: **bilaterality, smaller size (< 10 cm), ovarian surface involvement, nodular pattern of involvement and an infiltrative pattern of stromal invasion**
- **Immunohistochemical analysis** with antibodies such as **CK7, CK20, CDX-2, and p16 can be** useful for **identifying some metastatic mucinous carcinomas;** However, there is **overlapping of immunoprofiles of primary ovarian mucinous tumors with other mucinous tumors**
- **CA-125 is usually not elevated**
- **May be associated with Pseudomyxoma peritonei**

Extra edge

Pseudomyxoma peritonei

- *It is a clinicopathologic syndrome in which **mucinous ascites is accompanied by low-grade neoplastic mucinous epithelium***
- *Formerly thought to result from mucinous ovarian tumors*
- ***Currently believed to be derived from low-grade mucinous tumors of appendix; the ovarian involvement is secondary***

ENDOMETRIOID TUMOR

- Can be benign, borderline or malignant Mostly **malignant**
- Lining epithelium resembles that of endometrium
- Associated with **endometriosis in 10 - 40%** cases
- Associated with **endometrial cancer of an identical histologic variant in 10% cases** – majority are synchronous primary cancers rather than metastases. Adenoacanthoma is a well differentiated endometriod tumor with focal squamous metaplasia and has better prognosis.

CLEAR CELL TUMORS

- It can be benign/ borderline/ malignant. Malignant is most common (clear cell adenocarcinoma) also called mesonephroid tumor
- Occur in women 40–70 years of age
- Highly malignant and aggressive tumor
- About **50% are associated with endometriosis**
- **Microscopy**–contain cells with abundant glycogen termed **clear "hobnail" cells**
  - **Clear appearance of the cytoplasm results** from glycogen that has leaked when specimen is prepared for microscopic examination
  - **Hobnail cells**–bulbous nuclei protrude into the glandular lumen at the cytoplasmic limits of the cell

BRENNER TUMOR

- Account for 1–2% of all ovarian tumors
- 8–10% are bilateral
- Usually seen in **postmenopausal women**
- They are usually **benign** tumors
- Majority are **solid** and less than 2 cm in diameter
- Tumor secretes estrogen and the patient may present with abnormal vaginal bleeding or postmenopausal bleeding
- **Gross appearance–resembles fibroma of ovary**
- **Microscopy–Urothelial cells are seen.** The cells look like **"coffee bean"** as the nuclei have longitudinal grooves
- May be associated with **Pseudo-Meigs syndrome**–Brenner tumor in association with ascites and pleural effusion. Pseudo Meig's syndrome can also occur in Sex cord stromal tumors and Germ cell tumors

MIXED CARCINOMA

- **Mixed Carcinoma are** defined as a carcinoma in **which > 10% of the neoplasm exhibits a second histologic cell type**
- 10% of all epithelial ovarian tumor are mixed type
- Common **malignant combination is mixed clear cell carcinoma and endometrioid carcinoma, both related to endometriosis**

PRIMARY PERITONEAL SEROUS CARCINOMATOSIS (Primary Peritoneal Carcinoma)

- Papillary serous carcinoma of the peritoneum is a rare type of primary peritoneal adenocarcinoma (PPA)
- It constitutes 7–20% of all epithelial ovarian carcinoma.

Criteria for Diagnosis of Primary Peritoneal Carcinoma (Gynecologic oncology group (GOG) 1993)

- The ovaries are normal in size (< 4 cm diameter) or enlarged by benign processes
- Extra-ovarian sites are more involved than that of the ovarian surfaces
- Microscopically the ovaries are either not involved or exhibit cortical implants < 5 mm in depth
- The histologic and cytologic tumor character is serous type

- FIGO staging for ovarian carcinoma is followed
- The **pathology and response to treatment** of peritoneal serous carcinomas are **similar to that of ovarian serous carcinomas**
- Prognosis is generally poor
- It is recently apparent that the **tubal fimbriae may be the source of peritoneal carcinomatosis and high-grade serous carcinomas**

MALIGNANT EPITHELIAL OVARIAN TUMORS

- These may arise de novo as malignant or more commonly may result from malignant changes of benign cystic tumors
- These are **bilateral in about 50% cases**
- 75–85% of patients with epithelial ovarian cancer **are diagnosed in advanced stages**

Mode of Spread

Transcoelomic spread

- **Implantation of malignant cells can occur by:**
  - **Direct exfoliation of cells**–Ovarian carcinomas are distinctive by virtue of their propensity to exfoliate malignant cells into the peritoneal cavity
  - Penetration or rupture of tumor capsule

  The cells follow the normal circulation of peritoneal fluid up the right paracolic gutter and to the undersurface of the right hemidiaphragm -> Multiple secondary deposits are formed on the peritoneal surfaces specially in the pouch of Douglas, omentum, abdomino-pelvic organs, diaphragm and retroperitoneal nodes

Lymphatic spread

- The lymphatic spread occurs to the **draining paraaortic and superior gastric nodes** (Table 5.6)
- The **pelvic nodes** may be involved through peritoneal permeation into the subperitoneal lymphatics
- The **left supraclavicular nodes** may be enlarged due to obstruction of the efferent lymphatic channel of the nodes by the tumor emboli, as it enters the thoracic duct just prior to its drainage into the left subclavian vein
- Retrograde lymphatic spread in advanced disease may occur to the **inguinal nodes via the round ligament**

Table 5.6: Para aortic and pelvic lymph node involvement in epithelial ovarian tumors

Stage	*Paraaortic (%)*	*Pelvic (%)*
Stage I AND II	20	30
Stage III AND IV	65	67

- **Direct spread:** After the capsule is breached, the spread occurs directly to the adjacent organs such as tubes, broad ligament, intestines, omentum and uterus
- **Hematogenous spread:** The blood borne metastasis is late and involves organs like lungs, liver, bones, etc.

Clinical Features

Patient profile:

- More prevalent at >45 years of age, commonly occurs in **postmenopausal women**
- There is increased association with **nulliparity and family history**

Symptoms:

- Often asymptomatic in early stage
- The presenting symptoms are usually of **short duration and are not specific**
  - Feeling of abdominal distension and vague discomfort
  - Features of dyspepsia such as flatulence and eructations
  - Loss of appetite and bloating sensation after meals

- Gradually, more pronounced symptoms appear such as:
  - Rapid abdominal distension
  - Dull abdominal pain
  - Sudden loss of weight
  - Respiratory distress–may be due to ascites or pleural effusion
- **Menstrual abnormality is usually absent except in functional ovarian tumors**

Note
• *Even with symptoms of short duration, there may be extensive spread*
• *A huge tumor may be benign; conversely, an enlarged ovary may be malignant*

Clinical Examination

General Examination

- Cachexia and pallor of varying degree may be present
- Jaundice may be evident in late cases
- Left supraclavicular lymph node (Virchow's) may be enlarged
- Edema of the leg or vulva may be present

Abdominal examination

Palpation

- Liver may be enlarged, firm and nodular
- Mass may be felt in the hypogastrium; often bilateral with the following features:
  - Solid or heterogeneous in consistency
  - Irregular surface
  - Margins may be ill defined
  - Restricted mobility
  - Tenderness may be present

Percussion

- Usually dull over the tumor; may be resonant due to overlying intestinal adhesions
- Shifting dullness may be elicited in case of gross ascites

Bimanual Examination

- The uterus may be separately felt from the mass
- Nodules may be felt through the posterior fornix

Rectal Examination

- May reveal nodular deposits in the POD

Clinical Features Differentiating A Benign From A Malignant Ovarian Mass–Table 5.7

Table 5.7: Clinical Features Differentiating A Benign From A Malignant Ovarian Mass

Feature	Benign ovarian mass	Malignant ovarian mass
Age	Younger age group	Extremes of age (<20 and >50 years)
Duration of progression of illness	Slow	Rapid progression within a short period of few months
Cachectic symptoms (loss of eight and appetite)	Absent	Present
Palpation	Smooth surface, borders well defined, cystic consistency, mobile mass	Irregular surface, borders may be ill defined, variable consistency (due to presence of solid areas), restricted mobility or fixed mass

Contd.

Contd.

Site	Unilateral (80%)	Bilateral (70%)
Ascites	Absent	Present
POD deposits	Absent	May be present

Note

- *70% of cases with epithelial carcinomas have metastases outside the pelvis at the time of diagnosis*
- ***Most common sites of metastases are—peritoneum (85%), omentum (70%), contralateral ovary (70%), liver (35%), lung (25%) and uterus (20%)***

INVESTIGATIONS

Investigation are done to assess the following:

- To confirm nature of the mass
- To identify the extent of lesion.
- To detect any other primary site

To evaluate nature of the mass

Ultrasound of the abdomen and pelvis:

- Trans abdominal and trans vaginal ultrasonography (TAS and TVS) are performed
- TVS improves the detection rate
- Ultrasound features differentiating a benign from a malignant ovarian tumor are mentioned in the Table 5.8

Table 5.8: Ultrasound features differentiating a benign from a malignant ovarian tumor

Feature	Benign Ovarian	Malignant Ovarian
Bilaterality	Rare	Common
Solid areas	Rare	Common
Locularity	Unilocular	Multilocular
Cyst wall thickness	Thin	Thick
Septations	Thin septations	Thick septations
Surface papilla and intracystic papilla	Rare	common
Echogenicity	Anechoic (cystic)	Mixed echogenicity due to solid areas
Ascites	Rare	Common
Enlarged lymph nodes	Absent	Common
Hepatosplenomegaly and omental thickening	High-resistance flow pattern	May be present in advanced tumors
Doppler		Low-resistance flow pattern

Tumor marker CA 125:

- CA125 levels are usually elevated in nonmucinous epithelial ovarian tumors
- Levels are useful in differentiating benign from malignant lesions
- Sensitivity and specificity are high in postmenopausal women
- CA 125 is also useful to check response to therapy and for early diagnosis of recurrence

Extra Edge

TUMOR MARKER CA-125

- ***CA-125 is a high molecular weight glycoprotein***
- *Elevated in Breast, lung (pleural), Colon, Peritoneal, Gastric, Pancreatic, Endometrial and non mucinous epithelial ovarian cancers*
- ***Elevated in 50% of early and 90% of advanced stage ovarian cancers***
- *It is also elevated in several benign conditions such as Endometriosis, Pregnancy, PID, Fibroids, Cirrhosis, Benign breast diseases, Pancreatitis and Pleuritis*

CT and MRI:

- Performed if ultrasonography is not conclusive in detecting the origin of tumor
- Aids in identifying the spread of tumor and enlarged pelvic or para-aortic lymph nodes

Ascitic fluid for malignant cytology:

- Cytologic examination of the ascitic fluid collected by abdominal paracentesis or "cul-de-sac" aspiration
- Detection of malignant cells from the ascitic fluid is an indication of abdominal malignancies
- When this is combined with presence of a pelvic mass, it almost confirms ovarian malignancy

To identify the extent of lesion

- Complete blood count, renal and Liver function tests
- **Ultrasonography**– is of limited help in identifying the extent of lesion
- **Computed Tomography (CT) and Magnetic Resonance Imaging (MRI)**–helpful for:
  - Determination of the nature of ovarian mass
  - Assessment of retroperitoneal lymph nodes
  - Detection of metastasis (liver, omentum)
  - Detection of relapse of the tumor following initial treatment
- **Positron Emission Tomography (PET) scan** can differentiate normal from cancerous tissues. It is more sensitive than CT or MRI
- **Intravenous pyelography:** It is done in large tumors where normal anatomy may be distorted, to detect ureteric obstruction and deviation in course of ureters
- **Chest X-ray** to exclude pleural effusion and chest metastasis
- Cytologic examination of thoracentesis fluid
- **Pap smear** is a routine investigation

To detect any other primary site

- **Stool occult blood, upper GI endoscopy, Barium enema and colonoscopy:** These are done to rule out primary GIT malignancy
- **Mammography** is often recommended due to the association of ovarian cancer with breast cancer and because metastatic breast cancer can produce intra-abdominal carcinomatosis

DIAGNOSIS

- Nature of the tumor (benign or malignant) can be made out from history, clinical examination, ultrasonography other investigation modalities and with laparotomy findings
- Histological examination confirms the diagnosis and identifies the type and grade of malignancy

SURGICAL STAGING

Stage of the disease can be determined only following exploratory laparotomy and thorough evaluation of all intra abdominal organs

Principal steps of staging laparotomy are as follows (Table 5.9):

Table 5.9: Principal Steps of Staging Laparotomy

Incision	• Vertical midline skin incision is made (it minimizes chances of tumor rupture and facilitates better exploration of peritoneal cavity)
Aspiration cytology	• Aspiration of ascitic fluid or peritoneal washing for cytology is done (peritoneal washing is taken from paracolic gutters, pouch of Douglas, and undersurface of diaphragm by instilling 10–20 mL of normal saline or distilled water)
Pelvic exploration	• It is done to note the gross physical characteristics of the tumor and condition of the contralateral ovary, uterus, and tubes

Contd.

Contd.

Systematic palpation of entire peritoneal structures	• It is done starting from cecum, ascending colon, hepatic flexure, undersurface of diaphragm, transverse colon, splenic flexure, descending colon, sigmoid colon, omentum, liver, spleen, pelvic lymph nodes, and para-aortic lymph nodes. This is done for staging and assessment of operability of the tumor
Procedure done	• Total abdominal hysterectomy (TAH) with bilateral salpingo-ovariectomy (BSO) and infracolic omentectomy is performed
Peritoneal biopsies	• Multiple biopsies are taken from suspicious areas in peritoneal cavity (cul-de-sac, pelvic walls, paracolic gutters, mesentery), and scrapings are taken from the undersurface of the diaphragm
Lymph node sampling	• Pelvic and para-aortic lymph node sampling is done in all cases • Appendicectomy is performed in case of mucinous tumors

FIGO Staging of Carcinoma of Ovary, Fallopian Tube and Peritoneum (Revised surgical staging, 2014) – Table 5.10

Table 5.10: FIGO Staging Classification for Cancer of the Ovary, Fallopian Tube and Peritoneum

Stage I:	**Tumor confined to ovaries or fallopian tube(s)**
IA:	Tumor limited to 1 ovary (capsule intact) or fallopian tube; no tumor on ovarian or fallopian tube surface; no malignant cells in the ascites or peritoneal washings
IB:	Tumor limited to both ovaries (capsules intact) or fallopian tubes; no tumor on ovarian or fallopian tube surface; no malignant cells in the ascites or peritoneal washings
IC:	Tumor limited to 1 or both ovaries or fallopian tubes, with of the following
IC1:	Surgical spill
IC2:	Capsule ruptured before surgery or tumor on ovarian or fallopian tube surface
IC3:	Malignant cells in the ascites or peritoneal washings
Stage II:	Tumor involves 1 or both ovaries or fallopian tubes with pelvic extension (below pelvic brim) or peritoneal cancer
IIA:	Extension and/or implants on uterus and/or fallopian tubes and/or ovaries
IIB:	Extension to other pelvic intraperitoneal tissues
Stage III:	Tumor involves 1 or both ovaries or fallopian tubes, or peritoneal cancer, with cytologically or histologically confirmed spread to the peritoneum outside the pelvis and/or metastasis to the retroperitoneal lymph nodes
IIIA1:	Positive retroperitoneal lymph nodes only (cytologically or histologically proven):
IIIA1(i)	Metastasis up to 10 mm in greatest dimension
III A1(ii)	Metastasis more than 10 mm in greatest dimension
IIIA2:	Microscopic extrapelvic (above the pelvic brim) peritoneal involvement with or without positive retroperitoneal lymph nodes
IIIB:	Macroscopic peritoneal metastasis beyond the pelvis up to 2 cm in greatest dimension, with or without metastasis to the retroperitoneal lymph nodes
IIIC:	Macroscopic peritoneal metastasis beyond the pelvis more than 2 cm in greatest dimension with or without metastasis to the retroperitoneal lymph nodes (includes extension of tumor to capsule of liver and spleen without parenchymal involvement of either organ)
Stage IV:	Distant metastasis excluding peritoneal metastases
Stage IVA:	Pleural effusion with positive cytology
Stage IVB:	Parenchymal metastases and metastases to extra-abdominal organs (including inguinal lymph nodes and lymph nodes outside of the abdominal cavity)

NOTE

Modifications of the former staging system made in the revised FIGO staging 2014 are as follows:

- *Stage IC is now divided into three categories: IC1 (surgical spill)*
  - *IC2 (capsule ruptured before surgery or tumor on ovarian or fallopian tube surface); and IC3 (malignant cells in the ascites or peritoneal washings)*
- *Stage IIC has been eliminated*
- *Updated Stage III A –it is now subdivided into*
  - *IIIA1(i) (metastasis ≤10 mm in greatest dimension)*
  - *IIIA1(ii) (metastasis >10 mm in greatest dimension)*

- *Stage IIIA2 is now "microscopic extrapelvic peritoneal involvement with or without positive retroperitoneal lymph node" metastasis*
- *The wordings of Stage IIIB has been modified to reflect the lymph node status*
- *Stage IVB now includes metastases to the inguinal lymph nodes*

Clinicopathologic Explanation for Involvement of Various Sites in Ovarian Malignancy Table 5.11

Table 5.11: Clinicopathologic Explanation for Involvement of Various Sites in Ovarian Malignancy

Site	Clinicopathologic Explanation
Contralateral ovary	• In primary malignancy, the contralateral ovary involvement may be due to retrograde lymphatic spread through paraaortic nodes. • The contralateral ovary is involved in majority of metastatic ovarian malignancy
Uterus	Uterus is involved due to lymphatics or through direct transtubal spread
Ascites	Ascites is due to obstruction of peritoneal fluid outflow through the diaphragm. There is also increased transudation of serum across the peritoneal surfaces
Liver	Liver is usually involved by blood borne spread
Right-sided pleural effusion	**Explanations for right sided pleural effusion are as follows:** • More ascitic fluid reaches the right subdiaphragmatic space along the wider right paracolic gutter, facilitated by the increased negative suction created by liver during respiration ->The collected fluid can pass freely across the diaphragm because of free communication of sub mesothelial network of lymphatic capillaries with the corresponding plexuses on the thoracic surface of the diaphragm on the right side → right pleural effusion • Alternatively, there is more number of pleuroperitoneal sinuses on the right side and hence producing right pleural effusion.

MANAGEMENT OF MALIGNANT OVARIAN TUMORS

Surgery is the mainstay of treatment. Most of the patients require a staging laparotomy followed by chemotherapy (Table 5.12)

Table 5.12: Management Protocol for Ovarian Cancer

Early Stage Ovarian Cancer	
Stage IA (Grade 1)—low grade, low risk	Primary treatment is surgical staging and doing a TAH with BSO with infracolic omentectomy Patients with comprehensively staged stage IA grade 1 epithelial ovarian cancer need not receive postoperative chemotherapy In women who desire to preserve their fertility, **the uterus and contralateral ovary can be preserved in stage IA, Grade 1.** The patient must be periodically monitored with routine pelvic examination, USG, and determination of serum CA125 levels
Stages IA (Grades 2 and 3), IB, and IC: high grade, high risk	• Staging laparotomy is performed; TAH + BSO + infracolic omentectomy is performed followed by post operative adjuvant chemotherapy • High grade, high risk disease has a relapse risk of 20% that can be reduced with platinum-based chemotherapy • Paclitaxel/carboplatin for three to six cycles is the usual treatment
Advanced Epithelial Ovarian Cancer	
Stages II, III, and IV	• Primary debulking or cytoreductive surgery is performed which includes staging laparotomy with the removal of as much disease as possible (TAH + BSO + total omentectomy + resection of all macroscopic disease in abdomen) followed by postoperative chemotherapy • The standard regimen is six cycles of postoperative intravenous paclitaxel/carboplatin

Benefits of cytoreductive surgery in women with advanced epithelial ovarian cancer

- **Improves general condition:** Removal of the tumor bulk helps to rapidly improve the disease-related symptoms such as abdominal pain, abdominal distension, dyspnea, and early satiety and improves the quality of life
- **Increases chemosensitivity:** Removal of the tumor bulk reduces the tumor burden, there by maximizing the effect of chemotherapeutic agents (the residual lesions become well perfused and therefore mitotically active)
- **Improves immune function:** Removal of the tumor bulk may help to improve host immune competence by reducing the production of immune suppressive cytokines such as interleukin-10 by the tumor tissue

Note
• *When tumor masses <1 cm diameter are left behind, it is known as optimal debulking*
• *When large tumor masses of >1 cm in diameter are left behind, it is known as suboptimal debulking*

Interval Debulking

- This term is used to describe **surgery performed in the middle of a chemotherapy course, for patients in whom initial debulking surgery was attempted, but was unsuccessful, and whose disease appears to be responding to chemotherapy**
- Selected patients may benefit from interval debulking depending on the aggressiveness of the initial cytoreductive surgery and the response to chemotherapy

Chemotherapy in Ovarian Tumors (Table 5.13)

Table 5.13: Chemotherapy In Ovarian Cancers

Terminology	Description	Indications
Adjuvant chemotherapy	Chemotherapy given after surgery to destroy the remaining cancer cells, which couldn't be completely removed by surgery	• In stage IA, Grade 1, no chemotherapy is required • All other stages require postoperative chemotherapy
Neoadjuvant chemotherapy (NACT)	It refers to brief induction course of chemotherapy for 2-3 cycles prior to debulking surgery (chemotherapy for three cycles followed by interval cytoreductive surgery) Advantages of NACT • Rapid subjective improvement of symptoms • Increases the percentage of patients who will be successfully cytoreduced • Decreases operative morbidity	• Appropriate in patients who are poor surgical candidates at presentation • Stage III ovarian tumor with the following: – Irresectable pelvic mass – Extensive peritoneal disease – Perisplenic involvement – Nodes at portahepatis – Involvement of diaphragm • Whether NACT should be more universally applied remains controversial
Palliative chemotherapy	It refers to chemotherapy given to patients with stage IV cancer with distant metastasis.	Mainly palliative

Chemotherapy Agents

- **Platinum and taxane-based combination therapy is recommended as the first-line treatment for epithelial ovarian tumors**
- Chemotherapy agents usually administered are either cisplatin or carboplatin in combination with either paclitaxel or cyclophosphamide for three to six cycles

Platinum agents

- **Carboplatin and cisplatin** represent the most active group of chemotherapy drugs in the treatment of ovarian cancer
- There is no difference in efficacy between the two agents, carboplatin and cisplatin
- **Carboplatin is less emetogenic and produces less neurotoxicity and nephrotoxicity than cisplatin,** hence serves as the first-line platinum agent in the treatment of ovarian cancer
- **Dosage**–not to exceed 50 to 100 mg/m^2 every 3 weeks for cisplatin and AUC 5 - 7.5 every 3 weeks for carboplatin.
- **Oxaliplatin** use in ovarian cancer is **not shown to be superior** to or less toxic than carboplatin
- **Cisplatin** remains the standard platinum drug for **intraperitoneal administration**

Combination chemotherapy

- **Addition of a Taxane to Platinum Chemotherapy (Paclitaxel with cisplatin/carboplatin) prolongs progression-free and overall survival** and is found to be better than combination of cyclophosphamide with cisplatin/ carboplatin
- **Alternative taxanes–Docetaxel** was associated with **less neurotoxicity but more myelotoxicity.** It is an attractive option for patients at risk for neurotoxicity
- There are **no data to prove that the addition of any third cytotoxic agent** to front-line chemotherapy of ovarian cancer improves outcomes

Intraperitoneal Chemotherapy

- Intraperitoneal (IP) chemotherapy provides a means by which high concentrations of drugs and long duration of tissue exposure can be attained at the peritoneal surface
- As intraperitoneal progression of disease remains the main cause of morbidity and mortality in ovarian cancer, IP chemotherapy is a theoretically attractive approach in the treatment of ovarian cancers
- Intraperitoneal chemotherapy is administered through a specially designed port
- **Cisplatin can be used for intraperitoneal and intravenous therapy; carboplatin, which is less toxic and easier to administer is used as the standard agent for intravenous platinum therapy**
- **The theoretical benefit is only for very small tumor volume and is not useful in large-volume residual disease**
- **Agents that do not reach therapeutic systemic levels when given by the intraperitoneal route need to be administered intravenously as well** (peak concentrations are higher with IV cisplatin compared to the same doses of cisplatin given intraperitoneally, hence administered by both routes)

Clinical use of Intraperitoneal Therapy for Ovarian Cancer

- Numerous clinical trials have tested the benefits of intraperitoneal cisplatin in the treatment of ovarian cancer
- Despite the results, intraperitoneal therapy has not yet been consistently adopted for the treatment of optimally debulked ovarian cancer for the following reasons:
  - Intraperitoneal therapy is technically demanding
  - Use of Intaperitoneal catheters is not routine in many oncology practices
  - Associated complications such as intestinal injury, catheter blockage and infections
  - Intraperitoneal therapy may cause toxicity

Note

The option of intraperitoneal therapy should be discussed with patients who have had optimally debulked ovarian cancer. Trials are going on for identifying simplified, less toxic regimens

Newer Molecular Targeted Agents Combined with Chemotherapy–Bevacizumab

- The most promising agent **currently is Bevacizumab**–an **antiangiogenic agent**
- It is a **monoclonal antibody targeting vascular endothelial growth factor (VEGF)**
- It has produced single agent response rates of 20% in recurrent ovarian cancer
- It has improved survival when combined with chemotherapy in the treatment of metastatic colon cancer and lung cancer
- Currently not FDA approved for the treatment of ovarian cancer
- Very expensive
- Associated with a number of toxicities, including increased risk of bowel perforations
- **OCEANS trial (Ovarian Cancer Study Comparing Efficacy and Safety of Chemotherapy and Anti-Angiogenic Therapy in Platinum-Sensitive Recurrent Disease),** a randomized, double-blind, phase III trial, initiated to compare the efficacy and safety of Gemcitabine plus Bevacizumab (BV arm) and Gemcitabine plus placebo (PL arm) in patients with platinum-sensitive Recurrent ovarian cancers

Treatment Modalities Other Than Staging Laparotomy and Chemotherapy for Ovarian Tumors (Table 5.14)

Table 5.14: Treatment Modalities Other than Staging Laparotomy and Chemotherapy for Ovarian Tumors

Immunotherapy	• Use of cytokines, interferon, interleukin-2 is under trial • Monoclonal antibodies (Herceptin) when used along with chemotherapy improves response rate
Hormonal therapy	• Progesterones can be used in recurrent, well-differentiated endometrioid carcinoma • Tamoxifen, Leuprolide(GnRH agonist), Aromatase inhibitors are being studied in relapsed cases of ovarian tumor
Radiotherapy (salvage therapy)	• There is very little scope of radiotherapy as an adjunct to surgery because of the advent of chemotherapy • Radiotherapy can be used for palliation in advanced metastatic ovarian carcinoma–pulmonary, bone metastasis, etc.
Radioactive isotopes	• In early cases of ovarian cancer, radioactive phosphorus (32P) can be instilled into the peritoneal cavity. • The isotope emits β-rays and are taken up by macrophages and the radiation effects are limited to superficial 4–6 mm of peritoneal lining • Bowel complications are increased

IMPLICATIONS OF CLEAR CELL AND MUCINOUS HISTOLOGY

Clear Cell Tumors

- **Early stages at presentation is more common** than advanced stages
- **Do not respond well to platinum chemotherapy**
- Increased **risk of recurrence**
- More likely to have a **thromboembolic event**
- May also be associated with **hypercalcemia**

Mucinous Tumors

- **Early-stage mucinous tumors tend to be low-grade and have a good prognosis**
- Advanced-stage primary ovarian mucinous tumors are difficult to distinguish from metastatic mucinous tumors
- Advanced-stage mucinous tumors respond poorly to chemotherapy and associated with a reduced survival

Role of Prolongation of Primary Therapy/Consolidation of Therapy

- Many women with ovarian cancer have an excellent response to first-line chemotherapy, but most of the cases will have disease relapse
- Further therapy after a clinical complete remission would be warranted and several strategies are being tested in randomized trials
- The modalities studied include–whole abdominal radiotherapy, intraperitoneal P32, intraperitoneal cisplatin, greater than six cycles of primary therapy, consolidation with a different agent such as topotecan or epirubicin and high-dose chemotherapy with stem cell support. However, none of these approaches have produced any convincing survival benefit.

SECOND-LOOK LAPAROTOMY/LAPAROSCOPY

- ***Definition***–The term second-look laparotomy/laparoscopy refers to an abdominal procedure performed in a patient who has no clinical evidence of disease (on physical examination, CA 125, CT scan) after a prescribed course of therapy, to determine the response to therapy i.e., to assess whether or not residual disease remains

Procedure

- Second-look laparotomy is similar to surgical staging
- Multiple biopsies are taken
- Pelvic and para-aortic nodes are dissected, if not done previously

  Second-look laparoscopy is less invasive, but false-negative rates are high due to adhesions

Role of second-look laparotomy/laparoscopy

- Surgery is the most accurate way to assess response to therapy; but second look procedure is no longer in current standard of practice for the following reasons:
  - Not shown to influence patient survival–There is no evidence that any further therapy will prolong survival in patients who are clinically inapparent but with residual disease at second look laparotomy
  - Even patients with negative second-look laparotomy have a 50% recurrence risk
- To be performed only in research settings

FOLLOW-UP OF PATIENTS IN REMISSION

- Regular follow-up is essential for all patients with ovarian cancer who have clinical complete remission following treatment because of the high relapse risk
- Patients should be examined every 3 months for the first 2 years, and thereafter, every 4–6 months
- Recurrence **usually develops within the first 2 years** after treatment

Assessment during follow-up visits

- **Clinical assessment:** History and examination are done
- **Radiological assessment:** USG, CT, and MRI are done
- **CA 125 levels:**
  - Levels **usually become undetectable following initial surgery and with one or two cycles of chemotherapy**
  - CA125 levels will **rise before any symptoms suggestive of cancer recurrence develop**
  - Unlike the situation in screening, rise in **CA-125 after primary treatment for ovarian cancer is specific**
  - **Interpretation of CA 125 levels during follow-up visits is as follows:**

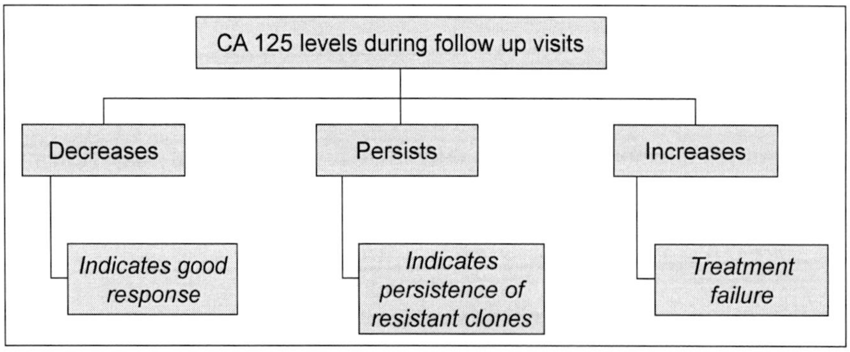

- If CA 125 level increases during the follow up visit, further evaluation such as CT scan and MRI may be performed

PERSISTENCE/RECURRENCE OF DISEASE

Terminologies

Terminology	Definition
Progressive/persistent disease	Disease-free interval of less than 6 months following primary therapy
Recurrence of disease	Disease-free interval of more than 6 months following primary therapy

Terminology	Definition
Platinum-refractory	Ovarian cancers with progression on platinum-based therapy
Platinum-resistant	Ovarian cancers which recur < 6 months after completion of platinum-based therapy
Platinum sensitive	Ovarian cancers which recur >6 months after completing treatment with a platinum-based regimen

Treatment of Persistent/recurrent Disease

Second-Line Chemotherapy

- Ovarian cancer that is resistant to primary chemotherapy is generally not curable. However, **patients who relapse after a substantial disease-free interval may benefit from further treatment**
- Women **with platinum-refractory therapy have a very poor prognosis, and response to any subsequent treatment is unlikely**

General principles of treating recurrent disease include the following:

- **Platinum compounds are the most active single agents in women with platinum-sensitive recurrent disease**
- Platinum-sensitive tumors are more sensitive than platinum resistant tumors to any cytotoxic agent
- **Platinum-based combinations** of cytotoxic agents **produce superior response rates and progression-free survival** compared with single agent platinum therapy in women with platinum-sensitive disease
- Combination therapy has not been shown to provide any benefit in women with platinum-resistant disease
- **Taxanes have consistently produced response rates over 20% in women with platinum-resistant disease.** No other agents have produced response in these patients
- Treatment is recognized as **primarily palliative,** and decisions about treatment regimens should include patient convenience, toxicity and efficacy

Treatment of Platinum-Sensitive Disease

- Platinum-containing combinations including paclitaxel, gemcitabine, and liposomal doxorubicin, produce superior progression-free survival to single agent platinum therapy in the setting of platinum-sensitive disease
- **Superior response rate and superior progression-free survival is observed with combination therapy**
- Results regarding overall survival are conflicting, and any such benefit is probably small
- Secondary debulking surgery has been hypothesized to be of benefit in this group and is under trial
- Repeated courses of carboplatin-based therapy increases the risk for hypersensitivity reactions. Not all patients allergic to carboplatin will be allergic to cisplatin
- The hypersensitivity reactions occur during drug infusion and are associated with flushing, nausea and hypertension.
- A number of desensitization protocols appear to be effective but are time-consuming
- Routine use of diphenhydramine premedication may produce a non-significant decrease in reaction rate

Treatment of Platinum-Resistant Disease

- Response rate to any single agent therapy in these women is about 10- 20%; Median overall survival is 9 to 12 months
- Agents with some activity in treatment of platinum-resistant recurrent ovarian cancer (Table 5.15)

Table 5.15: Agents in Treatment of Platinum-Resistant Ovarian Cancer

• Bevacizumab	• Etoposide
• Tamoxifen	• Gemcitabine
• Pegylated liposomal doxorubicin	• Ifosfamide
• Epirubicin	• Topotecan
• Docetaxel	• Irinotecan
• Weekly paclitaxel	• Vinorelbine
(contd..)	

- **Pegylated liposomal doxorubicin is one of the agents commonly used, based on the ease of administration and tolerable toxicity**

Flowchart 5.1: Summary of Management of Ovarian Cancer

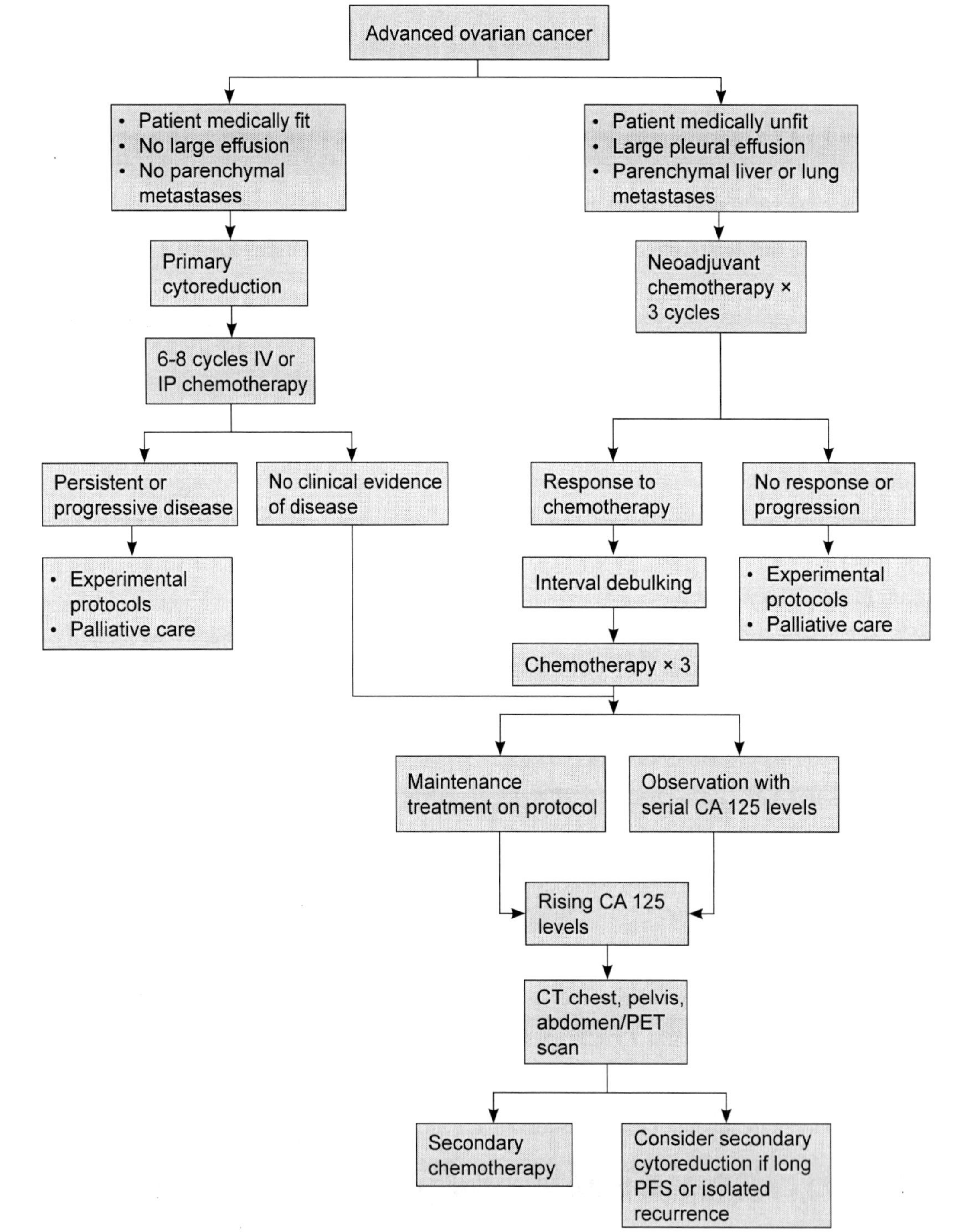

PFS–Progression Free Survival

Prognosis and 5 Year Survival (Table 5.16 and Table 5.17)

Table 5.16: Prognostic Factors In Ovarian Malignancy

Prognostic Variable	Prognosis
Surgical stage	Worse beyond stage II
Histological type	Endometrioid tumor has got a higher survival rate than serous type because the former tumor is highly well-differentiated
Histological grade	Higher the grade, poorer the prognosis

Contd.

Contd.

Tumor characteristics	Breach in capsule, surface excrescence, preoperative rupture and dense adherence
Peritoneal cytology	Positive malignant cells, higher the risk
Presence of ascites	Higher the risk
Presence of metastatic disease before cytoreductive surgery	Poor prognosis and survival rate
Volume of residual tumor after primary surgery	When < 5 mm better prognosis
Ploidy status	Diploid tumors are prognostically better compared to aneuploid tumors

Table 5.17: Five year survival rate

Stage	5-year survival (%)
I	75-90
II	60-70
III	20-40
IV	5-10

Reasons for Poor Outcome in Ovarian Cancer

- Late diagnosis
- No preinvasive stage of the disease
- No effective screening procedure
- No correlation of symptoms with the tumor size
- Extent of tumor spread is often unknown
- Limitations of cytoreductive surgery
- Variable chemosensitivity
- Radiation dose restriction by neighboring organs
- Tumor cells are freely mobile within the peritoneal cavity

BORDERLINE OVARIAN TUMORS/TUMORS OF LOW MALIGNANT POTENTIAL

Definition–Epithelial ovarian tumors having characteristics in between those of benign and malignant tumors are termed as borderline ovarian tumors (BOTs)

Features

- Approximately **10-20%** of all epithelial tumors are borderline ovarian tumors
- Most are of **serous or mucinous** variety
- Most are **diagnosed in early stages**
- Borderline tumors are likely to **affect young women (30-50 years),** in whom decisions regarding fertility-sparing, premature hormonal deprivation and adjuvant chemotherapeutic treatments are pertinent
- They are **slow growing even when presenting at advanced stages**
- They have **good prognosis;** 10 year survival rate for stage I is 99%
- **Recurrence is common after 15–20 years** and hence long term follow up is required

BOTs are differentiated from benign tumors by the following features (at least two features should be present to term as BOTs):

- Nuclear atypia
- Cellular pleomorphism
- Increased mitotic activity
- Microscopic papillary projections

Note

In BOTs, tumor cells display characteristic malignant histology, but do not have stromal invasion

Management

- Surgery is the **main treatment for early-stage and advanced-stage BOTs**
- Staging laparotomy is done
- The resected ovarian tumor is sent for frozen section; if BOT is identified, further management is as follows:

Flowchart 5.2: Management of Borderline epithelial ovarian tumors

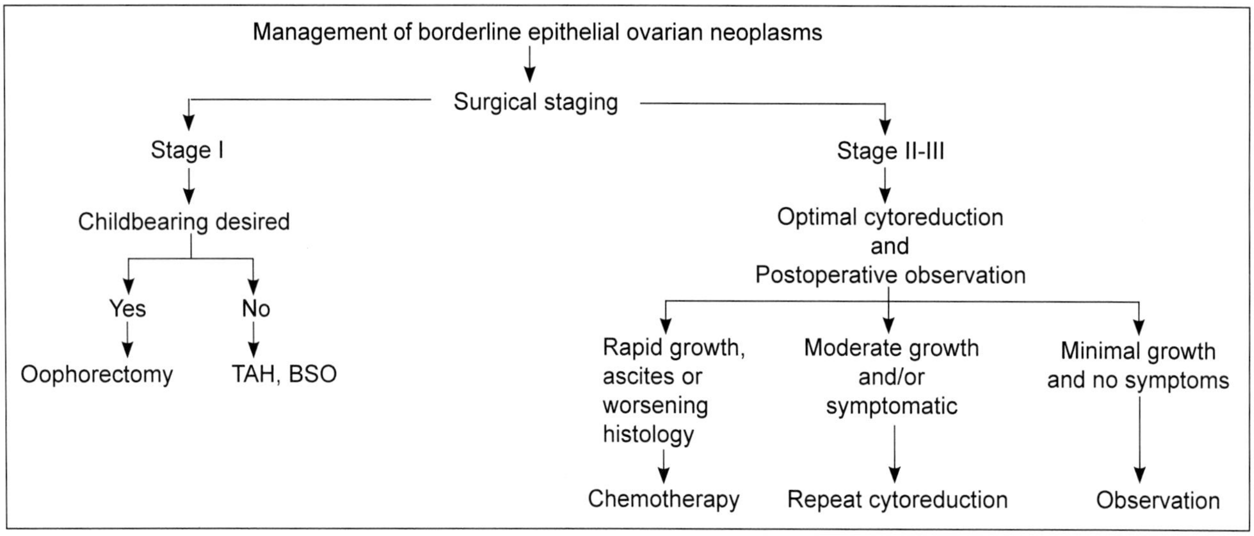

Note

- *In Stage I BOT patients in whom conservative surgical approach (U/L ovariotomy) has been performed, completion surgery (removal of other ovary and uterus) is done after completion of family*
- *Conservative surgical approach does not have an adverse effect on survival in patients with stage I borderline tumors*
- *As BOT have very slow growth, they are often* ***resistant to chemotherapy agents***
- *Serous borderline tumors have response rates of 15-60% to chemotherapy agents. However, there is no clear evidence that chemotherapy can decrease relapse or improve survival*
- *20-30% of ovarian tumors diagnosed as BOTs during frozen section examination may be reported as invasive carcinoma on final pathology report*

PREVENTIVE MEASURES FOR OVARIAN CANCERS

Primary Prevention

As the natural history of the disease is not well understood, primary prevention cannot be clearly formulated

Preventive measures include:

- **Genetic screening for BRCA 1 and 2** in women with high risk for ovarian and breast cancer
- **Periodic screening for other malignancies** (colonoscopy, endometrial biopsy) in women with Lynch II syndrome
- **Annual mammographic screening** in women with family history of breast cancer
- **Combined oral contraceptive pills** as a preventive measure is recommended in women belonging to Lynch II families.
- **Prophylactic oophorectomy is recommended** as a preventive measure against ovarian malignancy at completion of family or at > 35 years in 'high risk' women such as those with BRCA1/ 2 carriers and history of ovarian, endometrial or colonic cancers in first degree relatives. Periodic pelvic and ultrasound examinations and CA-125 levels on a regular basis are done until these women undergo prophylactic oophorectomy

Secondary Prevention (Screening for Ovarian Cancer)

Screening aims at detecting early ovarian malignancy in asymptomatic women. **No reliable procedures are currently available for early detection of ovarian cancer for the following reasons:**

- Natural history of the disease is not well understood

- There is no preinvasive stage like that of cervical intraepithelial neoplasia
- **Screening with pelvic examination, TVS , and CA-125 has not been shown to be effective including in those with BRCA mutations**

Screening Procedures

- **Clinical:** Regular and periodic clinical examination in an asymptomatic woman may detect an adnexal mass. However, clinical examination is not very specific
- **Tumor markers: CA 125** is a glycoprotein, which has been used for screening of epithelial cancers of the ovary
  - Normal value < 35 U/mL. Serum half-life of CA-125 is 20 days
  - Value > 35 U/mL may be suggestive of epithelial ovarian cancer
  - It is not a tumor specific antigen and there are several other conditions, where level of CA-125 is raised:
    - Normal woman (1%)
    - Carcinomas of the breast, lung, colon and endometrium
    - Endometriosis
    - Pelvic inflammatory disease
    - Peritonitis
  - It is used for monitoring a patient during chemotherapy and for follow up
  - The serum level of CA-125 falls after surgical resection of the tumor and following chemotherapy. Elevated level indicates residual disease or tumor recurrence or resistant clones to chemotherapy
- **Ultrasound imaging:**
  - Transvaginal color Doppler imaging has been able to differentiate benign from malignant tumors by assessment of its vascular supply and tumor blood flow. Increased neoangiogenesis in ovarian malignancy causes central neovascularity
  - **Vascular parameters -Pulsatility Index (PI) < 1.0 or Resistive Index (RI) < 0.4: Increases the risk of malignancy**
  - Three dimensional, contrast enhanced, power Doppler sonography is found to be more diagnostic
- **Risk of Malignancy Index (RMI):**
  - **RMI = U × M × CA 125**

    U = USG score (one point each for: multi-locular cyst; solid areas; metastasis; ascites; bilateral lesions)

    M = 3 (postmenopausal women)

    CA-125 level in U/mL

  The risk of cancer is 75% when the RMI value is > 250

Note

- ***Routine screening of the general population should not be performed*** *-A large multimodal screening trial* ***Prostate, Lung, Colorectal and Ovarian Cancer Screening Trial*** *concluded that screening with TVS and CA 125 has low positive predictive value in identifying the disease and may do more harm than good (complications from needless procedures)*
- ***In women with a family history of ovarian cancer or known BRCA mutations****, there is no evidence that screening can affect mortality due to this disease. Despite lack of evidence for benefit of screening in these high-risk women, it is prudent to follow up these patients with pelvic and ultrasound examinations and CA-125 levels on a regular basis until they undergo prophylactic oophorectomy*

Management in women with positive family history of ovarian cancer or BRCA 1/2 carriers:

- TVS and CA 125 done every 6 monthly
- OCPs are prescribed when not interested in fertility
- Prophylactic oophorectomy (as soon as family is completed or at 35 years of age)
- Annual mammography

GUIDELINES FOR MANAGEMENT OF AN ENLARGED OVARY

Premenopausal women frequently have palpable adnexal masses. Ovarian enlargement of size < 5cm are most often benign and are due to follicular or corpus luteum cysts

- An ovarian enlargement of size 5- 8 cm during childbearing period needs careful follow up
- In postmenopausal women, any ovarian enlargement should be assessed by transvaginal sonography and serum CA-125
- Surgical exploration is generally indicated in following cases
  - The ovary enlarges progressively beyond 8cm while under observation
  - Any symptomatic ovarian tumor regardless of size
  - Adnexal masses in postmenopausal women

Symptomatic ovarian cysts

- Symptomatic cysts of any size often need surgical intervention, as the symptoms are usually due to complications or large size of the cyst

Asymptomatic ovarian cysts

Management of asymptomatic ovarian cysts depends on the following:

- Age of the patient
- Menopausal status
- Size of the cyst
- Ultrasonography features
- Tumor marker levels

Management of asymptomatic ovarian cysts is outlined in the Flowchart 5.3

Flowchart 5.3: Management of asymptomatic ovarian cysts

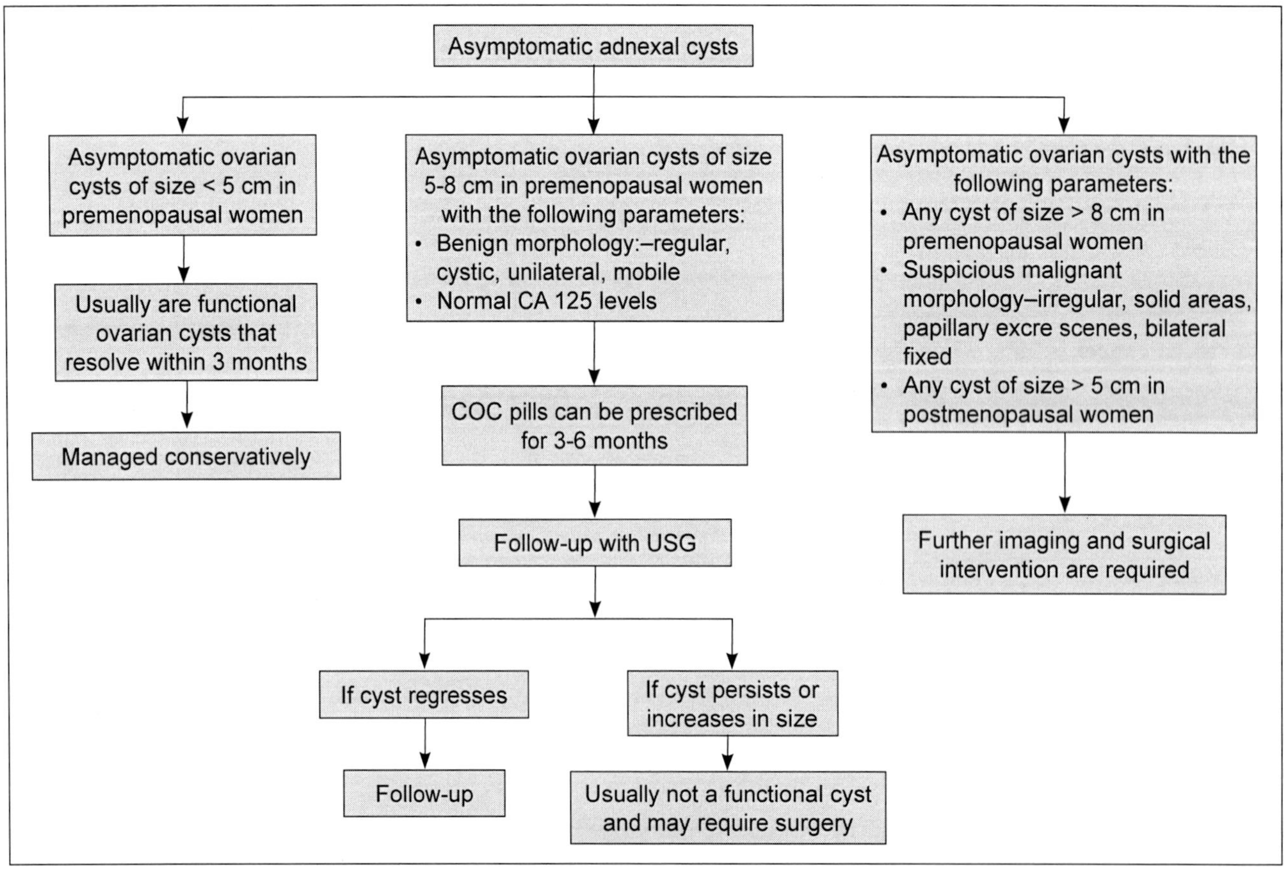

EXTRA EDGE–*Update on the various surgical procedures performed for ovarian tumors*

Primary cytoreductive surgery	Initial laparotomy to establish diagnosis, stage and attempt maximal tumor debulking to microscopic disease before the initiation of first-line chemotherapy. Also called "primary debulking" by some physicians
Interval cytoreduction or Interval debulking	Cytoreductive surgery after a biopsy only or a primary suboptimal debulking followed by induction chemotherapy
Second-look surgery	Surgery performed at the completion of primary chemotherapy in patients who do not have evidence of disease by CT scan or CA-125 to determine if there is residual disease in order to plan for additional chemotherapy. Currently rarely performed
Secondary cytoreductive surgery	Surgery in a patient with recurrent disease who has completed primary treatment, including primary debulking + chemotherapy, and had been without evidence of disease. The procedure is most commonly performed for platinum-sensitive patients with oligometastatic disease. Also called "primary debulking" by some physicians
Palliative surgery	Surgery performed to relieve symptoms, most commonly performed for a malignant bowel obstruction with the goal to remove the obstruction or perform a diversion. Not primarily intended to remove tumors
Complete debulking Result: no macroscopic disease	Complete resection: Cytoreduction of all tumors independent of preoperative tumor load to microscopic residual disease at the completion of surgery-no gross residual tumors left. R0 resection
Optimal debulking Result: macroscopic disease up to 1 cm	Minimal residual: Macroscopic disease up to 1 cm in diameter after primary surgery. Also called by some physicians "optimal cytoreduction". R1 resection
Sub-optimal debulking. Result: macroscopic disease > 1 cm	Gross residual: Primary cytoreduction resulting in macroscopic disease larger than 1 cm in size at the end of surgery. R2 resection

RECENT UPDATES

Hypothetical model of ovarian cancer dormancy and relapse after debulking surgery and potential stages of the disease where therapeutic intervention is envisioned –Shown in Figure 5.1

Figure 5.1: Hypothetical model of ovarian cancer dormancy and relapse after debulking surgery

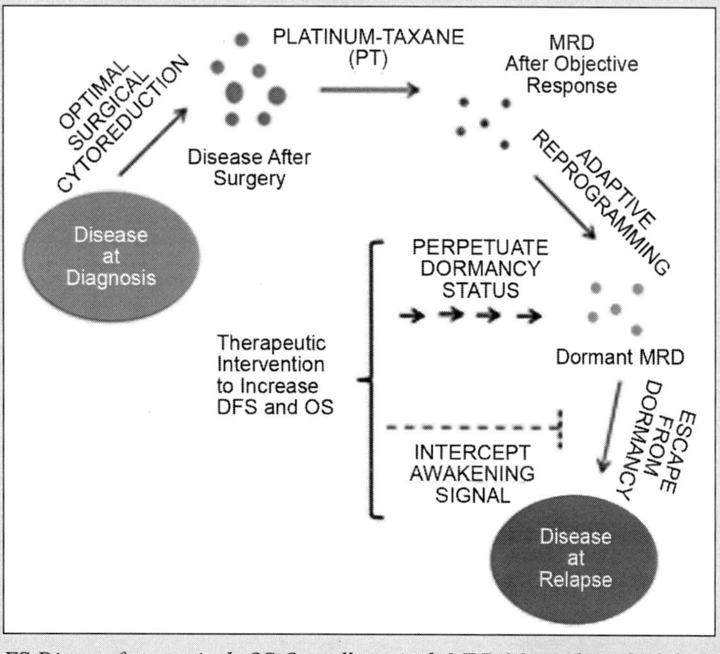

DFS-Disease free survival; OS-Overall survival. MRD-Minimal residual disease

ROLE OF VITAMIN D AND VITAMIN D RECEPTOR (VDR) IN GYNECOLOGICAL CANCERS (Figure 5.2)

- *Endogenous synthesis of vitamin D begins with the oxidation of cholesterol, resulting in pro-vitamin D3*

- *In the skin, ultraviolet B (UVB) radiation transforms pro-vitamin D3 to pre-vitamin D3. Pre-vitamin D3 isomerizes to vitamin D3, also named as cholecalciferol*
- *Two hydroxylation's by the enzymes vitamin D 25-hydroxylases (CYP27A1) and renal mitochondrial 1-hydroxylase (CYP27B1) are necessary to transform vitamin D3 into the active 1α, 25(OH)2D3*
- ***1α,25(OH)2 D3 binds to the vitamin D receptor which belongs to the family of nuclear receptors and forms a complex with retinoid X receptor (RXR) to regulate gene expression***
- ***Both vitamin D and its receptor have a protective role in gynecological cancers***
- ***Low levels of vitamin D are found in ovarian, cervical and vulvar cancer***
- As a response to cancer, the expression of the vitamin D receptor is up regulated in endometrial, ovarian, cervical and vulvar cancer
- ***Vitamin D receptor (VDR) is upregulated in all gynecological cancers, indicating its influence on cancer etiology***
- ***VDR polymorphism FokI seems to increase the risk of ovarian cancer (Figure 5.2). Other nuclear receptors, such as the RXR, also influence gynecological cancers***

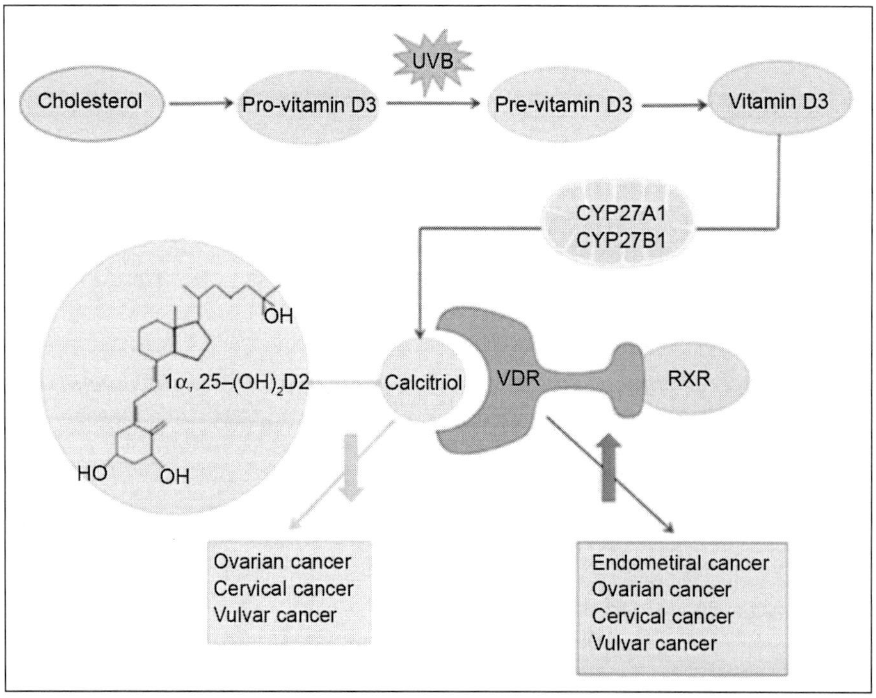

Figure 5.2: Role of Vitamin D and vitamin D receptor (VDR) in Gynecological Cancers

VITAMIN D RECEPTOR (VDR) GENE POLYMORPHISMS IN OVARIAN CANCER (Figure 5.3)

- ***The VDR gene is located on the chromosome 12q12-14***
- *Several VDR polymorphisms have been identified:* ***Fok1, Bsm1, Apa1, and Taq1***
- ***The restriction fragment polymorphism of Fok1 alters an ACG codon*** *resulting in an additional start codon and thereby generating a longer VDR protein.* ***The longer version of the VDR protein exerts less transcriptional activity***
- *The f allele indicates the absence of the restriction site encoding a 427–amino acid protein*
- *The F allele shows the presence of the restriction site encoding a 424–amino acid protein*
- ***Carrying the ff or Ff genotypes increases the risk of ovarian cancer***

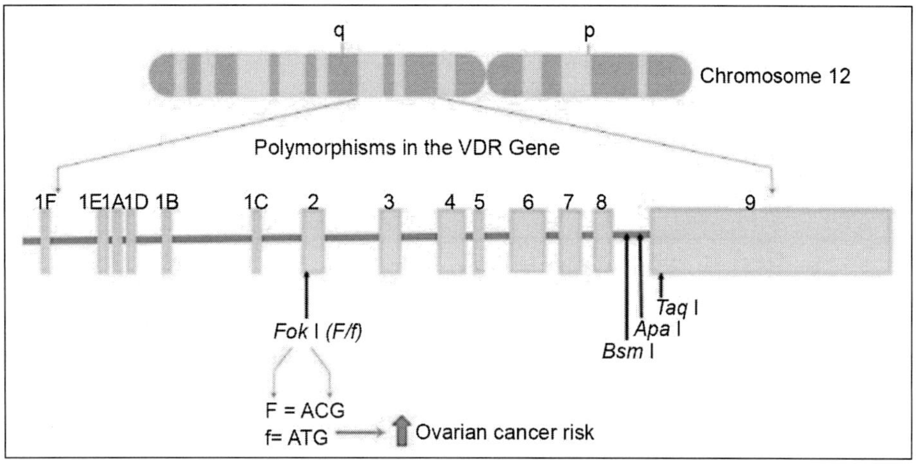

Figure 5.3: VDR gene polymorphisim in ovarian cancer

ROLE OF PARP1 INHIBITORS IN OVARIAN CANCER TREATMENT *(Figure 5.4)*

- ***Poly (ADP-ribose) polymerase (PARP) proteins are used by cells in several DNA repair processes***
- ***PARP inhibition can result in preferential death of cancer cells when another mechanism for repairing DNA is defective***
- ***Two PARP inhibitors, Olaparib and Rucaparib,*** *have been approved by the US Food and Drug Administration (FDA) for the treatment of recurrent, BRCA-associated ovarian cancer*
- *More recently,* ***a third PARP inhibitor, Niraparib,*** *was approved by the FDA as maintenance therapy following platinum-based chemotherapy for recurrent ovarian cancer*
- *PARP inhibitors has caused a paradigm shift in disease management and a challenge for clinicians, who must decide how best to use these agents in individualized treatment*
- *The oral formulation is attractive to patients, but has adverse effects such as* ***nausea and fatigue***
- *Treatment related adverse events reported are anemia (decreased hemoglobin concentration) and increase in alanine aminotransferase or aspartate aminotransferase concentration. Elevations in liver enzymes were generally transient, self-limiting, and not associated with other signs of liver toxicity*

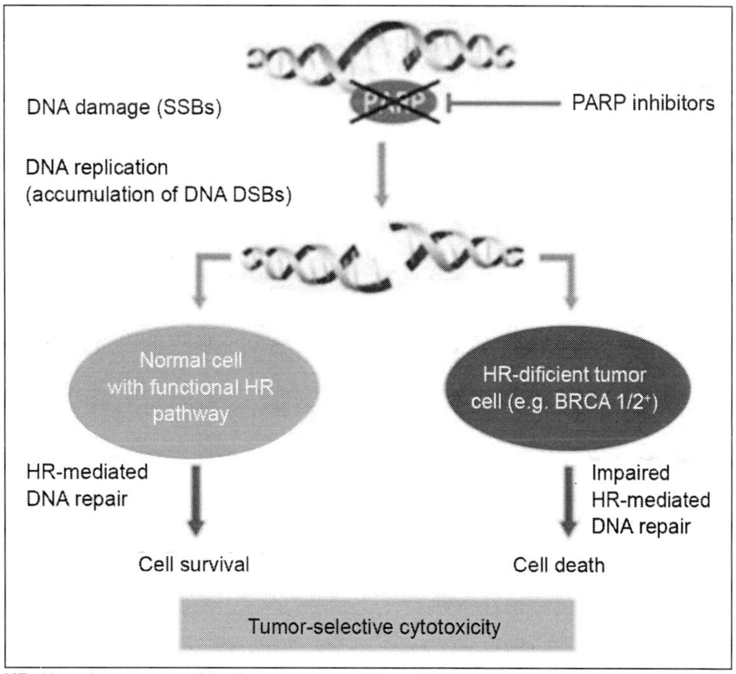

HR: Homologous recombination

Figure 5.4: Role of PARP inhibitors

- *Clinical research is now exploring the following major issues*
- *To find clinically predictive markers of response*
- *Reasons for resistance to parp inhibitor therapy*
- *If PARP inhibitors will be as beneficial in frontline therapy as in relapse setting*
- *Can we enhance efficacy of parp inhibitors in combination with anti-angiogenic drugs and in combination with immunotherapy*

Prediction of the Response to Immunotherapy

- *There is a growing evidence of immune checkpoint inhibitors as treatment for patients with ovarian cancer. However, immune checkpoint inhibitors have demonstrated clinical response only in a small subpopulation of patients with ovarian cancer*
- *Three major predictors for survival were identified so far, which include tumor infiltrating lymphocytes (TILs), Programmed death -Ligand 1 (PD-L1) expression and mutational burden*
- *Based on the study of melanoma, tumors have been classified into 4 groups based on the presence of TILs and PD-L1 expression: type I, adaptive immune resistance (TIL+/PD-L1+); type II, immunological ignorance (TIL−/PD-L1−); type III, intrinsic induction (TIL−/PD-L1+); type IV, tolerance (TIL+/PD-L1−)*
- *It was suggested that immune responses to ovarian cancer could be different among histologic subtypes. High-grade serous ovarian cancers (HGSOCs) are most likely associated with a favorable TIL response. They also showed that type I patterns were more common in HGSOCs*
- *In 2017, Ovarian Tumor Tissue Analysis Consortium published a large-scale multicenter observational, prospective survival cohort study in JAMA Oncology to evaluate histotype-specific survival associations with CD8+ TILs in epithelial ovarian cancer. This is the largest study on intraepithelial CD8+ TILs in ovarian cancer to date. The study showed a robust dose-response relationship between CD8+ TILs and overall survival (OS) in patients with HGSOC. It is essential to predict the response to immunotherapy*

  This study suggests that certain immunotherapy should be indicated in the HGSOC patients with high immune infiltration of CD8+ TILs.

Update on conventional treatment methods

Practice changeable update on lymphadenectomy for ovarian cancers

- *Current surgical treatment guidelines of advanced ovarian cancer include bilateral pelvic and para-aortic lymph node dissection*
- *Results of a large randomized trial, the Lymphadenectomy in Ovarian Neoplasms **(LION)** study (2017), did not support the current guidelines*
- *The conclusion of LION study was that patients with advanced ovarian cancer with clinically negative lymph nodes who undergo a complete resection need not undergo systematic lymphadenectomy because it has no effect on survival outcomes. Serious post-operative complications, including reoperation for complications, infections, and mortality within 60 days of surgery occurred more frequently in lymphadenectomy group than those in no-lymphadenectomy group. Therefore, it was indicated that lymphadenectomy can be safely omitted because it did not improve survival outcomes even if 50% patients had occult nodal disease.*

Role of secondary cytoreductive surgery in recurrent ovarian cancer

- *A phase III randomized trial The Descriptive Evaluation of preoperative Selection KriTeria for operability in recurrent ovarian cancer **(DESKTOP)** was conducted to evaluate the impact of secondary cytoreductive surgery in recurrent ovarian cancer. The interim analysis of the study in 2017 suggested secondary surgery in platinum-sensitive recurrent ovarian cancer in combination with chemotherapy as a viable option*
- *International Collaborative Ovarian Neoplasm **(ICON)** trial reaffirmed standard 3-week dosing schedule for paclitaxel rather than boosting up to a weekly dose-dense regimen. Triweekly carboplatin-paclitaxel is recommended to remain unmodified as a standard first-line regimen in ovarian cancer*

Non-platinum chemotherapy to prolong the progression free interval

- *The extension of progression free interval (PFI) by introducing non-platinum agents was hypothesized as a strategy to increase the platinum sensitivity, thus improving the outcome of partially sensitive disease*
- *The Multicenter Italian Trials in Ovarian Cancer (MITO), a randomized phase III trial concluded that platinum-based chemotherapy should not be delayed in partially sensitive recurrent ovarian cancer because there was nothing to be gained by using a non-platinum agent*

Effect of adding Bevacizumab to standard platinum-based chemotherapy in women with platinum-sensitive recurrent ovarian cancer (OCEANS trial)

- *A phase III randomized trial reported a clinically significant OS improvement by adding Bevacizumab to standard platinum-based chemotherapy*
- *The addition of Bevacizumab to standard chemotherapy and followed by maintenance therapy until progression might be an important therapeutic strategy which resulted in clinically meaningful OS improvement in patients with platinum-sensitive recurrent ovarian cancer.*

Screening of gynecologic cancer: Periodic pelvic examination

- *The pelvic examination is an important screening and diagnostic tool of gynecologic malignancy. However, there was a conflicting evidence regarding periodic pelvic examination in asymptomatic women*
- *In 2017, the US Preventive Services Task Force (USPSTF) released a statement about performing pelvic exams in primary care, "the current evidence is insufficient to assess the balance of benefits and harms of performing screening pelvic examinations in asymptomatic women" after a systematic review of available clinical evidence*

CHAPTER 6

NON EPITHELIAL OVARIAN TUMORS

INTRODUCTION

- Non-epithelial ovarian tumors such as Germ cell tumors (GCTs) and sex cord stromal tumors (SCSTs) account for approximately 10% of all ovarian malignancy
- Malignant GCTs represent 5% of all ovarian malignancy and 80% of the preadolescent malignant ovarian tumors
- SCSTs are rare neoplasms that account for approximately 3–5% of ovarian malignancies and the majority of ovarian tumors with endocrine manifestations
- Malignant germ cell tumors (GCTs) occur mainly in young women. Unlike GCTs, SCSTs occur over a wide range of age; granulosa cell tumors and thecomas are found mainly in peri- and
- Postmenopausal women, whereas juvenile granulosa cell tumors and Sertoli–Leydig cell tumors (SLCTs) usually develop in young females in whom maintenance of fertility is important

Staging System

- The staging system for non-epithelial ovarian cancers is generally adopted from the one for epithelial ovarian cancer originally defined by the International Federation of Gynecology and Obstetrics (FIGO, 2014) – (Refer chapter on Epithelial ovarian tumor)
- Adverse factors include age >45 years, > stage I, incomplete surgical resection and yolk sac tumor histology

GERM CELL TUMORS

- Benign and malignant tumors can arise from the germ cells of the ovary.
- **Most common germ cell tumor of the ovary is cystic teratoma,** which is a **benign** tumor
- **The most common malignant germ cell tumor** of the ovary is **dysgerminoma**

Characteristics of Malignant Germ Cell Tumors of The Ovary

- **About 20–25% of all ovarian tumors are germ cell tumors and 3% of these are malignant**
- Malignant germ cell tumors constitute **5% of all ovarian malignancies**
- 70% cases occur **before age of 20 years**
- **Mostly unilateral**
- Malignant germ cell tumors generally spread along the peritoneal surface or through lymphatic dissemination
- **Majority are stage I at diagnosis**
- Grow rapidly
- Majority are **highly chemo sensitive**
- Usually **have very good prognosis**

WHO classification of germ cell tumors (2014) – Table 6.1

Table 6.1: WHO classification of germ cell tumors (2014)

I.	Dysgerminoma
II.	Teratoma A. Immature B. Mature 1. Solid 2. Cystic a. Dermoid cyst (mature cystic teratoma b. Dermoid cyst with malignant transformation c. Monodermal and highly specialized 1. Struma ovarii 2. Carcinoid 3. Struma ovarii and carcinoid 4. Other
III.	Endodermal sinus tumor
IV.	Embryonal carcinoma
V.	Polyembryoma
VI.	Choriocarcinoma
VII.	Mixed forms

Histogenesis (Flowchart 6.1)

- Primordial germ cells migrate from the yolk sac through dorsal mesentery to the genital ridge
- **Dysgerminomas and embryonal carcinomas arise from these primitive germ cells**
- Dysgerminoma does not have the potential to differentiate further
- Embryonal carcinomas have totipotent cells that can differentiate into embryonic tissues such as ectoderm, endoderm and mesoderm and into e**xtraembryonic tissues** such as yolk sac and trophoblasts

Tumor markers secreted by germ cell tumors

- Many germ cell tumors possess the unique property of producing biologic tumor markers that are detectable in serum
- Measurement of tumor markers secreted by germ cell tumors may be useful in diagnosis, assessment of response to therapy and follow-up

  (see flowchart 6.1)

DYSGERMINOMA

- Dysgerminoma is the most common (30–40%) malignant germ cell tumor
- It arises from **undifferentiated germ cells**
- The counterpart of dysgerminoma in male is **seminoma**
- Majority (90%) of the tumors occur **at less than 20 years of age**
- Usually unilateral. **Bilateral in 10-20% of cases**
- It is the **most common malignant germ cell tumor associated with pregnancy** (20–30%)

Flowchart 6.1: Histogenesis of Ovarian Germ Cell Tumors and Tumor Markers

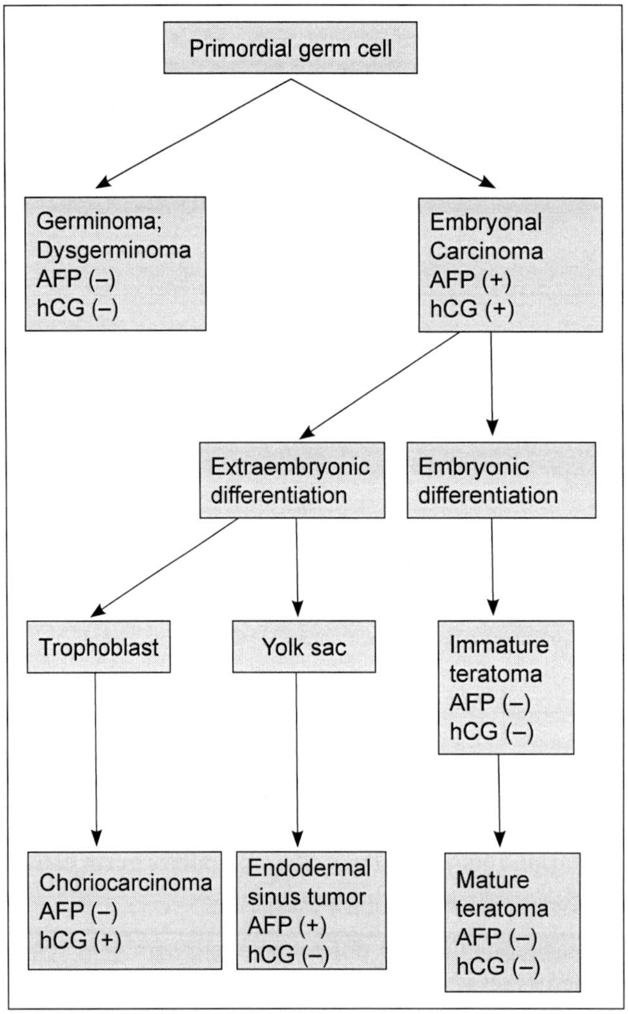

AFP = α-fetoprotein; hCG = human chorionic gonadotropin

- Dysgerminoma may be associated with choriocarcinoma or endodermal sinus tumor
- **Tumor markers: Secretes LDH and placenta-like alkaline phosphatase (PLAP). hCG assays may rarely be positive,** confusing the diagnosis with pregnancy. **Do not produce alpha fetoprotein (AFP)**
- **Dysgenetic gonad is a risk factor for dysgerminoma.** The risk is increased in dysgenesis containing Y-chromosome–Turner mosaic, Klinefelter syndrome, androgen-insensitivity syndrome, and pure and mixed gonadal dysgenesis. Karyotyping should be done when a premenarcheal girl presents with a pelvic mass
- Majority of dysgerminomas (75%) are confined to one ovary and are stage I at diagnosis
- Best prognosis of all germ cell tumors

Pathology

Gross appearance-Solid fleshy lobulated tumor with a **peculiar elastic rubbery consistency**

- **Microscopic appearance:** Characteristic histological appearance **similar to seminoma,** consisting **of nests and cords of primitive appearing germ cells with clear cytoplasm, prominent cytoplasmic borders and numerous mitoses.** The fibrous septae have **leucocytic infiltration**
- **The number of mitotic figures does not have any prognostic significance**

Immunohistochemistry

- Dysgerminomas stain positive for **c-kit** and **nuclear transcription factor OCT 3/4** that help in confirming the diagnosis
- Dysgerminoma is the **only ovarian germ cell tumor that displays c-kit staining**

- Both **dysgerminoma and embryonal carcinoma stain for OCT 3/4**
- In contrast to embryonal carcinoma, **dysgerminoma does not stain for CD30**

Clinical features

- Occur predominantly in girls younger than 20 years of age
- Asymptomatic in 25% cases, diagnosed incidentally on ultrasonography
- May present with acute abdominal pain (due to necrosis, hemorrhage, torsion or rupture), abdominal mass, abdominal distension or menstrual irregularities
- Examination reveals a solid lower abdominal mass, with/without ascites and metastasis to other sites

Investigations

- Ultrasonography–may reveal a complex ovarian mass
- Doppler–reveals low resistance flow index
- Tumor markers: AFP negative, LDH and PLAP positive and rarely hCG positive
- Karyotyping– done in premenarcheal girls

MANAGEMENT OF MALIGNANT GERM CELL TUMORS

Principles of management of malignant germ cell tumors

- The initial treatment approach for a patient suspected of malignant ovarian germ cell tumor is surgery, **both for diagnosis and for therapy**
- Germ cell tumors occur mostly in young girls,in whom preservation of fertility is a priority. Hence, **conservative surgery is planned-**minimizing the surgical resection while ensuring the removal of tumor bulk must be thoughtfully balanced
- The type of primary surgery depends upon the intraoperative findings
- **Germ cell tumors are most often Stage I at diagnosis and bilateral ovarian involvement is rare, except in 10-20% cases of pure dysgerminoma**
- Bilateral ovarian involvement may be found in cases of advanced germ cell tumors (stages II to IV), due to metastasis from one ovary to the opposite ovary
- **Fertility-sparing unilateral salpingo oophorectomy with preservation of the contralateral ovary and the uterus can be performed in most patients**
- **Contralateral ovary**
  - If the contralateral ovary appears grossly normal on careful inspection, it should be left undisturbed
  - In case of pure dysgerminoma, biopsy of contralateral ovary may be considered, as occult or microscopic tumor involvement occurs in 10% of patients
- With the advent of in vitro fertilization technology, traditional guidelines concerning surgical treatment in young patients with gynecologic tumors have to be revised

Surgical staging includes the following steps:

- Adequate midline incision
- Ascites (if present) or else peritoneal washings sent for cytology
- Systematic exploration of the peritoneal cavity and its structures are done
- The ovarian tumor and pelvis should be examined. Both ovaries should carefully be assessed for size, presence of obvious tumor involvement, capsular rupture, external excrescences or adherence to surrounding structures.
- **In young girls at any stage (reproductive function is desired)**
  - Perform Unilateral oophorectomy and send for frozen section
  - If frozen section is reported as dysgerminoma–Careful inspection and palpation of contralateral ovary and biopsy of suspicious areas is performed, as it is the only germ cell tumor that can be bilateral

- **If Reproductive function not desired**-Perform Hysterectomy with Bilateral salpingo-oophorectomy
- Multiple peritoneal and omental biopsies are taken
- Pelvic and para-aortic lymph node sampling is done
- If gross metastatic disease is present, it should be excised if feasible, or at least biopsied to document disease extent
- If widely spread tumor is encountered at initial surgery, perform a **cytoreductive surgery** where, as much of tumor should be removed as is technically feasible and safe. Even with extensive metastatic disease, it is possible to perform a fertility sparing procedure with preservation of a normal contralateral ovary

Adjuvant Therapy

- Germ cell tumors are extremely chemosensitive
- **Patients with stage IA dysgerminomas do not need adjuvant therapy**
- **For all other stages, adjuvant therapy with platinum-based combination chemotherapy is given.** Cure rate approaches 95%
- **Different chemotherapeutic agents are used either single or in combination for 3-4 cycles**

Single agent chemotherapy

- **Carboplatin** single agent therapy is used when the tumor has been removed completely

Combination chemotherapy regimens commonly used are as follows (Table 6.3)

- BEP (Bleomycin, Etoposide and Cisplatin)
- VBP (Vinblastin, Bleomycin and Cisplatin)
- VAC (Vincristine, Actinomycin and Cyclophosphamide)
  - Combination chemotherapy has significantly improved the survival rate following conservative surgery in germ cell tumors
  - Menstrual function, fertility and other endocrine functions have been found to be normal following use of these drugs
- Patient with Y chromosome as detected on karyotyping should have both the ovaries (gonads) removed

Table 6.3: Recommended Drugs and Doses for Chemotherapy in Germ cell tumors

Regimens and Drugs	Dosage and Schedule[a]
BEP	
Bleomycin	15 U/m²/week × 5; then on day 1 of course 4
Etoposide	100 mg/m²/d × 5 days every 3 week
Cisplatin	20 mg/m²/d × 5 days, or 100 mg/m²/d × 1 day every 3 weeks
VBP	
Vinblastine	0.15 mg/kg on days 1 and 2 every 3 weeks
Bleomycin	15 U/m²/week × 5; then on day 1 of course 4
Cisplatin	100 mg/m² on day 1 every 3 weeks
VAC	
Vincristine	1–15 mg/m² on day 1 every 4 weeks
Actinomycin D	0.5 mg × 5 days every 4 weeks
Cytoxan	150 mg/m²/d × 5 days every 4 weeks

a. All doses given intra-venously

RADIOTHERAPY: Dysgerminoma are highly radiosensitive but RT is not used in young patients due to loss of fertility

Recurrent Disease

- Treated either with combination chemotherapy or radiotherapy
- **POMB-ACE regimen** (Vincristine, bleomycin, methotrexate, cisplatin, etoposide, actinomycin D and cyclophosphamide) is the preferred combination chemotherapy for recurrence (Table 6.4)
- Radiotherapy is considered for patients treated with combination chemotherapy earlier

Table 6.4: POMB-ACE regimen for GCT	
POMB	
Day 1	Vincrinstine 1 mg/m² IV; methotrexate 300 mg/m² as a 12-hours infusion
Day2	Bleomycin 15 mg by 24-hours infusion; folinic acid rescue started 24 hours after the start of methotrexate in a dose of 15 mg every 12 hours for 4 doses
Day 3	Bleomycin 15 mg by 24 hours infusion
Day 4	Cisplatin 120 mg/m² as a 12-hours infusion, given together with hydration and 3 mg magnesium sulfate supplementation
ACE	
Days 1-5	Etoposide 100 mg/m², day 1 to 5
Days 3-5	Actinomycin D 0.5 mg IV, days 3, 4 and 5
Day 5	Cyclophosphamide 500 mg/m² IV, day 5
OMB	
Day 1	Vincristine 1 mg/m² IV; methotrexate 300 mg/m² as a 12-hours infusion
Day 2	Bleomycin 15 mg by 24-hours infusion, folinic acid rescue started at 24-hours
Day 3	Bleomycin 15 mg by 24-hours infusion

SURVIVAL RATE: Germ cell tumors have very good prognosis. Survival rate in dysgerminoma is as follows:

Stage I	**95%**
Stages II–IV	**85%**

IMMATURE TERATOMA

- Immature teratomas are derived from 3 germ layers–ectoderm, mesoderm and endoderm
- It is a rare tumor and constitutes<1% of ovarian teratomas
- It is common in women at 10 - 20 years of age and rarely seen after menopause
- Immature teratomas are almost often unilateral
- **Pathology:** Varying grades of undifferentiated tissue elements are present
- **Prognosis depends on the quantity of immature neural tissue elements**
- Prognosis depends mainly on **the tumor grade and stage of the disease. Serum AFP levels may be raised**
- Mature teratoma has excellent prognosis

Treatment

- **Unilateral oophorectomy with surgical staging** is the optimum treatment when the tumor is confined to one ovary
- **Elderly women in whom fertility is not desired-Hysterectomy with bilateral salpingo-oophorectomy is done**
- **Except stage Ia G1 immature teratoma, all other patients require adjuvant chemotherapy**
- **BEP or VAC regimen** is the preferred chemotherapy regimen

Survival rate

Stage I	**90%**
Stages II–IV	**75%**

ENDODERMAL SINUS TUMOR (YOLK SAC TUMOR)

- These tumors arise from the **primitive yolk sac**
- It occurs mostly between **15 and 20 years of age.**
- It accounts for **20% malignant germ cell tumor of the ovary (second most common malignant germ cell tumor)**
- Endodermal sinus tumors are 100% **unilateral, solid tumors** and cut section shows gelatinous or hemorrhagic areas

- **Characteristic histological feature is the presence of cystic spaces** lined by flattened epithelium. Within this space, a tuft of vascular tissue termed **Schiller-Duval body** is often seen. Eosinophilic, hyaline bodies containing **alpha-fetoprotein** and other proteins are also seen
- It is composed of **yolk sac endoderm and extra-embryonic mesoblasts**
- **The tumor produces alpha-fetoproteinand alpha 1 antitrypsin**
- It is **highly malignant** and spreads to the adjacent structures rapidly
- **Worst prognosis of all germ cell tumors.** May be associated with dysgerminoma

Treatment

- Surgical staging and unilateral salpingo-oophorectomy is the treatment of choice
- All patients need subsequent chemotherapy
- Different combination regimens (BEP, VBP, VAC and POMB–ACE) are used
- Combinations containing platinum-based compounds are associated with better response and survival
- Alpha feto protein titers are used to monitor regression of tumor and to detect recurrence

EMBRYONAL CARCINOMA

- Occurs in young females. **Median age of patients** with embryonal carcinoma is 15 years
- Most often, tumors are **unilateral** with explosive growth tendencies, leading to large tumor masses and acute abdominal pain
- **Causes precocious puberty in prepubertal girls**
- Tumors secretes both **AFP and hCG**
- Surgery and chemotherapy results in cure for approximately one-third of patients

POLYEMBRYOMA

- Rare cancer usually occurs in women of early reproductive age
- Rarely bilateral.
- **hCG and AFP** are often detectable in the serum of patients and act as tumor marker

NON-GESTATIONAL OVARIAN CHORIOCARCINOMA

- Ovarian choriocarcinoma may be gestational, arising from ovarian pregnancy or metastases from uterine choriocarcinoma
- **Primary Non-gestational ovarian choriocarcinoma is extremely rare. It is most often seen as a component of mixed germ cell tumors of the ovary**
- Most patients **present before 20 years of age**
- May present with **Isosexual precocious puberty**

Pathology

- Gross examination reveals abundant hemorrhage and necrosis
- Microscopic examination-revealsa plexiform pattern composed of both syncytiotrophoblast and cytotrophoblast cells with numerous mitoses
- Choriocarcinoma spreads by blood vessel invasion
- These tumors **secrete hCG** due to the presence of syncytiotrophoblast cells. Used as a marker in diagnosis and follow up
- Choriocarcinoma may stain for cytokeratins, epithelial membrane antigen and carcinoembryonic antigen
- Non gestational choriocarcinoma must be distinguished from gestational choriocarcinoma **because Non gestational choriocarcinoma has worse prognosis and requires aggressive therapy. The identification of paternal genetic material indicates that the tumor is of gestational origin**

Treatment

- Unlike gestational choriocarcinoma, it is **not very sensitive to methotrexate**
- **Surgery is the primary treatment** followed by chemotherapy
- Combination **chemotherapy (VAC, BEP)** is used
- Prognosis is poor

MIXED GERM CELL TUMORS

- Presence of more than one germ cell element (at least two) is considered as **mixed germ cell tumors**
- **Approximately 10% of germ cell tumors are composed of two or more subtypes of cancer.** Dysgerminoma is the most common (70–80%) tissue element
- Treatment and prognosis are based on the more severe element
- Treatment includes complete surgery followed by chemotherapy (VBP, MAC or VAC)

GONADOBLASTOMA

- It is a rare ovarian tumor
- It consists of **germ cells and gonadal stromal cells**
- **Dysgerminoma** is present in 50% of cases
- It is **bilateral in 30%** of cases
- Patients often present with **primary amenorrhea, virilism or genital abnormalities**
- **Occurs in dysgenic ovaries-commonly present in individuals with a Y chromosome or fragment such as mosaic genotype (46 X/46 XY) or testicular feminization (46 XY with androgen insensitivity)**
- **Treatment**–surgical removal of the tumor **and the contralateral ovary (as bilateral in 30% cases)**
- Prognosis is excellent

Flowchart 6.2: Summary of management of Germ Cell Tumors

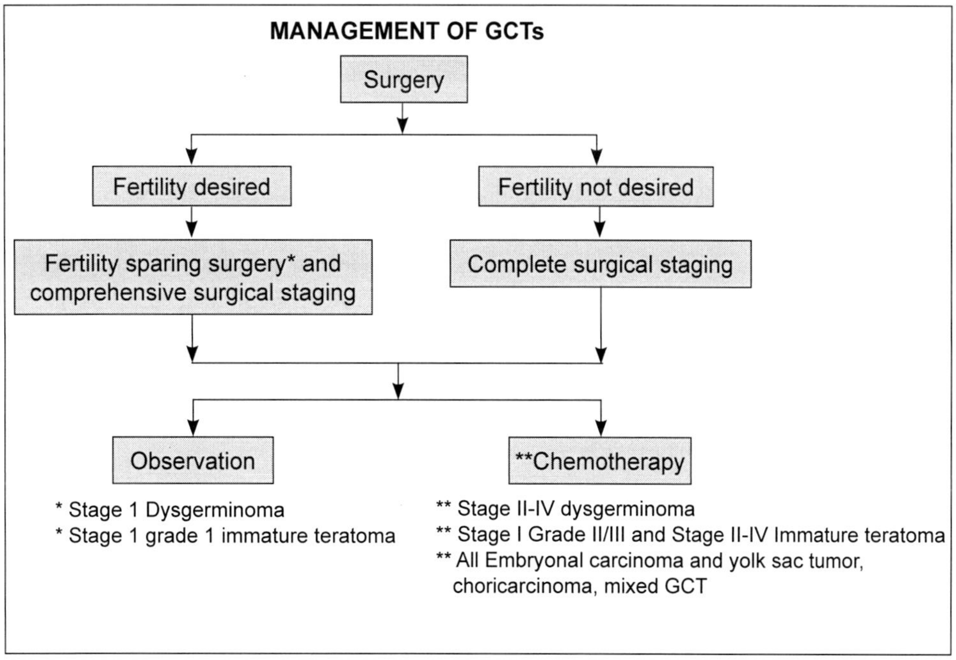

SEX CORD STROMAL TUMORS

- Sex cord stromal tumors constitute 6–10% of all ovarian neoplasms
- ***Most common age group involved-Perimenopausal women***

- Usually **unilateral**
- Confined to ovary for a long period
- **Diagnosed at an early stage**
- 15–30% of these tumors produce hormones, hence known as ***'functioning tumors'***
- Sex cord stromal tumors includes the following:

A.	Granulosa stromal cell tumors
	1. Granulosa cell tumor 2. Tumors in the thecoma-fibroma group a. Thecoma b. Fibroma c. Unclassified
B.	Androblastomas: Sertoli-Leydig cell tumors
	1. Well differentiated a. Sertoli cell tumor b. Sertoli-Leydig cell tumor c. Leydig cell tumor; hilus cell tumor 2. Moderately differentiated 3. Poorly differentiated (sarcomatoid) 4. With heterologous elements
C.	Gynandroblastoma
D.	Unclassified

GRANULOSA CELL TUMORS

- Granulosa cell tumors constitute 2% of all ovarian neoplasms
- The tumor originates from the 'rests' of primitive granulosa cells that are unused in folliculogenesis
- **It is the commonest ovarian stromal tumor**
- It occurs in all ages, 10% prior to puberty, 40% during childbearing period and 50% in postmenopausal women
- It is unilateral in 98% of cases and bilateral only in 2% of cases
- It is a slow growing tumor
- **Gross appearance**–The size varies and the consistency may be solid or cystic. **Cut section** is **characteristically yellow or orange due to its lipid content**
- **Microscopic appearance**–The cells are round or polygonal with granular eosinophilic cytoplasm and ill-defined borders. The tumor cell nuclei are pale, usually grooved or folded and are termed **"Coffee bean" nuclei**
- The large polyhedral lipid cells are arranged in a number of architectural pattern, commonly in folliculoid type, in which granulosa cells are arranged in small clusters around a central cavity termed **Call-Exner bodies that are pathognomonic of granulosa cell tumor**
- The tumor cells **secrete inhibin** which is a **marker for the tumor**
- The tumor produces estrogen and hence may be **associated with endometrial hyperplasia (50%) and endometrial carcinoma in 5–10% of cases**

Clinical Features

- The tumor produces **effects caused by hyperestrogenism which differs with ages**
  - Prior to puberty: Precocious puberty
  - Childbearing period: Abnormal uterine bleeding
  - Postmenopausal: Post menopausal Bleeding
- May present with **acute abdomen** as these tumors have the propensity to rupture

Treatment

- Laparotomy and surgical staging is done
- **Reproductive age/Before puberty-Unilateral salpingo-oophorectomy**
- **Post menopausal-TAH + BSO**
- **Not very sensitive to chemotherapy and radiotherapy**
- The features of precocious puberty revert back to normal after removal of the tumor
- Overall prognosis is good
- Metastatic disease and recurrences are treated with BEP chemotherapy regimen
- **Life time follow up is essential as recurrence can occur as late as 30 years after treatment**

JUVENILE GRANULOSA CELL TUMORS

- Occur in premenarchal girls
- Induces abnormal bleeding and breast development
- Juvenile tumor has less number of Call-Exner bodies and "Coffee bean" nuclei compared to the adult variety
- Early–stage disease is curable with surgery
- Prognosis for disease spread beyond ovary is poor

THECOMA

- The coma predominantly occurs in **postmenopausal age group**
- It is mostly benign
- It may occur as a distinct entity or **mixed with granulosa cell tumor**
- **Gross appearance**–External appearance looks like a fibroma. Cut surface shows islands of yellow tissue separated by grey fibrous septa
- **Microscopic examination**–reveals cells like that of cortical stroma with areas of granulosa cells
- **Estrogen producing tumor**–Due to excess estrogen production, associated with **endometrial hyperplasia and endometrial carcinoma**
- **Clinical features**–It presents with postmenopausal bleeding. Rarely it may cause ascites and cause Pseudo Meig's syndrome
- **Treatment**
  - Post menopausal women–Total hysterectomy with bilateral salpingo-oophorectomy
  - In younger age group–conservative surgery may be done as it mostly benign

FIBROMA

- Usually occurs in the **postmenopausal women**
- It is derived from the stromal cells and are similar to thecomas
- Less than 10% are bilateral
- **Meig's syndrome (Ascites, pleural effusion and ovarian fibroma) is seen in about 1% of cases**
- Presence of Call-Exner bodies (micro follicular pattern) are diagnostic

SERTOLI-LEYDIG CELL TUMOR (ANDROBLASTOMA, ARRHENOBLASTOMA)

- Rare tumor of **mesenchymal origin**
- Accounts for <0.5% of all ovarian tumors
- **Also termed as Arrhenoblastoma/Androblastoma**

- **Affects the age group of 10-35 years**
- The tumor produces **predominantly androgens (80%)** and in some cases estrogen
- **Gross appearance**–The tumors are small, usually unilateral (90%) and solid in consistency. Cut surface shows yellowish tinge with areas of hemorrhage and necrosis
- **Microscopic examination**–resembles various testicular cells such as Sertoliand Leydig cells
- **Clinical features:** The androgens produced by the tumor initially leads to **defeminization**–atrophy of the breasts and uterus and amenorrhea, followed by **masculinization (50%)**–hirsutism, acne, receding hairline, clitoromegaly and deepening of the voice
- Serum testosterone level is elevated
- **Treatment** is surgical removal of the tumor
  - Younger age group–Unilateral oophorectomy is optimum
  - Older women–Total hysterectomy with bilateralsalpingo-oophorectomy is performed
- Removal of the tumor results in rapid resolution of most hormonal effects except deepening of voice and clitoromegaly
- **Prognosis is based on the extent of differentiation. Adjuvant therapy** is needed for poorly differentiated tumor
- Combination chemotherapy (VAC or VBP) is given for recurrent disease

LEYDIG CELL TUMOR/ HILUS CELL TUMOR

- Rare, derived from Hilar cells of ovary
- Almost always unilateral and benign tumor
- **Clinical features**–virilization, elevated 17-ketosteroid excretion and unresponsive to cortisol suppression
- **Microscopic examination**–large lipid laden cells with distinct borders; **Reinke's crystals are common**

GYNANDROBLASTOMA

- This is a very rare type of tumor
- It contains both granulosa cell (estrogenic) and Sertoli-Leydig cell (androgenic) components
- Usually it has got a benign course
- Treatment–Surgical removal is the optimal treatment

METASTATIC TUMORS

- About 5-6% of ovarian tumors are metastatic from other organs, most frequently from tumors of the female genital tract, breast, or the gastrointestinal tract
- The metastasis may occur from direct extension of another pelvic neoplasm, by hematogenous spread, lymphatic, or by transcoelomic spread
- Prior to exploration of an adnexal tumor in a woman > 40 years, a barium enema is indicated to exclude a primary gastrointestinal carcinoma with metastases to the ovaries
- Metastatic colon cancer can mimic a mucinous cystadenocarcinoma of the ovary
- Tubal carcinomas involve the ovaries usually by direct extension. Sometimes, it is difficult to ascertain whether the tumor originates in the tube or in the ovary when both are involved
- Cervical cancer spreads to the ovary only in rare cases (less than 1%), and most of these are of advanced clinical stage or of adenocarcinoma histotype
- Adenocarcinoma of the endometrium can spread directly to the ovaries in 5% cases, but two synchronous primaries, usually an endometrioid carcinoma of the ovary associated with the adenocarcinoma of the endometrium can occur
- Malignant melanoma rarely can metastasize to the ovaries
- Metastatic breast carcinoma to the ovaries occur in about 25% cases

KRUKENBERG TUMOR

- Accounts for **30–40% of metastatic cancer to the ovary**
- Arises in the ovarian stroma and has **characteristic mucin-filled signet ring cells**
- **Primary is most frequently located in stomach** and less commonly in colon, breast, or biliary tract
- **Usually bilateral**
- Ovaries **are enlarged and have a smooth surface**
- **Shape of the ovary is maintained**
- **No tendency of adhesion and capsule remains intact**
- Cut surface shows **waxy consistency** with cystic spaces due to degeneration
- The lesions may not be discovered until the primary disease is advanced, and **hence survival is poor.** In some cases, a primary tumor is not found

NOTE: In other cases of metastasis from the gastrointestinal tract to the ovary, the tumor does not have the classic histologic appearance of Krukenberg tumor

Features differentiating **Krukenberg's tumor and other metastatic tumors to the ovary are mentioned in Table 6.5**

Table 6.5: Differentiating Features Between Krukenberg's Tumor and Other Metastatic Tumorsto Ovary

Metastatic Tumors to Ovary	Krukenberg Tumor
Metastatic tumorsfrom intestine, Gall bladder, pancreas, uterus and cervix	Metastatic tumorsfrom stomach, large bowel and breast
Most commonly bilateral	Always bilateral
Irregular surface	Smooth surface
Spreads by surface/retrograde implantation	Always arise by retrograde lymphatic spread

Extra Edge

Specific histopathology cell types in ovarian tumor

- **Papillary cystadenoma:** Psammoma bodies
- **Brenner tumor:** Walthard's inclusion bodies
- **Clear cell tumor:** Hobnail cells
- **Granulosa cell tumor:** Call-Exner bodies and coffee bean nuclei
- **Leydig cell tumor:** Reinke crystal
- **Yolk sac tumor:** Schiller-Duval bodies
- **Krukenberg tumor:** Signet ring cells

RECENT UPDATES

- *Correct pathological diagnosis is essential in cases with non epithelial ovarian tumors because of their chemosensitivity and the increasing adoption of fertility-sparing surgery*
- *Diagnosis can be made on conventional histological material. Due to the multiplicity of morphological features, immune histochemical markers and fluorescent in situ hybridisation (FISH) can be used to confirm the diagnosis in difficult cases (Table 6.6)*
- ***SALL4 and OCT4 are widely used; more recently, it has been recognised that SOX2 is expressed in embryonal carcinoma and primitive neuroectodermal tumors of teratomatous origin***
- *An immune panel of* ***inhibin alpha, calretinin and FOXL2, together with FOXL2 mutational analysis is useful to confirm the diagnosis of adult granulosa cell tumors (AGCTs),*** *in morphologically ambiguous cases*
- ***Activin A*** *is another molecule involved in the tumorigenesis of AGCTs is*
- ***Sex cord stromal tumors (SCSTs) is negative for FOXL2 on immunostaining but these tumors usually express inhibin alpha and/or calretinin***
- *Another recent finding about SCST has been the* ***occurrence of DICER1 mutations***

Table 6.6: Immunohistochemistry of Primitive GCTs

	Sall4	OCT 3/4	SOX2
Dys	+	+	–
YST	+	–	–
EC	+	+	+
Dys, dysgerminoma; EC, embryonal carcinoma; GCT germ cell tumor; YST, yolk sac tumor			

Small cell carcinomas of the ovary hypercalcemic type (SCCOHTs)

- *These are the most common form of ovarian undifferentiated carcinomas in women < 40 years*
- *Most common ovarian tumor associated with hypercalcaemia (70%)*
- *This tumor is typically unilateral and should be distinguished from primitive GCTs and granulosa cell tumors (mainly juvenile)*
- *Although its histogenesis is unknown, recent reports suggest that it may represent an ovarian malignant rhabdoid tumor*
- *Recent studies have identified mutations in the SWItch/Sucrose Non-Fermentable (SWI/SNF) chromatin-remodelling gene, SMARCA4 encoding BRG1. These mutations represent a frequent event occurring in 75–100% of SCCOHTs*
- *Germline mutations in SMARCA4 or SMARCB1 were already known to predispose to the development of pediatric tumours, namely atypical teratoid/rhabdoid tumours*
- *SMARCA4 immunohistochemistry is highly sensitive and specific for a diagnosis of SCCOHT [loss of SMARCA4 (BRG1) protein expression] and is useful in the differential diagnosis of poorly differentiated ovarian tumors*
- *Differential diagnosis includes juvenile or adult granulosa tumors, metastatic melanoma, dysgerminoma, Ewing tumor and undifferentiated carcinoma*

Updated Guidelines on Non-Epithelial Ovarian Cancer–Summary of The Recommendation By European Society For Medical Oncology (ESMO) 2018

(Ref: ESMO Clinical Practice Guidelines for diagnosis, treatment and follow-up-*ESMO Guidelines Committee-Annals of Oncology, Oct. 2018)*

Diagnosis and pathology/molecular biology

- *Diagnostic work-up should include pelvic ultrasound, abdomino-pelvic CT scan and chest X-ray and PET scan in selected cases (GCTs) [III, B]*
- *In youngpatients, hCG, AFP, LDH and Inhibin B levels, full blood count, liver and renal function tests should be carried out*
- *In case of suspected gonadoblastomas, a preoperative karyotype should be obtained on all premenarchal girls*
- *Histological second opinion by an expert pathologist should always be considered. Diagnosis can be made on conventional histological material [V, B]*
- *Neoplasms of pure ovarian stroma: in morphologically ambiguous cases, an immune panel of inhibin alpha, calretinin and FOXL2, plus mutational analysis for FOXL2, is useful to confirm AGCTs [V, B]*

Staging and risk assessment

- *A surgical approach can be carried out through open route or, in selected cases, by laparoscopy and robotics approaches, thereby avoiding tumor rupture during surgery*
- *A careful examination of the abdominal cavity is required*
- *The staging procedure includes infracolicomentectomy, biopsy of the diaphragmatic peritoneum, paracolic gutters, pelvic peritoneum and peritonealwashings (macroscopic stage I disease)*
- *Unilateral salpingo-oophorectomy with preservation of the contralateral ovary and the uterus is considered an adequate surgical treatment for patientswith GCTs. This should be considered even in advanced disease because of the sensitivity of the tumor to Chemotherapy [IV, B]*
- *No systematic ovarian biopsy isnecessary when the contralateral ovary is macroscopically normal [III, A]*
- *Given the very high chemosensitivity of GCTs, potential nodal metastasis should be cured by adjuvant chemotherapyin these patients [III, A]*
- *Nodal dissection should be carried out only if evidence of nodal abnormality [III, A]*
- *For SCSTs, retroperitoneal evaluation is not mandatory [III, A]*
- *An endometrial curettage must be carried out to rule out concomitant uterine cancers in patients with granulosa cell tumors [IV, B]*
- *Conservative surgery is also an acceptable approach in young patients with stage I SCSTs [IV, B]*

Contd.

Contd.

- *In postmenopausal women and patients with advanced-stage disease or with bilateral ovarian involvement, abdominal hysterectomy and bilateralsalpingo-oophorectomy should be carried out with careful surgical staging for SCST [III, A]*

Early-stage GCTs: management

- *Stage IA pure dysgerminoma should be treated with surgery only [III, A]*
- *Patients with stage IA grade 1 immature teratoma do not require further adjuvant ChT after adequate surgical staging [III, A]*
- *Adjuvant ChT in stage IA-IC G2-G3 immature teratoma, stage IA-IB YST with negative postoperative tumor markers and IB-IC dysgerminomas is recommended but active surveillance is an option [III, B]*
- *5-day BEP is the most used regimen [III, A]*
- *The close surveillance schedule involves regular clinical review with clinical examination, radiological imaging including abdomen-pelvic vaginalsonography at regular intervals and the monitoring of tumor markers to detect relapse over a period of 10 years, with a gradual increase of the interval between clinical appointments [III, C]*

Advanced-stage and recurrent GCTs: management

- *Fertility-sparing surgery should be considered also in advanced stages [IV, B]. The aim of surgery is to remove as much gross tumor as possible; however,the procedure should be moderated to avoid delays in postoperative ChT and long-term morbidity*
- *In postmenopausal women with advanced-stage disease or with bilateral ovarian involvement, abdominal hysterectomy and bilateral salpingo-oophorectomy could be carried out with careful surgical staging [III, A]*
- *Platinum-based regimens are the treatment of choice with the BEP regimen being the most widely used, generally, three cycles of 5-day BEP regimen incompletely resected disease and four cycles (bleomycin should be omitted to reduce the risk of lung toxicity after the third cycle) for patients with macroscopic residual disease [III, A]*
- *In patients previously treated with platinum, with platinum-sensitive relapse (progression > 4–6 weeks after completion of ChT), combinations withplatinum should be considered [IV, C]*
- *Patients resistant to a cisplatin-based combination may receive VAC or paclitaxel/gemcitabine or gemcitabine/oxaliplatin as salvage therapy [IV, C]*
- *HDCT for recurrent ovarian GCTs may result in durable and prolonged remissions [IV, C]*
- *Any resectable residual disease should be removed, particularly for patients with normal serum marker and for patients with immature teratoma in orderto avoid the growing teratoma syndrome [III, A]*

Early-stage SCSTs: management

- *Stage IA granulosa cell tumor disease has an excellent prognosis after surgery alone and does not require adjuvant therapy [III, A]*
- *Adjuvant therapy should be considered for juvenile granulosa tumor stage IC patients [IV, B] or for AGCT stage IC2-IC3 patients [IV, C]. In these cases, platinum-based ChT is the treatment of choice [III, A]*
- *For SLCTs, postoperative adjuvant ChT should be considered for patients with stage I poorly differentiated or heterologous elements (mesenchymal type)[IV, B]*
- *BEP is the most commonly used regimen [III, A]. Alternative ChT options include paclitaxel and carboplatin [III, B], EP, CAP or platinum agent alone [III, A]*

Advanced-stage and recurrent SCSTs: management

- *Debulking surgery remains the most effective treatment of advanced or recurrent granulosa cell tumor [III, A]*
- *Platinum-based ChT is currently used for patients with advanced-stage SCSTs or recurrent disease [III, A]*
- *BEP regimen for three cycles or six cycles of carboplatin/paclitaxel is recommended for postoperative ChT and patients with recurrent SCSTs [III, A]*
- *Patients with steroid cell tumors that are pleomorphic, large, at an advanced stage or with an increased mitotic count should be treated with additional postoperative platinum-based ChT, either BEP (if not previously used) or a taxane–platinum combination [IV, C]*
- *Response to GnRH agonists, tamoxifen, progestin and AIs has been reported and could be an interesting option specifically for adult GCT [IV, B]*

For patients with persistent SLCTs, adjuvant ChT should be considered [III, B]

- *Early and advanced SCCOHT: management*
- *All suspected cases should benefit from a review by an expert pathologist and be discussed in a specialised tumor board [V, A]*
- *Optimal treatment: a multimodal approach including ChT [III, B], radical surgery [IV, A], HDCT [II, C] and RT [IV, C]*
- *Debulking surgery (initial or interval) remains the most effective treatment [IV, A]*
- *Combination of a cisplatin–and etoposide-based therapy is the most appropriate for all stages [III, B]*

Contd.

Contd.

- *The use of pelvic RT, either concurrently or sequentially to HDCT and ASCT, may be considered for patients after surgery [IV, C]*
- *Efforts should be made to treat patients in a more homogeneous way through national and international networks [V, A]*
- *Response evaluation and follow-up after initial treatment*
- *Serum tumor markers (hCG, a-FP, LDH, CA 125 and inhibin B) can correlate with tumor response during ChT [V, A]*
- *A CT scan of the abdomen, pelvis and chest (in case of suspected lung metastases) and pelvic ultrasound are the most common and useful imaging techniques to evaluate the response to ChT [V, A]*
- *For GCT, follow-up visits must include history, physical examination with pelvic examination and tumor markers every 3 months for the first 2 years,then every 6 months during the third year and then yearly until progression [V, A]*
- *For SCSTs, follow-up visits including physical exam and tumor markers must be carried out every 6 months starting from the third year and this frequency should be maintained indefinitely [V, B]*
- *A pelvic ultrasound should be carried out every 6 months in those patients who have undergone fertility-sparing surgery, whereas a CT scan of theabdomen and pelvis is carried out according to clinical indication*
- *PET scan for tumor response evaluation or follow-up is not yet recommended [V, D]*

Fertility and hormone replacement

- *Oocyte cryopreservation is an option for patients scheduled to receive ChT [V, C]*
- *Hyperstimulation followed by oocyte cryopreservation 12 months after the end of ChT is another option [V, C]*
- *Fertility preservation should not jeopardise the oncological management*
- *HRT may be used safely for many GCTs [V, A]*
- *An HRT approach should be avoided for SCST [V, D]*

α-FP, alpha foetoprotein; AGCT, adult granulosa cell tumor; AI, aromatase inhibitor; ASCT, autologous stem cell transplantation; BEP, bleomycin/etoposide/cisplatin; CA 125, cancer antigen 125; CAP, cyclophosphamide/doxorubicin/cisplatin; ChT, chemotherapy; CT, computed tomography; EP, etoposide/cisplatin

GCT, germ cell tumor; GnRH, gonadotropin-releasing hormone; hCG, human chorionic gonadotropin; HDCT, high-dose chemotherapy; HRT, hormone replacement therapy; LDH, lactate dehydrogenase; PET, positron emission tomography; RT, radiotherapy; SCCOHT, small cell carcinoma of the ovary hypercalcemic type; SCST, sex cord-stromal tumor; SLCT, Sertoli-Leydig cell tumor; VAC, vincristine/actinomycin D/ cyclophosphamide; YST, yolk sac tumor

Table of levels of evidence and grades of recommendation (adapted from the Infectious Diseases Society of America-United States Public Health Service Grading System) (Table 6.7, 6.8)

Table 6.7: Levels of evidence

I	*Evidence from at least one large randomised, controlled trial of good methodological quality (low potential for bias) or meta-analyses of well-conducted randomised trials without heterogeneity*
II	*Small randomised trials or large randomised trials with a suspicion of bias (lower methodological quality) or meta-analyses of such trials or of trials demonstrated heterogeneity*
III	*Prospective cohort studies*
IV	*Retrospective cohort studies or case–control studies*
V	*Studies without control group, case reports, expert opinions*

Table 6.8: Grades of recommendation

A	*Strong evidence for efficacy with a substantial clinical benefit, strongly recommended*
B	*Strong or moderate evidence for efficacy but with a limited clinical benefit, generally recommended*
C	*Insufficient evidence for efficacy or benefit does not outweigh the risk or the disadvantages (adverse events, costs, ...), optional*
D	*Moderate evidence against efficacy or for adverse outcome, generally not recommended*
E	*Strong evidence against efficacy or for adverse outcome, never recommended*

IMMUNO HISTOCHEMISTRY (IHC) OF OVARIAN TUMORS

Epithelial Ovarian Tumors

1. **Serous ovarian carcinoma-Low grade (LGSC)**
   - *P53 imunostaining-wild type nuclear positivity*

- *WT1-nuclear statining*
- *ER, PR-nuclear staining*
- *CK7, CA 125- cytoplasmic staining*
- *EMA-membranous staining*
- *CK20, Calretinin-negative*

2. **High Grade Serous Carcinoma of Ovary (HSGC)**
   - *P53-aberrant nuclear immunostaining positivity*
   - *WT-1-nuclear staining*
   - *CAM5.2, CK7- cytoplasmic staining*
   - *EMA-membranous staining*
   - *ER-alpha–Majority are positive*
   - *BRCA 1 and P16-cytoplasmic staining-majority positive*
   - *Inhibin, p63, h-caldesmon, thrombomodulin-negative*
3. **Primary Mucinous ovarian carcinoma**
   - *CK7-diffuse cytoplasmic expression*
   - *CK20-variable expression-majority being patchy positive*
   - *P16, ER, PR, CDX2-negative*
   - *LGALS4(galectin 40)-increased expression*
4. **Seromucinous Ovarian Tumor**
   - *CK7, CA125, ER, PR, Mesothelin-positive*
   - *CK20, CDX2, WT1-Negative*
   - *BAF250a(ARID1a) expression- lost*
5. **Endometrioid Carcinoma**
   - *CK7, PAX8, PAX-2-positive*
   - *EMA-positive*
   - *ER, PR-nuclear staining*
   - *BRCA1- usually positive*
   - *HNF1beta-NUCLEAR POSITIVE-50% cases*
   - *BAF250a(ARID1a) expression –retained*
   - *WT1, p16, Napsin A-negative*
   - *CDX2, CK20, SATB2-negative (to diff from metastatic colonic adenocarcinoma)*

   MLH1, MSH2, MSH6, PMS2 proteins-anyone shows negative in Lynch syndrome associated MSI-high endometrioid carcinoma
6. **Clear Cell Carcinoma**
   - *CK7, CAM5.2, EMA, LeuM1, B72.3, 34beta E12, mesothelin-positive*
   - *HNF1beta, Napsin A, AMACR, OC125-positive*
   - *P53-wild type nuclear staining*
   - *BAF250a (ARID 1a) expression-lost*
   - *ER, PR, CK10, CK20, AFP-negative*
   - *CD10, RCCma-negative (to differentiated from RCC)*

7. **Benign And Malignant Brenner Tumor:**
   - *CK7, EMA, GATA3, CEA, CA 19-9-Positive*
   - *Urothelin markers-uroplakin III luminal pattern positive and thrombomodulin is strong membranous staining*
   - *P53-wild type immunostaining*
   - *CK20, WT1, PAX8, PAX 2, SALL4, P16, ER, PR, Calretinin-negative*
8. **Undifferentiated Carcinoma**
   - *EMA, CAM5.2, B72.3, CK7-positive*
   - *CK20-negative*

Sex Cord Stromal Tumors

1. **Granulosa Cell Tumor**
   - *Inhibin, Calretinin-Positive*
   - *New sexcord markers- FOXL2 (marker of granulosa cell), SF-1, CD56-positive*
   - *Estradiol, vimentin, CD99, Follicle regulatory protein-positive*
   - *EMA-negative*
   - *Reticulin special stain surround tumour cell nests*
2. **Sertoli Cell Tumor And Sex cord Tumor with Annular Tubules**
   - *Testosterone, inhibin, calretinin-positive*
   - *Sex cord markers–positive*
   - *SOX9-marker of sertoli cell-positive*
3. **Fibroma**
   - *WT1, CD56, FOXL2, SF-1-Positive*
   - *Inhibin, calretinin-negative*
4. **Thecoma**
   - *Sexcord markers-positive*
5. **Sclerosing Stromal Tumor**
   - *Sexcord markers-positive*
   - *Smoothmuscle actin, desmin, ligandin-positive*
6. **Signet Ring Stromal Tumor**
   - *Sexcord markers-positive*
   - *Focal cytokeratin-positive*
   - *EMA-negative*
7. **Microcystic Stromal Tumor**
   - *FOXL2, SF-1, WT-1-Positive*
   - *Nuclear beta catenin, CD10, vimentin-positive, uniform expression*
   - *Inhibin, calretinin, CD56-negative*
   - *Betacatenin gene CTNNB1 mutation*
8. **Steroid Cell/Lipid Cell Tumor**
   - *Inhibin, calretini, SF-1 and Melan A–positive*
   - *FOXL2,WT-1–negative*
9. **Gynandroblastoma**
   - FOXL2, DICER1 mutation-present

10. Primary Small Cell Carcinoma of Ovary, Hypercalcemic Type

- *SMARCA4 Protein expression lost due to mutation in same gene*

Germ Cell Tumours of Ovary

1. Dysgerminoma

- *SALL4-primitive germcell marker-positive*
- *PLAP–membranous positivity*
- *CD117(c-kit), D2-40(podoplanin), OCT 4 (nuclear staining), NANOG-positive*

2. Yolk Sac Tumour (Primitive Endodermal Tumor)

- *AFP, Glypican-3, SALL4, HNF-1-positive*
- *CK7, EMA, Napsin A, AMACR-negative*
- *Differentiated pattern markers-TTF-1, CDX2, HepPAR1, GATA3*

3. Embryonal Carcinoma

- *OCT-4, NANOG, CD30, Cytokeratin-positive*
- *CD117, D2-40-negative*
- *EMA-Negative*
- *Chromosome 12p abnormalities-present*

4. Polyembryoma

- *Embryoid bodies*
- *AFP-yolk sac cell positive*
- *hCG-in syncytiotrophoblasts*
- *CD30, OCT 4 in embryonic disk-positive*

5. Choriocarcinoma

- *Beta hCG-positive*

6. Immature Teratoma

- *SOX2, SALL4-Immature neuroepithelium*
- *OCT4 in higher grade immature teratoma*

7. Struma Ovarii

- TTF-1, Thyroglobulin positive

8. Carcinoid Tumor of Ovary

- *Synaptophysin, chromogranin-strong and diffuse positive*
- *pancytokeratin, low molecular weight cytokeratin (CK8/CK18)-positive*
- *EMA, CK7, ER, PR-negative*
- *Inhibin, calretinin-negative*

Gonadoblatoma

- *Sexcord tumour cells-inhibin, FOXL2, SF-1, SOX9- positive*
- *Germcell tumour-CD117, SALL4, OCT4-positive*

Metastatic Tumours of Ovary

1. Metastatic Colonic Adenocarcinoma

- *CDX2, CK20, SATB2-POSITIVE*

- *CK7, PAX8, ER-negative*
- *SATB2-positive in ovarian mucinous carcinoma of teratomatous origin*

2. **Metastatic Pancreatic Adenocarcinoma**
   - *Mesothelin, fascin, prostate stem cell antigen-positive pancreatic markers*
   - *Lack of reactivity for Dpc4-pancreatic adenoca*
   - *CK7, CK20, CDX2-not useful*
3. **Metastatic Breast Ca**
   - *GATA-3-highly sensitive, positive*
   - *GCDFP-15-positive*
4. **Metastatic Renal Cell Carcinoma**
   - *CD10, Renal cell carcinoma marker (RCCma), PAX8-positive*
   - *CK7, Mesothelin-negative*
5. **Metastatic Bladder Transitional Cell Carcinoma**
   - *Urothelin, Thrombomodulin, CK20-Positive*
   - *WT-1-Negative (Opposite immunoprofile in primary transitional cell carcinoma of ovary)*
6. **Metastatic Malignant Melanoma of Ovary**
   - *S-100, HMB-45, Melan-A, SOX10, MART-1, MITF-Positive*
7. **Metastatic Lung Carcinoma**
   - *TTF-1, Napsin A, CK7-POSITIVE*
   - *CK20 negative*

CHAPTER 7

FALLOPIAN TUBE CANCER

INTRODUCTION

- Primary carcinoma of fallopian tube is **a rare malignancy of the female genital tract**
- Incidence is **< 0.5% of all gynecological malignancies**
- Most commonly affected age group is **50-60 years**
- More common among **white women**

Note
• *Current Concept is that, the papillary serous tumors of the ovary may arise from epithelial lining of the fallopian tube fimbria*

FALLOPIAN TUBE CARCINOMA

Predisposing Factors

- Infertility
- Nulliparity, early menarche, and late menopause
- Family H/o ovarian cancer
- Women with BRCA1 or BRCA2 mutations

Protective Factors

- Oral contraceptive pill usage
- Multiparity
- Breastfeeding
- Tubal ligation

Hereditary Fallopian Tube Cancer

- Lifetime risk of fallopian tubal cancer **in BRCA mutation carriers is 0.6 - 3%**
- **BRCA1 > BRCA2 in association with tubal cancer**
- Precancerous changes of fallopian tube without the presence of cancer, have been noted with increased frequency in high-risk women

Pathology

- Common site–**Distal portion of the tube**
- Most frequent site of origin is the **ampulla of fallopian tube,** followed by the infundibulum.
- Mucosa is commonly affected.
- The fimbrial end usually gets blocked resulting in hydrosalpinx or hematosalpinx
- It is mostly **unilateral (80%)**
- Tumor is bilateral in one-third of cases

- Most common type is **papillary serous adenocarcinoma** arising from within the lumen of the tube **in 90%**
- Tubal walls are so thin that they are rapidly invaded and the growth encroaches on the peritoneal cavity either directly or by sprouting through abdominal ostium.

Spread

- More than 50% cases present with Stage I or II disease
- In contrast to patients with ovarian cancer, the majority of patients with tubal cancers are diagnosed when disease is confined to tubes and pelvic structures.
- Most common mode of spread is direct spread, followed by lymphatic spread to regional lymph nodes (paraaortic nodes). Blood borne spread to distant organs can occur in late stages
- **Peritoneum is the most frequent site of metastatic spread**
- Higher propensity for retroperitoneal lymph node spread
- Suburethral vaginal metastases represent venous embolism either directly from tubes or via uterus

Clinical Features

- Usually occurs in nulliparous post-menopausal women
- May be asymptomatic
- May present with Postmenopausal bleeding.
- **Hydrops tubae profluens–characterized by colicky lower abdominal pain relieved by intermittent profuse watery vaginal discharge, occurs in few cases**
- Colicky lower abdominal pain–Tubal distention produces more intense pain than those reported in ovarian cancer
- Bimanual examination reveals a unilateral mass which may be tender.
- On compression of the adnexal mass, if it reduces in size, along with passage of watery discharge through the cervix, it is suspicious of fallopian tube cancer.

Triad of Fallopian Tube Cancer

- Watery vaginal discharge-**hydrops tubae profulens**
- Pelvic pain
- Pelvic mass

Diagnosis

- Most often diagnosed accidentally on laparotomy and histologic examination of the excised tube.
- **Suspected features** are:
  - Persistent postmenopausal bleeding without any uterine pathology (Endometrial sampling and hysteroscopic examination are negative)
  - Persistent positive Papanicolaou smear with a negative cervical and endometrial pathology
- **Ultrasound–A fluid filled sausage shaped mass** separate from the uterus and ovary is seen. Ascites may be present
- **Laparoscopy** done in cases of persistent postmenopausal bleeding with a negative uterine pathology
  - May reveal an adnexal mass that resembles pyosalpinx or tubercular lesion
  - When the tumor is confined to mucosa, the tube is generally soft on palpation, and the initial impression is often hematosalpinx, pyosalpinx, or hydrosalpinx
- **Doppler flow velocity** shows low-resistance blood flow
- **Serum level of CA-125 is raised** in 85% cases of **adenocarcinoma**

Classification

Hu pathologic criteria to aid in the distinction of the primary Fallopian tube cancer:

On gross inspection:

- The main tumor is in the fallopian tube
- On microscopic inspection, the mucosa is involved and shows a papillary pattern
- If the tubal wall is involved extensively, transition between benign and malignant epithelium should be demonstrable

Sedlis modification of Hu criteria of fallopian cancer

- The tumor arises from the endosalpinx
- The histologic pattern reproduces the epithelium of tubal mucosa
- There is transition from benign to malignant epithelium
- Ovary and endometrium are either normal or with a tumor that is smaller than tumor in the tube

NOTE–*Main criterion used to* ***differentiate a primary fallopian tube cancer from metastatic carcinoma*** *in fallopian tube is histologic proven transition between in situ carcinoma and invasive malignancy within fallopian tube epithelium*

STAGING OF FALLOPIAN TUBE CANCER

FIGO staging (2014)

- **The updated, revised FIGO staging system (2014) combines the classification for ovarian, fallopian tube, and peritoneum cancer, based on findings made mainly through surgical exploration** ***(Refer chapter on Epithelial ovarian tumor for FIGO staging system)***
- Erez staging scheme based on the relationship of the tumor to the histologic layers of the tubal wall was used earlier (Table 7.1)

Table 7.1: Erez Classification (used earlier)

Stage I	The tumor is limited to the mucosa and muscle
Stage IIA	The serosa is breached but the tumor has not spread to other organs
Stage IIB	The tumor invades the pelvic organs
Stage III	Metastasis outside the pelvis but within the abdominal cavity
Stage IV	Extra-abdominal metastasis is present. Para-aortic lymph nodes are involved in the advanced stages

Management

- Surgical staging and surgical management of fallopian tube carcinoma is similar to that of epithelial ovarian cancer
- **Procedure**–Total hysterectomy with bilateral salpingo-oophorectomy along with infracolic omentectomy followed by platinum based combination chemotherapy as an adjuvant therapy. In advanced cases, radiotherapy is considered
- **Prophylactic surgery in patients with hereditary predisposition**–Bilateral salpingo-oophorectomy following completion of family

Recent Advances

Occult tubal cancers: SEE-FIM (Sectioning and Extensive examination of fimbrial end) is done to identify occult tubal cancers

Procedure–Fallopian tube are sectioned at 2-3 mm intervals and examined histologically with lengthwise sectioning of fimbrial protion to maximize exposure of tubal plicae.

All cases of **high grade serous carcinoma and Serous tubal intraepithelial carcinoma (STIC)** should be sampled by this method

Prognostic Factors

Five Year survival depends on the following:

- Degree of invasion of the fallopian tube wall
- Location of the tumor within the tube

- Depth of invasion of primary lesion
- Histologic differentiation
- Lymphatic involvement

Survival Rate (Table 7.2)

Table 7.2: Five year survival depending on degree of invasion of tubal wall in fallopian tube cancer

Lesion	5 Year Survival
Intramucosal lesions	90%
Invaded muscular wall	50%
Penetrated tubal serosa	<25%

Table 7.3: Five year survival in fallopian tube cancer

Stage	Survival
Stage I	60%
Stage II	40%
Advanced stage	10%

Follow up

- Patient is Followed-up every 2-4 months for the first 2 years, every 3-6 months for the following 3 years and then annually after 5 years

Secondary fallopian tube carcinoma

- **Metastasis to fallopian tube is more common** (90%) than primary cancer
- **Common primary sites are** ovary, uterus, breast and gastrointestinal tract
- **Mode of spread** from the ovary or uterus is probably by lymphatics rather than a direct one

Other malignancies of fallopian tube

- **Choriocarcinoma:** Choriocarcinoma can occur in the fallopian tube following ectopic pregnancy or tubal hydatidiform mole
- **Sarcoma** can occur as mesodermal mixed tumor

RECENT UPDATES

Genetics Related to Fallopian Tube Cancer

- *Genetics related to fallopian tube cancers are similar to ovarian cancers*
- *Gene mutations include **ERBB-2 (HER-2/neu), TP53 (p53), and K-RAS (K-ras) mutations***
- ***Most frequent Genetic changes detected in fallopian tube carcinoma are gains at 3q (70%) and 8q (75%), with high-level amplifications***
- *Loss of heterozygosity at **13q** has been reported in BRCA-related fallopian tube and ovarian cancers*
- ***Mutation of tumor suppressor gene TP53 is the most frequent genetic abnormality associated with fallopian tube cancer***
- *p53 mutations are also **present in tubal dysplasia** associated with fallopian tube cancer*
- *HER-2/neu has been shown to be overexpressed in >50% of advanced-stage disease, suggesting a role in progression of disease*
- *Benign, normal-appearing tubal mucosal areas with high nuclear staining for p53 are called as **p53 signatures.** However, cells displaying these signatures do not invariably progress to malignancy*
- ***Li-Fraumeni syndrome contains abundant regions with p53 signatures in distal fallopian tube.** But these patients rarely develop fallopian tubal cancer, implicating that additional genetic events are required in addition to p53 over expression to produce a malignant phenotype*
- *Events such as BRCA mutation or reduced expression of cyclin-dependent kinase inhibitor p27 are required to facilitate transit from precursor cells to cancer*

C H A P T E R 8

PREMALIGNANT LESIONS OF VULVA AND VULVAR CARCINOMA

INTRODUCTION

- Vulvar cancer accounts for 3-5% of gynecological malignancy primarily affecting postmenopausal women
- There is no specific screening tool and the most effective strategy to reduce incidence of vulval cancer is the treatment of predisposing and premalignant lesions associated with vulvar cancers
- Vulvar cancer may be asymptomatic; women present with vulvar pruritus, pain, lump or ulcer. Therefore, any suspicious vulvar lesion should be biopsied to exclude cancer
- The most common subtype is squamous cell carcinoma
- Treatment depends primarily on histology and surgical staging. Treatment is predominantly surgical, although concurrent chemoradiation is an effective alternative, particularly for advanced tumors
- Management should be individualized, and carried out by a multidisciplinary team in a cancer center experienced in the treatment of these tumors

Recap of Anatomy of External Genitalia (Figure 8.1)

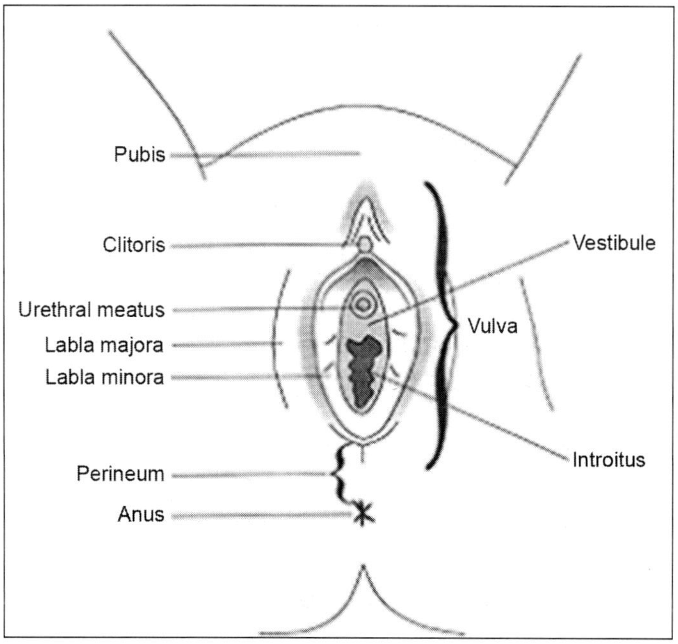

Figure 8.1: Anatomy of external genitalia

Vulva (Pudendum)–[Mons veneris (pubis) + Labia Majora + Labia Minora + Clitoris + Vestibule] + Perineum

- **Mons pubis**–subcutaneous adipose connective tissue lying in front of the pubis
- **Labia Majora**
  - Elevation of skin on either side of vulva; labia majora join posteriorly to form the posterior commissure
  - Composed of **squamous epithelium, apocrine sweat glands (modified sweat glands),** sebaceous glands and hair follicles; Inner surface is hairless (NOTE: **Hydradenoma of vulva arises from apocrine sweat glands**)

- **Homologous to male scrotum**
- **The round ligament terminates at the anterior third of labia majora**

- **Labia Minora**
  - Folds of skin **devoid of fat** lies within the labia majora
  - Do not contain hair follicles
  - **Anteriorly** they unite with each other to enclose the clitoris and form the prepuce (anterior to clitoris) and frenulum (posterior to clitoris)
  - **Posteriorly** they fuse in midline to form **fourchette. Between the fourchette and vaginal orifice is the fossa navicularis**
  - **Homologous to the ventral aspect of penis**
- **Clitoris**
  - Attached to undersurface of the pubis by **Suspensory Ligament**
  - **Homologous to penis in male**
  - **Lymphatics drain into Cloquet's Lymph node/Rosenmuller's Lymph node** in femoral triangle
- **Vestibule**
  - **Triangular space** bounded by clitoris anteriorly, fourchette posteriorly and labia minora laterally
  - It has four major openings–**urethral opening, vaginal opening/hymen, Bartholin's ducts and Skene's ducts (Paraurethral glands)**
- During childbirth the hymen is subjected to lacerations which later form cicatrized nodules termed **Carunculae myrtiformes / hymen tags**

Blood supply of vulva–**Internal pudendal artery and superficial and deep external pudendal arteries**

Nerve supply of vulva–**pudendal nerve, ilioinguinal nerve and genital branch of genitofemoral nerve**

Lymphatic Drainage of Vulva - Table 8.1; Fig 8.2

Table 8.1: Lymphatic Drainage of Vulva

Site	Lymphatic Drainage
L. Majora (anterior half)	Superficial inguinal nodes
L. Majora (posterior half)	Superficial inguinal → deep inguinal → external iliac nodes
L. Minora and prepuce of clitoris	Superficial inguinal nodes
Glans of clitoris	Deep inguinal nodes (Lymph node of Cloquet)
Bartholin's glands	Superficial inguinal and anorectal nodes

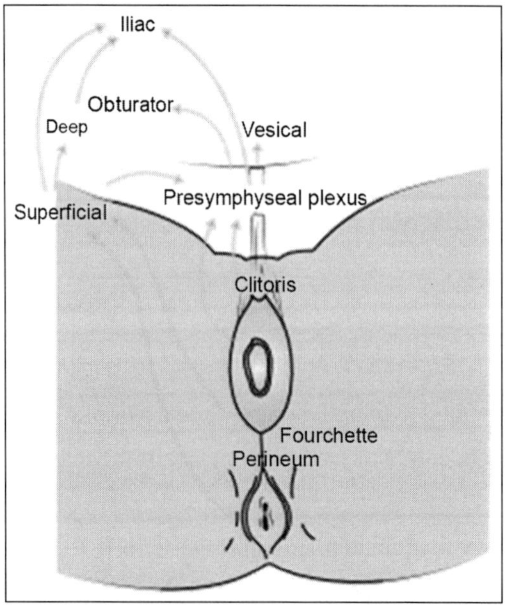

Figure 8.2: Lymphatic drainage of vulva

VULVAR LESIONS (Table 8.2, 8.3)

Table 8.2: Classification of Vulvar Epithelial Disorders

Non neoplastic epithelial disorders	Vulvar Intra epithelial neoplasia (VIN) Neoplastic epithelial disorders
• Lichen sclerosis • Squamous hyperplasia (Hyperplastic dystrophy or Lichen simplex chronicus)	**Squamous Intra epithelial neoplasia** • VIN I, II, III **Non Squamous Intra epithelial neoplasia** • Paget's disease • Non invasive tumor of melanocyte **Invasive tumor**

Table 8.3: Premalignant and Malignant Diseases of The Vulva

Premalignant diseases of the vulva	Vulvar malignancies
• Vulvar intraepithelial neoplasia (VIN)–**most common** • Paget's disease of vulva • Bowen's disease • Erythroplasia of Queyrat • Melanoma in situ	• Squamous cell carcinoma–most common • Melanoma • Adenocarcinoma (Bartholin's gland) • Basal cell carcinoma • Sarcoma • Secondaries (from primary sites in other genital organs)

VULVAR INTRAEPITHELIAL NEOPLASIA

- The term VIN along with grade VIN 1, 2, 3 was adopted from CIN terminology (Table 8.4)
- VIN includes cellular atypia of epithelium **without stromal invasion**

Table 8.4: VIN Grades

VIN–I	VIN–II	VIN–III
Mild cellular atypia	Moderate cellular atypia	Severe cellular atypia or CIS
Loss of maturation limited to lower 1/3rd of epithelium.	Loss of maturation involving lower 2/3rd of epithelium	Loss of maturation of whole thickness of epithelium

International Society for the Study of Vulvovaginal Disease (ISSVD) 2004 Classification of Squamous vulvar intraepithelial neoplasia

Recently, ISSVD classified VIN into a Two–category system (Table 8.5 and Table 8.6)

- Usual type VIN–HPV associated
- Differentiated VIN–not associated with HPV

Table 8.5: Squamous Vulvar Intraepithelial Neoplasia (VIN) Types

VIN usual type	VIN differentiated type
• VIN warty type • VIN basaloid type • VIN mixed type	

Table 8.6: Differentiation Between Two Categories of Squamous Vulvar Intraepithelial Neoplasia

	VIN usual type (Warty- basaloid type)	VIN differentiated type (simplex)
Age	Premenopausal (30-40 years)	Postmenopausal (>65 years)
% of VIN	95%	5%
HPV association	Driven by HPV: HPV 16, 18	Develops independently of HPV
HIV association	Yes	No
Risk factors	Smoking, immunosuppression	Not identified

Contd.

Contd.

Distribution	Multifocal	Unifocal, unicentric
Background histology	–	Lichen sclerosus
Progression to	Warty/basaloid Squamous cell carcinoma	Keratinizing squamous cell carcinoma
Immunohistochemistry findings	p16+, p53-, Ki67+	p16-, p53+, Ki67+
Prognosis	Less aggressive; 90% regress and 10% progress to invasive cancer	More aggressive and more likely to progress to invasive carcinoma

Epidemiology and risk factors for VIN

- Occurs in **30–40 years age group (younger age compared to vulvar carcinoma)**
- **Associated with**
  - **Chronic vulvar irritation**
  - **HPV 16, 18, 31, 35 infection**
  - **HIV infection**
  - **Condylomas**
  - **Vulvar dystrophies**
- **Associated CIN and concomitant neoplasia of genital tract may be present (due to similar exogenous risk factors)**
- **VIN Progression to invasive vulvar carcinoma is < 10% (less than CIN), occurs over a period of 20–30 years (CIN 10–15 years)**
- Unlike cervical cancers where majority are associated with a CIN lesion, only one third of invasive vulvar squamous carcinoma cases have co existing VIN III

Clinical Features

Symptoms

- May be asymptomatic
- Pruritis vulvae (Most common symptom)
- Dysuria, dyspareunia, soreness of vulva
- Burning pain in perineum

Local examination

- **Multifocal lesions are common**
- Raised or verrucous vulvar lesion may be present
- Often misdiagnosed initially
- Application of 5% acetic acid–may reveal acetowhite lesions with punctuation, mosaic pattern and vascular abnormalities

Diagnosis

- Confirmed by biopsy. **Multiple biopsies** are taken after 5% acetic acid or toluidine blue dye application (Monsel's solution (Ferric subsulphate) is used to control profuse bleeding following biopsy)
- Cytologic evaluation should also be done to exclude VAIN and CIN as they may co-exist together
- Cytologic screening for VIN is unreliable and usually not done

Cytology features of atypical cells

- Loss of polarity
- Cellular immaturity
- Nuclear abnormalities
- Increased mitotic activity
- Hyperkeratosis, acanthosis and chronic inflammatory cell infiltration
- Koilocytes may be present

NOTE:

In VIN:

- *Basement membrane is intact*
- *No involvement of the dermis*

Management of VIN (Table 8.7)

- **VIN–low malignant potential, risk of progression to invasive disease is < 10%. Conservative management is acceptable**
- Observe young women with HPV positive VIN lesions for 6 months. Persistent lesions require treatment
- **Medical treatment–preferred in young women**

Table 8.7: Treatment Options For VIN

Medical	Excision	Ablative	Surgery
Local application of dinitrochlorobenzene, **Topical 5-fluorouracil cream**	**Local excision**–Wide local excision with 1 cm margin **Skinning vulvectomy**–for more extensive or diffuse lesions, especially in postmenopausal women	**CO2 laser vaporization**–for multi focal lesions; has better cosmetic results, lower recurrence rate	**Simple vulvectomy** in older women and in Bowen's disease

Long term follow up is needed following treatment–as there is high risk of recurrence

PAGET'S DISEASE OF VULVA

- **A special type of VIN, common in post menopausal women**
- Accounts for 1-5% of vulvar neoplasms.
- **Mostly confined to epithelium. The lesion grows horizontally within the epidermis**
- **Symptoms**–Pruritus, vulvar soreness or bleeding
- **Examination**–Erythematous, raised, velvety, hyperemic, well-demarcated, thick lesions with induration and excoriation
- **Usually HPV negative**
- **Paget's disease may be associated with underlying adenocarcinoma of vulva**–About 5-10% of newly diagnosed Paget lesions are associated with underlying adenocarcinoma arising locally in vulvar vestibular gland or skin appendage **(apocrine gland)** or from a distant site such as the **breast, genito urinary tract or colon BL1> Classification of Paget's disease of vulva (Table 8.8)**

Table 8.8: Classification of Paget's Disease

Primary Paget's disease of the vulva	Secondary Paget's disease of the vulva
a. Intraepithelial Paget's disease	a. Secondary to anorectal adenocarcinoma
b. Intraepithelial Paget's disease with stromal invasion	b. Secondary to urothelial carcinoma
c. As a manifestation of underlying adenocarcinoma of skin appendage or vulvar vestibular gland	c. As a manifestation of another non-cutaneous adenocarcinoma (e.g., endocervical, endometrial, ovarian cancer)

- **Histology-Paget cells in epidermis**–large, oval shaped cells with abundant pale cytoplasm
  - **Two types in histology–Intra epithelial and invasive Paget's disease**

Treatment

- **Intraepithelial Paget's**–Radical Wide local excision
- **Invasive Paget's**–Radical vulvectomy + LN dissection
- **Recurrence is high. Recurrence is** treated with **Laser ablation**

BOWEN'S DISEASE

- It is a rare Intraepithelial vulvar carcinoma
- Most common symptom–Pruritis

- Appears as a slow growing reddish indurated patch
- Histopathology reveals prickle cells invading epidermis, **Giant Cells and Corps Rond (Corps ronds** refer to cells with small pyknotic nuclei, perinuclear halo and eosinophilic cytoplasm) **are characteristic**
- **Associated malignancies of genital tract may be present**
- **Treatment**–Simple vulvectomy

VULVAR DYSTROPHIES–NON NEOPLASTIC EPITHELIAL DISORDERS

Vulvar dystrophies include the following:

- **Atrophic dystrophy–Lichen sclerosis**
- **Hyperplastic dystrophy - Sq. Cell Hyperplasia/Leukoplakia/Lichen Simplex Chronicus/Neurodermatitis**

Lichen Sclerosis

- Occurs in Post menopausal age group
- Symptoms–pruritus (most common), discomfort, dyspareunia, dysuria
- Examination findings
  - Atrophy of vulva-skin is papery thin and atrophic
  - Narrowing and contracture of introitus and labial fusion
  - **Hour-glass involvement** of external genitalia
- Associated with autoimmune diseases
- Associated with VIN–differentiated type
- Malignant change in 1-5% cases
- May be present adjacent to vulvar squamous cell carcinoma in 15-40% of cases

Diagnosis–Histopathology examination of vulvar biopsy reveals **flattening of rete pegs** and thinning of epithelium with dermal fibrosis

Treatment–Steroid cream (Clobetasol cream)

Squamous Cell Hyperplasia / Lichen Simplex Chronicus

- Common in **postmenopausal** women
- **Symptoms**–pruritus (most common), soreness, dyspareunia, discharge
- **Examination**–Involves labia, introitus and perianal region. Skin is thick, rubbery and hyperkeratotic
- Associated with autoimmune diseases
- Malignant change–10-30% cases
- **Diagnosis**–Histopathology examination of Vulvar Biopsy reveals:
  - Heavy accumulation of keratin on surface
  - Increased **thickening of prickle cell layer**
  - Irregular **down growth of rete pegs deep into dermis**
- **Treatment–Steroid cream** (Clobetasol cream)

VULVAR CANCERS

- Vulvar cancers constitute **3-5% of genital malignancies**
- Usually occurs in **postmenopausal women**; Median age is 60 years
- Usually presents with **non resolving pruritus,** irritation, pain or a mass lesion; **diagnosis is often delayed**

- **Most common malignancy of vulva is squamous cell carcinoma (90%)**
- Second most common vulvar malignancy is melanoma

Etiology and Risk Factors

- Commonly occurs in postmenopausal women
- Human papilloma virus DNA (type 16, 18) has been detected in patients with invasive vulvar cancer
  - **HPV can be identified in 80% vulvar intraepithelial lesions, 50 % of invasive vulvar cancers**
  - HPV type 16, 18–detected in invasive cancer **(most common is HPV 16)**
- **VIN lesions,** if left untreated -> invasive carcinoma; **Unlike cervical cancers where majority are associated with a CIN lesion, only 1/3rd of vulvar squamous carcinoma have co existing VIN III**
- **Associated with HIV, HSV-2**
- Vulvar cancer may have causal relation with condyloma accuminata (HPV 6, 11), herpes simplex virus and lymphogranuloma venereum.
- **Vulvar dystrophies** can undergo malignant change to form vulvar cancers
- **Prior cervical cancer** is a risk factor for vulvar carcinoma
- Associated with low socioeconomic status, poor hygiene

NOTE-20% cases with vulvar cancers have other synchronous primary malignancies; Carcinoma cervix is the most common associated malignancy

Pathology (Table 8.9)

- Most common site is **labium majora (50%),** followed by clitoris and labium minora
- **Anterior two-third of vulva** is commonly affected

Table 8.9: Types of Vulvar Cancer

Type	Percent
Squamous cell carcinoma **(most common)**	92
Melanoma	2-4 Whilst melanoma is rightly the 2nd MC malignancy, percentages of upto 7 and even 10% is given in various sources like Williams and Medscape, ma'am.
Basal cell carcinoma	2-3
Bartholin gland tumor (adenocarcinoma, squamous cell, transitional cell, adenoid cystic)	1
Metastatic carcinoma	1
Verrucous carcinoma	< 1
Sarcoma	< 1
Tumors from Appendage (e.g., hidradenocarcinoma)	Rare

- **60% of cases have adjacent vulvar intraepithelial neoplasia (VIN)**
- **Lichen sclerosus adjacent to vulvar squamous cell carcinoma is seen in 15 - 40% of cases.**
- **Vulvar squamous cell carcinoma can be considered in two distinct groups (Table 8.10)**
  - **Associated with HPV**
  - **Not associated with HPV**

Table 8.10: Vulvar Cancer Groups based on HPV Association

HPV Positive Vulvar Cancers	HPV Negative Vulvar Cancers
• Comparatively younger women • Associated with VIN • Multifocal • Basaloid/warty, contain less keratin	• Older women • Associated with chronic inflammation/Lichen sclerosus • Unifocal • Exuberant keratin • Associated with p53 mutations

> ***NOTE– Presence of Desmoplasia (a fibroblastic stromal tumor response), has been correlated with a high risk of lymph node metastasis and poorer survival in vulvar cancer***

Clinical Features

Symptoms

- May be asymptomatic
- **Most common symptom–Pruritus vulvae**
- Long-term pruritus or a lump/mass on the vulva is present in > 50% of cases with invasive vulvar cancer
- Other symptoms–Difficulty in urination, vulvar ulceration, pain, bleeding, inguinal mass, offensive discharge

Clinical examination

- Vulvar inspection reveals an ulcer or a fungating mass on the vulva
- Ulcer has sloughing base with raised, everted and irregular edges and bleeds on touch. Surrounding tissue may be edematous and indurated
- Clinical examination of cervix, vagina, urethra, rectum should be done **(coexistence of other primary cancers)**
- Inguinal nodes may be enlarged

Diagnosis

- Diagnosis is made by **biopsy.** Tissue biopsies should include the cutaneous lesion with underlying stroma along with contiguous area, so that the presence and depth of invasion can be accurately assessed
- Immediate evaluation with biopsy helps to avoid the delay in starting appropriate therapy
- In case of **diffuse lesion-**Biopsy is taken from **multiple sites** or following toluidine blue test or acetic acid application
- **Pap smear, Colposcopy, Cystourethroscopy, Proctoscopy** are done to rule out other synchronous carcinoma
- Lymph nodes can be assessed by CT/MRI scan, sentinel node lymphoscintigraphy and PET scan

Extra Edge

Indications for excisional biopsy of vulvar lesion

- *Change in surface area of nevus*
- *Change in elevation of a lesion: Raised, thickened, or nodular*
- *Change in color: Especially brown to black*
- *Change in surface: Smooth to scaly or ulcerated*
- *Change in sensation: Itching or tingling*

Staging of Vulvar Cancers

Vulvar cancer has been surgically staged and final diagnosis is based on histological evaluation of the vulvar and lymph node specimens

The FIGO revised staging of vulvar carcinoma (2009) is applicable for most of the malignancies arising from the vulva, except melanoma

FIGO staging (updated 2009)– Surgical staging system -Table 8.11

Table 8.11: FIGO Staging of Vulvar Cancer

Stage I	**Tumor confined to the vulva**
IA	Lesions ≤ 2 cm in size, confined to the vulva or perineum and with stromal invasion ≤ 1.0 mm, with negative nodes
IB	Lesions > 2 cm in size or with stromal invasion > 1.0 mm, confined to the vulva or perineum, with negative nodes
Stage II	**Tumor of any size with extension to adjacent perineal structures (1/3 lower urethra, 1/3 lower vagina, anus) with negative nodes**

Contd.

Contd.

Stage III	**Tumor of any size with or without extension to adjacent perineal structure (1/3 lower urethra, 1/3 lower vagina, anus) with positive inguino-femoral lymph nodes**
IIIA	(i) With 1 lymph node metastasis (≥ 5 mm), or (ii) 1-2 lymph node metastatis(es) (< 5 mm)
IIIB	(i) With 2 or more lymph node metastases (≥ 5 mm), or (ii) 3 or more lymph node metastases (< 5 mm)
IIIC	With positive nodes with extracapsular spread
Stage IV	**Tumor invades other regional (2/3 upper urethra, 2/3 upper vagina), or distant structures**
IVA	Tumor invades any of the following: (i) Upper urethral and/or vaginal mucosa, bladder mucosa, rectal mucosa, or fixed to pelvic bone, or (ii) Fixed or ulcerated inguino-femoral lymph nodes
IVB	Any distant metastasis **including pelvic lymph nodes**

Note

- *Tumors with a depth or thickness of 1 mm or less, have little or no risk of lymph node metastasis*
- *The depth of invasion is defined as the measurement of the tumor from the epithelial stromal junction of the adjacent, most superficial dermal papilla to the deepest point of invasion*
- *Inguinal nodes involvement – Stage III*
- *Pelvic nodes involvement – Stage IV*

(In cervical and endometrial cancers, pelvic nodes involvement is Stage III)

Mode of Spread

- **Commonest mode of spread is direct spread followed by lymphatics**
- Direct spread occurs to the urethra, vagina, rectum and even to pelvic bones
- Hematogenous spread is rare, occurs in advanced cases. **Most common site of hematogenous spread is lung**
- **Pares Jones described lymphatic spread in vulvar malignancy**

Facts about Lymphatic Spread

- 50% of lymphatics are involved by the time the patient attends consultation.
- Nodal status is determined by the surgical evaluation of the groin region
- **Incidence of lymph node involvement is directly related to site, size of lesion and depth of stromal invasion (Table 8.12)**
- The **superficial inguinal nodes** are the most frequent site of lymphatic metastasis
- Lymphatic spread is primarily by embolization and only at later stage; spreads by permeation to fill lymphatic channels
- Metastasis to the contralateral groin nodes or deep pelvic nodes is unusual in the absence of ipsilateral groin metastases
- **LN involvement follows a sequential pattern: lymphatics of labia→superficial inguinal lymph nodes→deep inguinal lymph nodes→pelvic nodes**
- Spread beyond the inguinal lymph nodes is considered distant metastasis
- **Bilateral lymph node involvement increases when midline structures (clitoris, perineum) are involved**
- **Contralateral metastases is present in 25% cases if midline structures involved**
- Pelvic nodes are secondarily involved in 20% cases with affected inguinal nodes
- **Lymphatics of clitoris drain directly into pelvic nodes**

- **Sentinel lymph node**–More recent experience with intraoperative mapping has demonstrated that lymphatic drainage from most vulvar sites proceeds initially to a "sentinel" node located within the superficial inguinal group

Table 8.12: Depth of Stromal Invasion and Groin Lymph Node Involvement in Squamous Cell Carcinoma of Vulva

Depth of invasion (mm)	Percent with positive groin nodes
< 1	0
1-2	7.5
2.1-3	10.0
3.1-5	30

Causes of Death

- Uremia–ureteric obstruction due to enlarged common iliac and para-aortic nodes
- Rupture of the femoral vessels by the overlying involved inguinal lymph glands
- Sepsis

TREATMENT OF VULVAR CANCERS (Refer flowchart 8.1, 8.2, 8.3 and Table 8.13)

Flowchart 8.1: Management of Stage I and II lateralized vulvar cancers

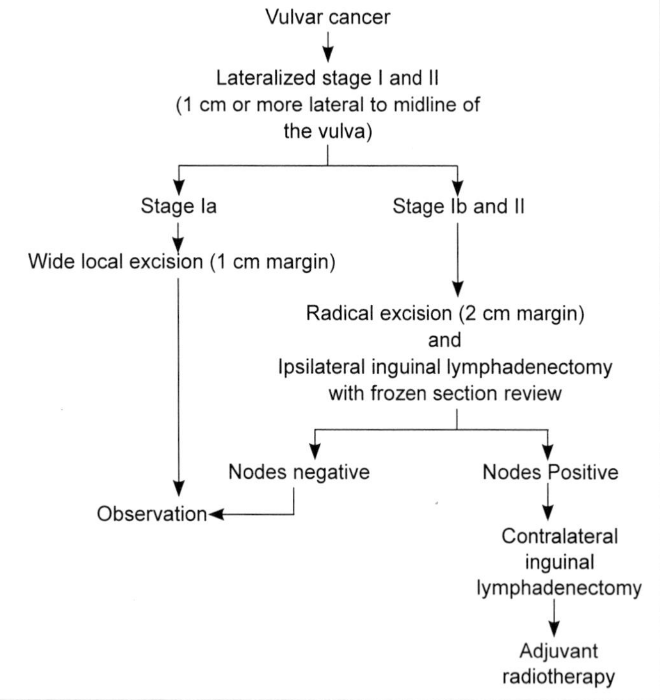

Flowchart 8.2: Management of Stage I and II central vulvar cancers

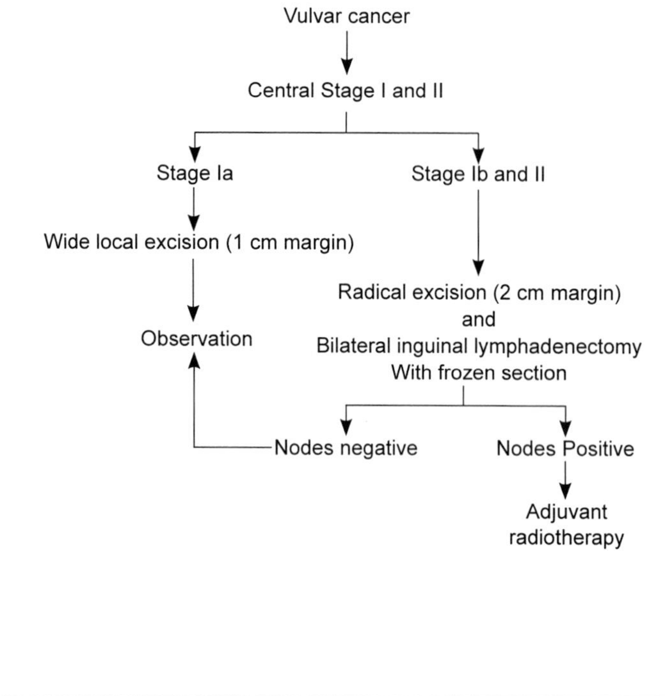

Note

- *Microinvasive cancer, i.e., Stage IA or stromal invasion < 1 mm: wide local excision/ simple partial vulvectomy, no need for lymphadenectomy.*
- *Stage IB and II–Radical vulvectomy with inguinofemoral lymphadenectomy*
- *If lesion is central bilateral lymph node dissection is performed*
- *If lesion is > 2 cm from midline (lateral lesion), ipsilateral lymph node dissection is performed*
- *Postoperative radiotherapy to be given if*
  - *2 or more groin nodes are involved or*
  - *disease free margin is < 8 mm*

Flowchart 8.3: Management of stage III and IV vulvar cancer

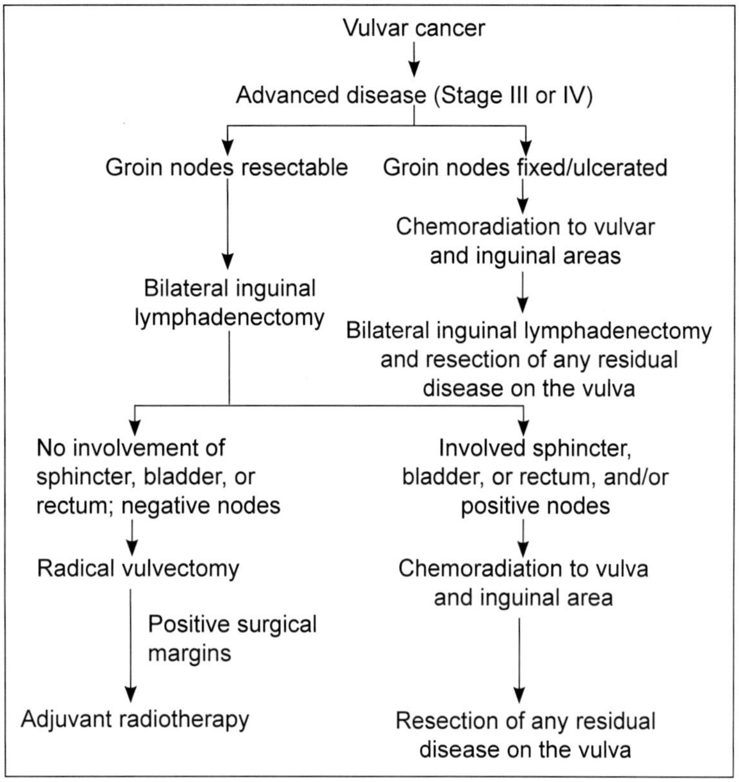

NOTE

- *Tumor free surgical margin of atleast 1 cm is required to prevent recurrence*
- *Chemotherapy agents used–cisplatin, bleomycin, 5-FU*

Table 8.13: Summary of Treatment for Vulvar Carcinoma

Disease State	Description	Treatment
Early disease (stage I and II)	Lesions with less than 1 mm stromal invasion (FIGO Stage Ia)	Wide local excision -> follow up Inguinal Lymph Node dissection not done
	Truly lateralized small vulvar lesions (FIGO Stage Ib and few cases of stage II)	Wide radical excision + ipsilateral inguinal lymph node dissection initially • If nodes are negative -> follow up • If nodes are positive -> proceed with contralateral LN dissection and/ or RT
	Centrally located small vulvar lesions (FIGO Stage Ib and few cases of stage II)	Wide Radical excision + bilateral inguinal lymph node dissection initially • If nodes are negative -> follow up • If nodes are positive -> RT
Advanced disease (Stage III)	Groin nodes resectable	B/L inguinal LN node dissection and surgical debulking of tumor with post-op chemoradiation or Primary chemoradiation followed by surgery
	Nodes fixed /ulcerated	Chemoradiation ->surgical Debulking of enlarged nodes and tumor
Metastatic disease (Stage IV)		Individualized treatment may include surgery, radiation, and chemotherapy Pelvic RT is recommended for patients with involved nodes. Survival is poor

Note

- *Current recommendation in case of small vulvar cancers of Stage 1B and stage II - to do a wide radical excision, also termed as partial radical vulvectomy in order to reduce surgical morbidity associated with radical vulvectomy (earlier radical vulvectomy was performed for these cases)*
- ***Wide local excision–1 cm normal tissue margin***
- ***Wide radical excision–2 cm normal tissue margin***

Incision Techniques for Resection of Vulvar Cancers (Figure 8.3)

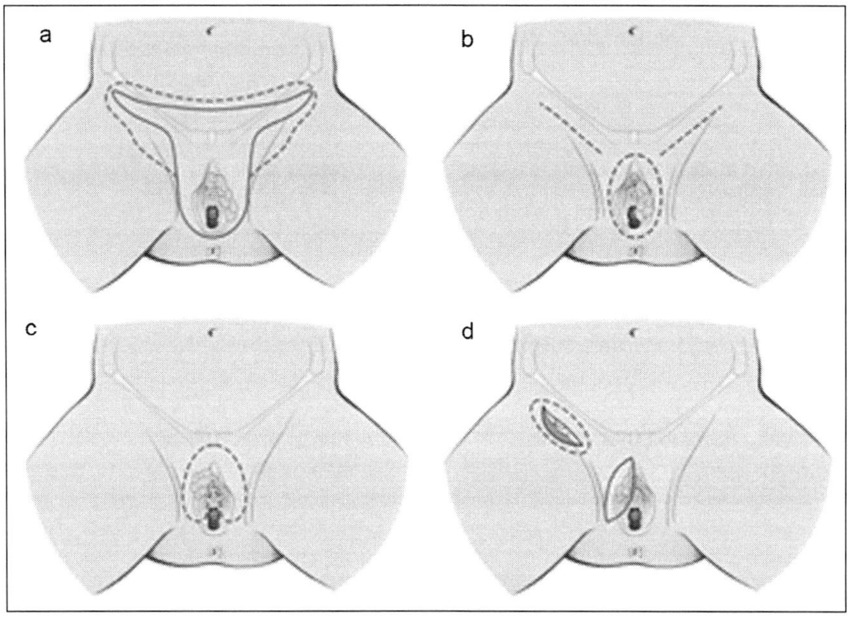

Figure 8.3: Approach to resection of vulvar cancer (a) Modified butterfly incision. (b) Triple incision method preserving skin along the inner thighs. (c) Anterior horseshoe incision. (d) Unilateral incision in the groin and elliptical excision of the primary vulvar lesion

RADICAL VULVECTOMY

- **This procedure was earlier performed for Stage IB and Stage II vulvar cancers**
- **"Butterfly" or "longhorn" approach is** the traditional incision for radical vulvectomy and bilateral lymphadenectomy
- **This technique has been abandoned lately**
- **Radical vulvectomy traditionally involves removal of the following:**
  - Primary tumor with wide margin of normal skin and remaining vulva
  - Dermal lymphatics
  - Bilateral Inguinal lymph node dissection

Complications of radical vulvectomy

- Loss of normal vulvar tissue
- Alteration in appearance of vulva
- Sexual dysfunction
- Wound breakdown
- Groin complication–breakdown, lymphocyst formation, lymphangitis
- Lymphedema of lower extremities

RADICAL WIDE EXCISION/ PARTIAL RADICAL VULVECTOMY

- **Currently preferred surgical option to resect small vulvar cancers**

- Wide excision of primary lesion with 2 cm margin and dissection is carried upto deep perineal fascia
- Unilateral inguinal node dissection in lateral lesion or bilateral inguinal node dissection in near midline lesion is done
- **Inguinal lymphadenectomy is performed through separate incisions (Triple Incision Techniques)**
- **Lesser incidence of wound breakdown**

Triple Incision Techniques

- Three separate incisions given
- One incision to remove the lesion with 2 cm normal skin margins
- Two separate incisions, parallel to the inguinal ligament to perform Bilateral inguinofemoral lymphadenectomy
- This technique preserves the radicality of the vulvar resection while retaining the skin over the groin
- Reduces the incidence of major wound breakdown

INGUINAL LYMPHADENECTOMY

Superficial Inguinal Lymphadenectomy

- This involves removal of 8-10 lymph nodes that lie superficial to the cribriform fascia, surrounding the branches of saphenous vein

Deep Inguinal (Femoral) Lymphadenectomy

- The deep inguinal (femoral) lymph nodes are 3-5 in number, that lie beneath the cribriform fascia medial to femoral vein
- **The most superior deep inguinal node is known as lymph node of Cloquet**

Sentinel Lymph Node Mapping

- **Sentinel lymph node is the first lymph node in the lymphatic pathway and the main site of metastasis**
- **Sentinel lymph node identification**–Intraoperative toluidene blue dye staining technique along with **radioactive 99mTc lymphoscintigraphy** administered shortly before surgery, combined with intraoperative use of a handheld gamma probe aids in Sentinel lymph node detection
- Sentinel lymph node biopsy can allow for the detection of smaller tumor foci compared to complete groin node dissection and traditional pathologic examination
- **The prognosis associated with groin relapse is poor, and sentinel lymph node identification should be confirmed by a prospective randomized controlled trial before considering it as part of standard surgical care for vulva carcinoma**

RECURRENT VULVAR CANCER

- Local vulvar recurrences correlate with number of positive groin nodes (≥ 3) and size of primary tumor (> 4 cm)
- Recurrence occur in 30% cases within 2 years
- Recurrence can be local (vulva) in the groin, and/or distant
- Local recurrence is seen in 75% cases
- **Common site of local recurrence is the clitoral hood and perineal skin**
- Regional and distant recurrences have a poor prognosis

Management of recurrent cancers (Table 8.14)

Table 8.14: Management of Recurrent Cancers

Local recurrence	• Can be excised and covered with myocutaneous flap, e.g. gracilis • Radiotherapy (external beam with interstitial needles) can also be used, but may have delayed sequelae of necrosis
Regional recurrence	Chemoradiation and/or palliative surgical resection
Distant metastases	Chemotherapy

Survival Rate (Table 8.15)

Lymph node involvement is the single most important prognostic factor

Prognostic factors

- Clinical stage
- Site of the tumour
- Depth of stromal invasion
- Lymph node involvement (most important prognostic factor)
- Tumor histology and differentiation
- DNA ploidy status

Table 8.15: Survival Rate in Vulvar Cancer

Survival By Stage		Survival By Node Status (5 Years)	
Stage I	100	**Negative nodes**	80-100%
Stage II	65-75	**Positive inguinal femoral nodes**	30-50%
Stage III	35-45	**Positive pelvic nodes**	10-20%
Stage IV	20-30		

Prevention

- **Screening for VIN is not reliable and hence not done**
- **HPV vaccination prevents half of vulvar cancers and 2/3rd of VIN**

OTHER MALIGNANT VULVAR TUMORS

MALIGNANT MELANOMA

- **Second most common vulvar cancer; accounts for 2-4% of vulvar cancers**
- Vulvar melanoma accounts for 5% of all melanoma
- **Most common sites–clitoris and labia minora**
- **May arise from a junctional nevus**
- **Radical vulvectomy and bilateral regional lymphadenectomy is the preferred treatment**
- **Pelvic lymphadenectomy does not alter the prognosis**
- **Radiotherapy, chemotherapy or immunotherapy are ineffective**
- **Poor prognosis**

High-Risk Group for Development of Melanoma

Increased risk with one or more of the following:

- *Family history of melanoma*
- *Poor or no tanning ability, often with a history of sunburn in adolescence*
- *Unusual moles with any of the following characteristics:*
  - Dark (blue-black) look
  - Speckled color pattern
  - Jagged or fuzzy border
  - Recent change in size, shape, or color of a mole
  - Any mole larger than 1 cm

BASAL CELL CARCINOMA

- **Accounts for 2-3 % of vulvar malignancies**

- Presents as an ulcer invading deeper tissues of vulva
- Most common site **is labia**
- **Locally malignant and metastasis is rare**
- **Responds well to wide local excision with 1 cm margin**
- **If lesions are Unresectable -> Radiotherapy**

BARTHOLIN GLAND ADENOCARCINOMA

- 1% of all vulvar malignancies
- **Most primary adenocarcinomas of the vulva arise in the Bartholin's gland**
- Invasive vulvar Paget disease can give rise to adenocarcinoma
- Primary malignant Bartholin gland tumors include adenocarcinoma and squamous cell carcinoma
- Generally occurs in older women
- It is generally advisable to excise an enlarged Bartholin gland at >50 years of age, especially if there is no history of prior Bartholin's cyst
- Primary Bartholin gland cancers are characteristically deep in location and difficult to detect in early stages
- 20% of women with primary carcinoma of Bartholin gland have metastasis to the inguino femoral lymph nodes at the time of diagnosis
- Treatment–radical vulvectomy with Lymph node dissection +/- Post op Radiotherapy

Honan Criteria for Bartholin Gland Adenocarcinoma

- The tumor is in correct anatomic position
- The tumor is located deep in the labium majus
- The overlying skin is intact
- There is some recognizable normal gland present

VERRUCOUS CARCINOMA OF THE VULVA

- Incidence <1%
- It is an exophytic-appearing growth that can be locally destructive
- Clinically, it may resemble condyloma acuminatum
- Excellent prognosis
- Verrucous tumors may be associated with HPV 6 or its variants
- **Verrucous carcinomas are locally invasive and rarely metastasize**
- Treatment by **radical wide excision is usually curative**
- **Local recurrence** can occur, especially when the tumor has been inadequately resected
- Radiotherapy is not recommended for verrucous carcinoma (there are reports of anaplastic transformation and widespread metastasis following RT)

VULVAR SARCOMA

- Incidence < 1% of all vulvar malignancies.
- Common sarcomas in vulva–leiomyosarcoma, malignant fibrous histiocytoma and rhabdomyosarcoma
- **Blood borne spread is common**
- Metastasis is common
- Treatment is by **chemoradiation with surgical resection**
- **Rhabdomyosarcomas respond well to both chemotherapy and radiotherapy**
- Prognosis is poor

RECENT UPDATES

Focus on Sentinel Lymph Node Testing

- *Different techniques to identify sentinel lymph nodes have been used in trials, based on experience with different cancer types such as breast cancer and cutaneous melanoma*
- *The best detection rates for sentinel nodes identification are seen when a combination of blue dye and technetium-based tests are used*
- *The **GROINSS-VI trial** concluded that patients with early stage vulvar cancer and negative sentinel node have low rates of groin recurrence (2-3%), excellent survival rates at 3 years (97%) and minimal morbidity*
- *The GROINSS-VII trial seeks to treat patients with metastatic sentinel lymph nodes directly with radiotherapy instead of inguino-femoral lymphadenectomy followed by radiotherapy, thus theoretically reducing the morbidity of dual modality treatment*

Impact of HPV Vaccine

- *HPV vaccine has been projected to decrease the incidence and morbidity of pre-cancerous and cancerous genital disease*
- *The **Future II trial,** a randomised control trial which compared women given a HPV vaccine to placebo, showed a vaccine efficacy of 75% for low grade warty or basaloid VIN*
- *HPV is the main etiological cause in only 30-40% of invasive vulval cancers. The predicted decrease in incidence of cervical cancer following the introduction of the vaccine may not have such significant effects on the prevalence of vulval cancer, particularly in the aging population*
- *Topical treatments such as Imiquimod and Cidofovir are being investigated to determine their efficacy in treating VIN so the morbidity of surgery can be reduced*

The Influence of HPV Status on Mechanisms of Carcinogenesis

- *Despite sharing common pathways of dysregulation, HPV-associated and HPV-independent VSCC are characterized by unique genetic, epigenetic and immune factors that are important considerations in the development of novel approaches to anti-cancer therapy. The mechanisms specific to each distinct VSCC etiology are detailed below*

HPV-associated VSCC

- *Nearly half of all VSCC is associated with HPV infection, with HPV-16 being the dominant subtype*
- *Its precancerous lesion, usual or undifferentiated VIN (uVIN), is characterized by a high ki-67 proliferative index and diffuse staining of p16*
- *As with other HPV-related cancers, there is significant interplay between HPV and the immune system, with the host immune response playing an important role in the development and progression of HPV-associated VSCC. This is underscored by the high prevalence of HPV in pre-neoplastic lesions (80%) when compared with invasive disease (40%) which suggests a better immune response to uVIN*
- *Studies have shown that the HPV-independent precancerous lesion, differentiated VIN (dVIN), has a higher risk of progression compared with uVIN*
- *As toll-like receptor (TLR)-mediated host response are involved in immune responses to HPV infection, their targeting may be a potential therapeutic strategy in HPV-associated VSCC*
- *Exploitation of the immune system's role in the pathogenesis of cancer of HPV-associated VSCC through enhancement of host immunity and direct targeting of HPV oncogenic proteins E6/E7 warrant further research in the management of HPV-associated VSCC*

HPV-independent VSCC

- *Up to two-thirds of patients with HPV- independent VSCC have genomic mutations*
- *High mutation rates in PTEN and TP53 have been noted in the precursor lesion, dVIN*

- *A number of other somatic mutations have been implicated in the development of HPV-independent VSCC such as CDKN2A, HRAS and PI3KCA*
- *Adverse survival has been reported in patients carrying somatic mutations in HPV-independent VSCC and hence there may be a unique opportunity to improve their outcomes with targeted therapies*

Molecularly targeted therapies in VSCC

- *The goal of targeted therapies in VSCC is to minimize surgical morbidity and expand systemic treatment options in advanced disease*
- *Molecular targeted therapies currently in clinical development that are of general relevance to the management of VSCC, and those of specific importance to HPV-associated and HPV-independent disease, are detailed in Figure 8.4 and 8.5)*
- *On-going trials open to patients with VSCC are presented in Table 8.16.*

Table 8.16: On-going trials open to patients with VSCC

All VSCC			
Agent	**Target**	**Phase**	**Disease**
Erlotinib	EGFR	II	VSCC
Triapine	Ribonucleotide reductase	I	Cervical/vaginal/Pelvic malignancies
Mk-3475 (Pembrolizumab) + Ziv-Aflibercept	PD-1; VEGF	I	Advanced solid tumors
Atelolizumab	PD-L1	I	Advanced solid tumors
Durvalumab	PD-L1	I/II	Advanced solid tumors
Pembrolizumab	PD-1	II	Advanced solid tumors
HPV-associated VSCC			
HPV-16/18	E6/E7-specific T lymphocytes	I	HPV-associated cancers
Nivolumab	PD-1	I/II	Virus-associated tumors
p16INK4a-peptide with Montanide ISA-51VG	P16^{ink4a}-based vaccine	I/II	HPV-induced cancers

VSCC, vulvar squamous cell carcinoma; PD-L1, Programmed death Ligand 1; EGFR, Epidermal growth factor receptor; VEGF, Vascular endothelial growth factor

Molecular Targets in vulvar squamous cell carcinoma

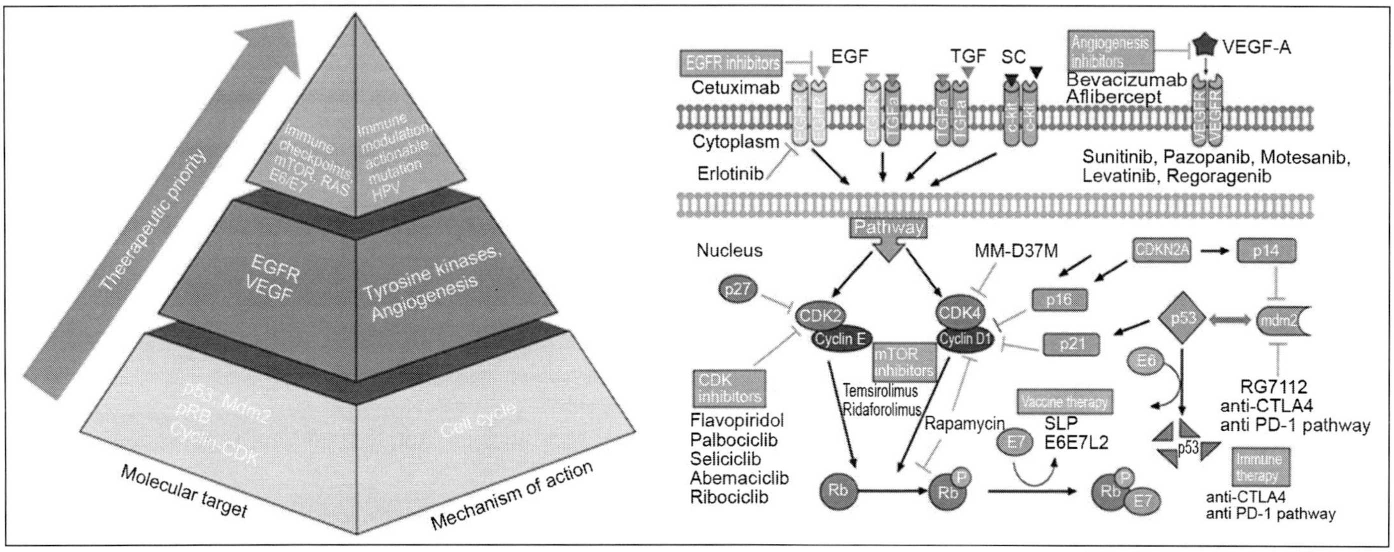

Figures 8.4 and 8.5: Molecular Targets in vulvar squamous cell carcinoma

CHAPTER 9

VAGINAL CANCER

INTRODUCTION

- Primary vaginal cancer is a rare malignancy accounting for about 2% female genital malignancies
- Occurs in women often >60 years of age

Recap of Anatomy

- Vagina is a fibromuscular structure that extends from cervix to vulva, forms a communicating channel between the uterine cavity and exterior
- It is the organ of copulation and forms the birth canal
- **Vaginal canal is directed upwards and backwards, forming an angle of 45° with the horizontal plane in erect posture**
- Appears **'H'** shaped in transverse section; anterior wall is 8 cm in length; posterior wall is 10 cm
- **Diameter of vaginal canal is 2.5 cm; narrowest at the introitus**
- **It has four fornices: Anterior, posterior and 2 lateral fornices; shallowest is anterior; deepest is posterior**
- Vaginal wall is composed of three layers: the mucosa, muscularis and adventitia. Lined by **stratified squamous non–keratinized epithelium**
- **Vaginal epithelium of newborn is transitional type**
- **Vaginal pH is acidic (pH 4-5) during reproductive years due to the presence of Doderlein's bacilli (Gram-positive anaerobic Lactobacillus)** that produces lactic acid from glycogen of exfoliated cells
- Doderlein's bacilli begin to appear during **reproductive period**
- **Before puberty and after menopause the pH of vagina is around 7 (Table 9.1)**

Table 9.1: pH of Vaginal Secretion at Different Phases of Life

Period	pH of Vaginal Secretions
Birth–2 weeks postnatal	4–5
2 weeks postnatal-Prepuberty	>7
Puberty	Shifts from alkaline to acidic pH
Reproductive period	4–5
Postmenopausal	Alkaline: 6 to >7

- Vaginal rugosities are evidence of estrogenization
- Vagina does not contain any mucous secreting glands. Hence vaginal secretions are not derived from vagina and are derived from endocervical, endometrial and Bartholin's glands
- For **hormonal cytology, scrapings from lateral wall of upper third of vagina is preferred as it is most sensitive to hormonal influence**

Table 9.2: Relationship of Vagina to Surrounding Structures

Anteriorly	Bladder (upper 2/3rd) Urethra (lower 1/3rd)

Contd.

Contd.

Posteriorly	Pouch of Douglas (upper 1/3rd) Ampulla of rectum (middle 1/3rd) Perineal Body (lower 1/3rd)
Laterally	Mackenrodt's Ligament (upper 1/3rd) Levator ani (middle 1/3rd) Bulbocavernosus Vestibular bulb Bartholin's glands

- **Vagina has no serosal covering except the area covered by Cul de sac posteriorly**
- **Transverse vaginal sulcus is a landmark for location of neck of bladder**
- **Blood supply: Vaginal artery (anterior division of internal iliac artery),** cervico vaginal branch of uterine artery, middle rectal artery and internal pudendal artery
- **Venous drainage into internal iliac vein**
- **Nerve supply:** Pudendal nerve and sympathetic and parasympathetic from **S_2 to S_4**
- **Lymphatic drainage of vagina (Table 9.3; Fig 9.1)**

Table 9.3: Lymphatic Drainage of Vagina

Upper vagina	Lymphatics follow lymphatic drainageof cervix	Anterior vaginal wall drains into obturator and hypogastric nodes Posterior vaginal wall drains into inferior gluteal, presacral, and anorectal nodes
Middle vagina	–	Internal iliacnodes
Distal vagina	Lymphatics follow drainage patterns of the vulva	Inguino femoral nodes and then to the pelvic nodes

- Near the lateral fornix of vagina, uterine artery crosses above the ureter ('water under the bridge')

MATURATION INDEX (Table 9.4)

- **Indicates the ratio of basal/parabasal: Intermediate cells: Superficial cells in the vaginal epithelium**
- **Parabasal cells-predominant when there is no hormonal dominance: Menopause**
- **Intermediate cells–basophilic cells, predominant under progesterone influence: Luteal phase**
- **Superficial cells – eosinophilic cells, predominant under estrogen influence: Follicular phase**

Table 9. 4 Maturation index during various phases of life

Period	**Maturation index**
Newborn	0/95/5
Children	80/20/0
Ovulation	0/30/70
Menopause	10/90/0
Post partum	100/0/0

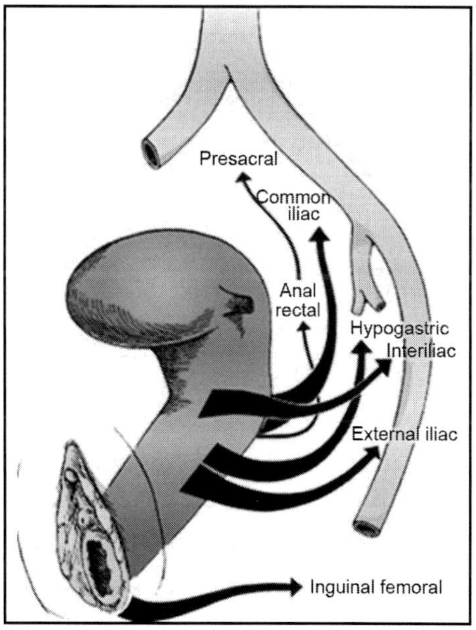

Figure 9.1: Lymphatic drainage of vagina

PREMALIGNANT LESIONS OF VAGINA–VAGINAL INTRAEPITHELIAL NEOPLASIA (VAIN)

- Etiologic agent is oncogenic **Human papilloma virus (HPV)**
- 70% cases of VAIN are **associated with CIN**
- Most VAIN lesions involve **upper vagina**
- Women with persistent positive Pap smear findings following treatment of CIN should be examined for VAIN
- Smokers and immuno compromised individuals are at increased risk of VAIN

Pathology

VAIN is of 3 grades of severity similar to CIN (Table 9.5)

Table 9.5: Grades of VAIN

VAIN	Description
VAIN–I	There is loss of stratification and polarity of the cells limited to one third of epithelium
VAIN–II	Epithelial abnormality extends onto the middle-third of the epithelium
VAIN–III	Carcinoma-in-situ–There is loss of polarity and stratification involving entire thickness of epithelium. Basement membrane remains intact

Diagnosis

- Vaginal scrape cytology
- Colposcopy
- Biopsy

Management

- VAIN 1 lesions may regress spontaneously and often require no treatment
- Local excision is diagnostic as well as therapeutic for small vaginal lesions
- Ablation therapy
  - Electrocautery under colposcopic guidance
  - LASER ablation
- **Intravaginal 5-Fluorouracil (5-FU)** can be used to treat patients for persistent disease after resection. 5-FU cream is applied at night for 5-10 days and repeated every 2 weeks for 2-3 courses
- **Topical 5% imiquimod: Imiquimod** (applied topically either in creams or drug-embedded tampons) is an immune response modulator that activates the innate immune response and subsequently induces pro-inflammatory factors such as interferons. It provides an alternative noninvasive and safe method of treating women with VAIN, especially young women with multifocal lesions

VAGINAL CARCINOMA

Introduction

- Primary vaginal cancer is rare and accounts for < 0.2% of all cancers in women
- It constitutes about 2% of genital malignancies in women
- Occurs in women >60 years of age
- 80-90% vaginal cancers represent metastasis from other primary gynecologic (cervix or vulva) and non gynecologic sites, involving the vagina either by direct extension or lymphatics or hematogenous routes

Primary vaginal carcinoma should fulfill the following criteria:

- The primary site of growth is in the vagina
- The cervix and the vulva must not be involved
- There must not be clinical evidence of metastatic disease to vagina

Etiology and Risk Factors

Exact etiology is unknown. Following factors are often related:

- **HPV** may have a causal relationship
  - HPV is detected in 80% of VAIN and 60% of invasive Squamous cell carcinoma of vagina
  - HPV-induced vaginal lesions are thought to arise in areas of squamous metaplasia that develop during healing of mucosal abrasions caused by coitus, tampon use, chronic pessary use, or other trauma

  - High-risk HPV are noted in 95% of VAIN III lesions. **HPV Type 16** is the most common
- Progression from **vaginal intraepithelial neoplasia**
- Women with history of **cervical cancer** (multicentric neoplasia)
- **Diethyl stilbesterol (DES) exposure is related with clear cell adenocarcinoma of the vagina. This is found in women with history of intrauterine exposure to Diethyl Stilbesterol**
- Previous irradiation therapy to the vagina or immunosuppression
- Prolonged use of pessary
- More common amongst whites than blacks

Pathology

- **Commonest site is the upper-third of the posterior wall**
- The growth may be ulcerative or exophytic
- **Squamous cell carcinoma accounts for > 90%** of the cases. Others are adenocarcinoma, melanoma, fibrosarcoma, sarcoma botryoides and malignant mixed mullerian tumors
- **Spread is by direct continuity, lymphatics** and rarely, blood borne
- **Inguino-femoral lymph nodes and pelvic lymph nodes** are commonly involved
- Most frequent site of hematogenous metastasis is the lung. Less frequently, vaginal cancers may metastasize to liver, bone, or other sites

Clinical features

Symptoms

- May be asymptomatic, discovered during routine screening procedures
- Abnormal vaginal bleeding
- Postcoital bleeding is an early symptom
- Foul smelling discharge per vaginum

Clinical examination

- Lesions are often multifocal and usually involve the upper-third of the posterior wall
- Speculum examination reveals an ulcerative, nodular or exophytic growth
- The cervix looks apparently normal

Diagnosis

- Cytology screening procedure reveals abnormal cells
- Investigation of choice is **colposcopic examination and targeted biopsy** in patients with abnormal cytology or unexplained vaginal bleeding
- Local application of estrogen in the form of cream? Specific preparation may be mentioned in old women enhances colposcopic view
- Biopsy should be taken from clinically suspicious lesion
- A non healing decubitus ulcer should be biopsied
- Cystourethroscopy, proctosigmoidoscopy, CT/MRI are done to assess the extent of spread

Staging of vaginal cancer (Table 9.6; Fig 9.2)

- Vaginal carcinoma is primarily **clinically staged,** based on the results of a physical examination, biopsy, and imaging tests performed before treatment selection
- The 2009 FIGO staging for primary vaginal cancer is described in Table 9.6

Table 9.6: FIGO staging of vaginal cancer	
Stage I	Cancer limited to the vaginal wall
Stage II	Cancer with involvement of the subvaginal tissue but no extension to the pelvic sidewall
Stage III	Cancer with extension to the pelvic wall
Stage IV	Cancer with extension beyond the true pelvis or involvement of the mucosa of the bladder or rectum not including bullous edema
Stage IVA	Invasion of the bladder or rectal mucosa and/or direct invasion beyond the true pelvis
Stage IVB	Distant metastasis

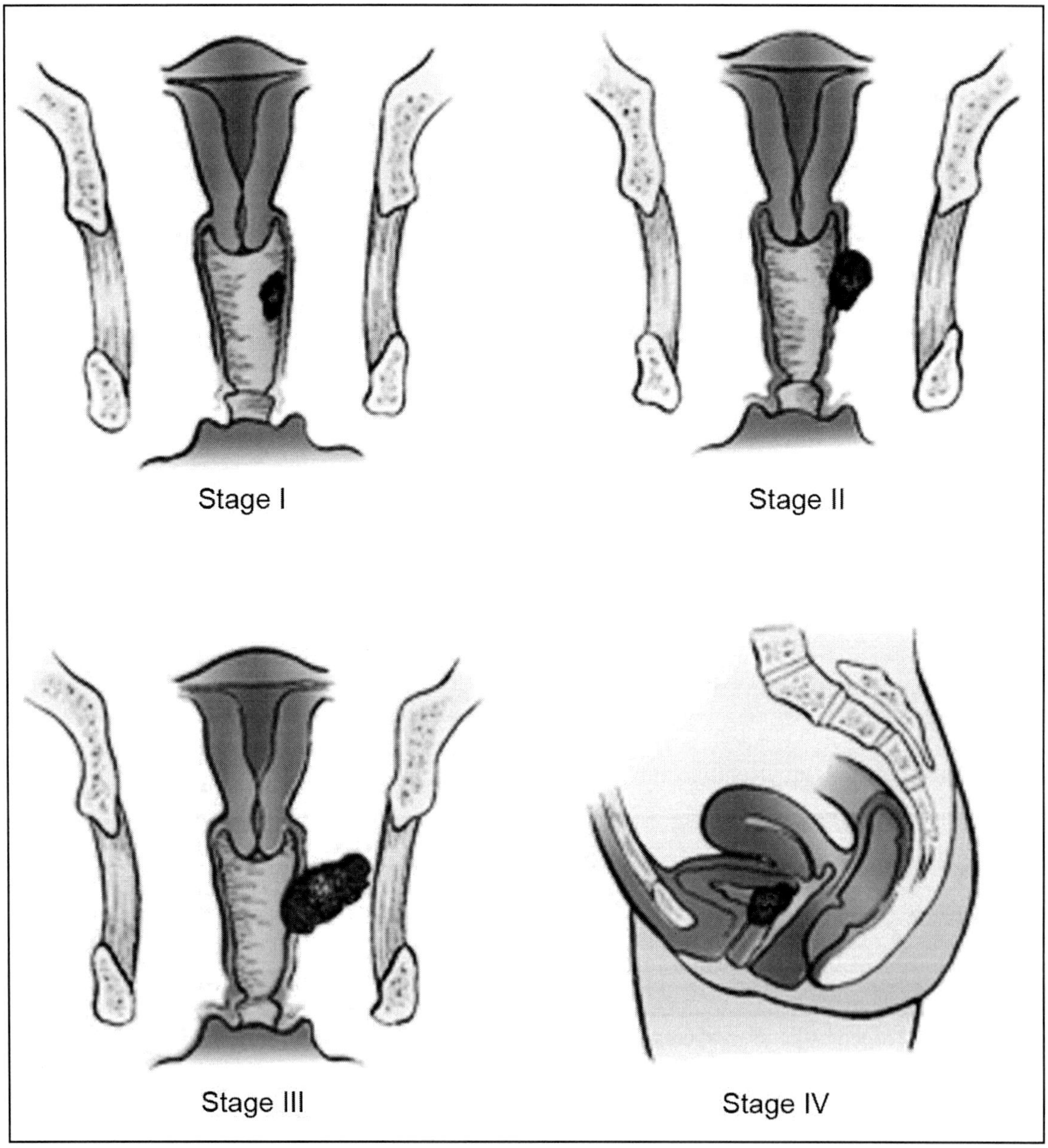

Figure 9.2: Staging of vaginal cancer

ROLE OF IMAGING TECHNIQUES

- Vaginal cancer is currently staged clinically, as is cervical cancer
- Modern imaging techniques such as computed tomography (CT), magnetic resonance imaging (MRI), and positron emission tomography (PET) are encouraged to guide management; however, these tests should not be used to change the initial clinical staging

- FIGO Gynecologic Oncology Committee recommends that wherever available, imaging should be used to better define tumor volume and extension of disease
- The Committee encourages registering of imaging findings and their influence on therapeutic decisions which will allow further analyses that could change the current staging system
- MRI is highly sensitive in detecting tumor size, as well as paravaginal or parametrial involvement
- In primary vaginal tumors, clinical assessment may be difficult and MRI may be a useful tool due to its superior soft tissue resolution

Treatment

- **Radiotherapy or surgery or combination of both** is used as therapy for invasive primary carcinoma of the vagina
- Choice depends on the clinical stage, anatomical location and size of the lesion (Table 9.7)
- The role of surgery is limited in primary vaginal cancer since the primary tumor is in close proximity to the bladder, urethra, and rectum
- Primary treatment with surgery is limited to early and small lesions confined to the vaginal mucosa (less than 2 cm)

Table 9.7: Treatment for Vaginal Cancer

Stage	Extent of lesion	Treatment
Stage I	Growth limited to the upper-third of vagina	**RT or surgery** (Radical hysterectomy, Radical vaginectomy and bilateral pelvic lymphadenectomy)
	Growth limited to the lower-third of vagina	**RT or surgery** (Radical vulvectomy, Radical vaginectomy and bilateral inguinofemoral lymphadenectomy)
	Middle one third of vagina	Radiation by external beam therapy and Brachytherapy
Stage II–IV		• **RT is the treatment of choice** • Radiation by external beam RTand Brachytherapy • Pelvic exenteration operation in selected cases

NOTE

- *Radiotherapy is widely used as primary treatment for invasive vaginal cancer*
- *Radiotherapy is preferred over surgery as total vaginectomy/exenteration is required to obtain satisfactory resection of margins*
- *In cases of small stage IVA cancers, pelvic exenteration can be done, particularly if a rectovaginal or vesicovaginal fistula is present, followed by radiotherapy*
- *In case of pelvic exenteration surgery, vaginal reconstruction is done using a gracilis myocutaneous flap or rectus abdominis myocutaneous flap*

Radiotherapy

- In the majority of cases and especially in advanced stages, radiation is the cornerstone of treatment for this disease
- This is a combination of external beam radiation (EBRT) and intracavitary radiotherapy or brachytherapy (ICRT)
- MRI imaging is done for defining tumor volume and the spatial relationship of the tumor with neighboring organs during treatment planning
- EBRT to the pelvis includes the external iliac and obturator nodes. In addition, the inguinal nodes may be included if the tumor is in the distal vagina
- Usually, **EBRT of 4500 to 5000 cGy** is administered to the pelvis encompassing the vagina. Additional **3000 to 4000 cGy is delivered in the form of brachytherapy** with iridium or cobalt
- The optimal threshold dose is 70 Gy. Doses higher than 70 Gy results in toxicity
- Intensity modulated radiation therapy (IMRT) is an advanced form of radiation that allows for higher dosages of radiation to be delivered to the cancer site, with fewer adverse effects because dose to the adjacent structures is limited
- **Complications of radiotherapy to pelvis**–Vaginal stenosis, Bladder and rectal fistula

Concurrent chemotherapy with radiation

- Modern management of vaginal cancer often include concurrent chemotherapy such as cisplatin or 5FU along with RT, extrapolated from the successful outcomes of this treatment with cervical cancer

Prognosis

- Stage of disease is an important prognostic factor
- Tumor size also is an important predictor of outcome. Tumor that involves the entire vagina tends to be associated with a poor prognosis
- Exophytic tumors have better prognosis than infiltrating/necrotic lesions
- Recurrence can occur and majority of the recurrences will be confined to pelvis and vagina
- Median time from treatment to recurrence is 6-12 months

Survival Rate (Table 9.8)

Table 9.8: Survival rate of vaginal cancer

STAGE	5 year survival rate
Stage I	80%
Stage II	60%
Stage III	40%
Stage IV	10%

CLEAR CELL ADENOCARCINOMA

- Primary vaginal adenocarcinoma is rare-accounts for 8-10% of cases
- Clear cell adenocarcinoma (cervix/vagina) is seen in adolescent girls who had history of intrauterine exposure to **diethyl stilbestrol** during first trimester of pregnancy
- These patients are more likely to develop **vaginal adenosis** and rarely clear cell adenocarcinoma
- Risk of an offspring to develop clear cell adenocarcinoma of the vagina following DES exposure is 1 in 1000 or less
- Most of these cases were diagnosed between the ages of 14 and 22 years
- The lesion **usually involves the upper-third of the anterior vaginal wall.** The cervix may also be involved
- Women with history of intrauterine exposure to DES require close follow-up with annual cytology and careful visualization of both the cervix and vagina (including colposcopy)
- **Non-DES adenocarcinoma** is exceptionally rare and is identified as a different entity with a different natural history.
- **Treatment**–Most vaginal adenocarcinomas are treated in the same manner as squamous cell carcinomas
- **Poor prognostic features** are primary adenocarcinoma, large tumor bulk, tumor site (lower vaginal lesions have worse prognosis), and posterior vaginal wall involvement

Secondary Vaginal Carcinoma

- Secondary vaginal carcinoma follows direct spread from carcinoma vulva, cervix or urethra
- **Metastases to the lower-third of the anterior vaginal wall or vault occurs in Choriocarcinoma and Endometrial carcinoma**

OTHERS RARE VAGINAL TUMORS

MELANOMA

- Primary vaginal melanomas represent <20% of genital melanomas

- Account for 3% of primary vaginal cancers
- **Usually originate in distal third of the vagina**
- Mean age is about 55 years
- **Vaginal melanomas tend to be associated with poorer prognosis than vulvar melanomas**
- **Treated with wide excision followed by RT.** Distant disease is the predominant cause of treatment failure in patients with vaginal melanoma
- Poor prognosis: 5-year survival rates-15-20% after treatment with surgery, radiation or both

SARCOMA

- About 3% of vaginal cancers are sarcomas
- About two-thirds of these are leiomyosarcomas
- **Embryonal rhabdomyosarcoma (sarcoma botryoides) is a highly malignant sarcoma that occurs in young girls, usually below 6 years of age**

Sarcoma Botryoides

- Rhabdomyosarcomas are the most common soft tissue cancers in children and adolescents
- Accounts for 4-6% of all malignancies in this age group
- Twenty percent of these occur in the lower genital tract, and embryonal histologic subtype is the most common subtype
- The 2013 WHO classification of tumors of soft tissue and bone classified rhabdomyosarcomas into four main histologic subtypes:
  - Typical embryonal variant (most common accounting for 60% of cases)–comprises the classic botryoides
  - Spindle cell/sclerosing variant
  - Alveolar variant
  - Pleomorphic variant
- Rhabdomyosarcomas in children mostly occur in the vagina, where as adolescents have predominantly cervical lesions
- Sarcoma botryoides often presents in the first few years of life with bleeding and nodular lesions (grape like) filling and protruding from the vagina

Treatment

- It is recommended that a multidisciplinary team be involved in decisions regarding treatment, especially when this involves children and adolescents
- Treatment previously involved extensive surgery but it is now suggested that less radical surgery can be done with good outcomes in terms of survival as well as quality of life
- Wide local excision and chemotherapy have been used with good success rates
- Unfavorable factors such as - cervix as the primary site, large lesion size and extent of the disease may require radical surgical intervention or chemotherapy
- Neoadjuvant chemotherapy is another option that can be given, followed by surgical resection
- Radiotherapy should be avoided if possible, as there are long-term adverse effects

Pseudosarcoma Botryoides

- Pseudosarcoma botryoides refers to rare **benign vaginal polyp** that resembles sarcoma botryoides. It can be found in the **vagina of infants and pregnant women**
- Although large atypical cells may be present microscopically, **strap cells are absent**
- Grossly, these polyps resemble the grapelike appearance of sarcoma botryoides and are therefore called **"pseudosarcoma botryoides"**
- Treatment by **local excision is effective**

SMALL CELL CARCINOMA

- 5% of small cell carcinomas arise in extrapulmonary sites
- **Most common site in genital tract is cervix** > Ovary, Endometrium, vagina, vulva
- Small cell carcinoma of vagina has **poor prognosis**

VERRUCOUS CARCINOMA

- These are Large, warty tumors that **are locally aggressive with minimal tendency to metastasize**
- Treatment of choice–**Wide surgical excision of the tumor**
- **Regional lymphadenectomy is usually not required**

Extra Edge
Vaginal tumors in infants and children
• Endodermal sinus tumors
• Embryonal rhabdomyosarcoma (Sarcoma botryoides)

Table 9.11 Summary of the age Group and Clinical Correlation of Vaginal Cancers

Tumor type	**Predominant age (years)**	**Clinical correlations**
Endodermal sinus tumor (adenocarcinoma)	< 2	Extremely rare; α-fetoprotein secretion; often fatal; multimodality therapy
Sarcoma botryoides	< 8	Aggressive malignancy; multimodality therapy
Clear cell adenocarcinoma	> 14	Associated with intrauterine exposure to Diethylstilbestrol
Melanoma	> 50	Very rare, poor survival
Squamous cell carcinoma	> 50	**Most common** primary vaginal cancer

CHAPTER 10

GESTATIONAL TROPHOBLASTIC DISEASES

INTRODUCTION

- The terminologies Gestational Trophoblastic Diseases and Gestational Trophoblastic Neoplasia are described in Table 10.1

Table 10.1: Terminologies in Gestational Trophoblastic Diseases

Terminology	Definition	Includes the following
Gestational Trophoblastic Diseases (GTD)	This term is used to describe a group of tumors derived from abnormal proliferation of gestational trophoblastic tissue	**Includes:** Hydatidiform mole and Gestational trophoblastic neoplasias (GTNs)
Gestational Trophoblastic Neoplasia (GTN)	This term is applied to a subset of GTDs that are locally invasive and have capability to metastasize outside uterus	It includes **all GTDs except hydatidiform mole** and are as follows: • **Invasive mole** • **Choriocarcinoma** • **Placental site trophoblastic tumor (PSTT)** • **Epithelioid trophoblastic tumor (ETT)**

Classification of GTD (Flowchart 10.1 and Table 10.2)

Flowchart 10.1: Classification of GTD

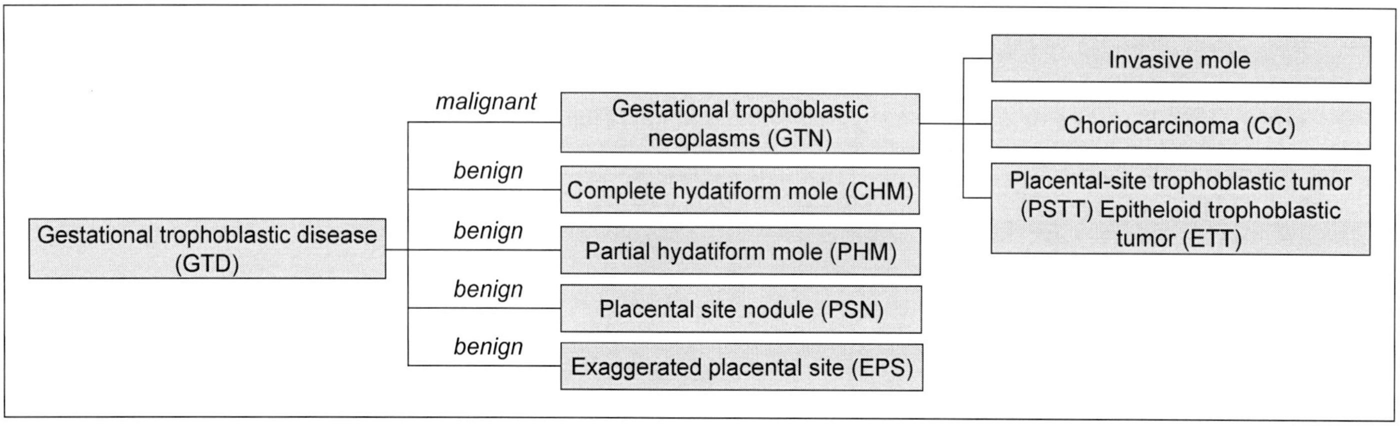

WHO Classification of GTD (2014) (Table 10.2)

Table 10.2: WHO Classification of GTD (2014)

Molar pregnancies
Hydatidiform mole
Complete
Partial
Invasive mole
Trophoblastic tumors
Choriocarcinoma
Placental site trophoblastic tumor
Epithelioid trophoblastic tumor
GTD=gestational trophoblastic disease; WHO=World Health Organization

GESTATIONAL TROPHOBLASTIC DISEASES

Incidence

- Incidence of GTD varies from 1/1000 in North America and Europe to **12/1000** in India and Indonesia. The difference in incidence may be due to socioeconomic and nutritional factors

Risk factors–See Table 10.3

Table 10.3 Risk factors in Gestational trophoblastic diseases

Risk factor	Remark
Race	Incidence is highest in the Southeast Asian countries
Maternal age <20 years and >35 years	Increases incidence of complete mole. No association between age and partial mole The degree of risk is higher for the older women than younger women
Previous history of abortion	Increases incidence of GTD
Previous history of hydatidiform mole	Increases incidence of GTD Women with a prior history of GTD should undergo Ist trimester sonographic examination in subsequent pregnancies
Combined oral contraceptive pills	Increases risk of GTD
Vitamin A and Carotene deficiency	Increases incidence of complete mole
Smoking Irregular menstrual cycles	Increases incidence of partial mole
Women of group A and AB	Elevated relative risk (RR) of benign mole

HYDATIDIFORM MOLE

Definition: It is a benign neoplasm of the trophoblast which involves both cytotrophoblast and syncytiotrophoblast in different proportions in different cases. Proliferation and hydropic degeneration of the chorionic villi give rise to the typical **vesicles which is characteristic of hydatidiform mole**

- Hydatidiform mole generally resolves after uterine evacuation, but they have the potential to persist despite treatment and can become invasive and hence requires follow up

It is of two types:

- Complete mole
- Partial mole

Pathology RECAP (Table 10.4)

Table 10.4 Placenta consists of three types of trophoblasts

Trophoblasts	Type	HCG secretion
Syncytiotrophoblasts (also termed as the hormonal factory of placenta)	Highly differentiated cells	Secrete HCG
Cytotrophoblasts	Primitive trophoblasts with mitotic activity	Do not secrete HCG
Intermediate trophoblasts	Invade the decidua, myometrium and blood vessels	Secrete HCG, but not to the same extent as syncytiotrophoblasts

Complete Hydatidiform Mole

Complete mole is **more common than partial mole**

Origin

- In **90% of cases,** an **"empty" ovum** containing no genomic DNA is fertilized by one sperm, which duplicates its DNA, leading to an abnormal 46, XX karyotype, with all DNA paternal in origin (Fig. 10.1)
- In the remaining 10% of cases, the "empty" ovum is fertilized by two sperm, resulting in an abnormal 46, XX or 46, XY karyotype, again with all DNA of paternal origin
- Thus, in complete mole all the chromosomes are paternally derived

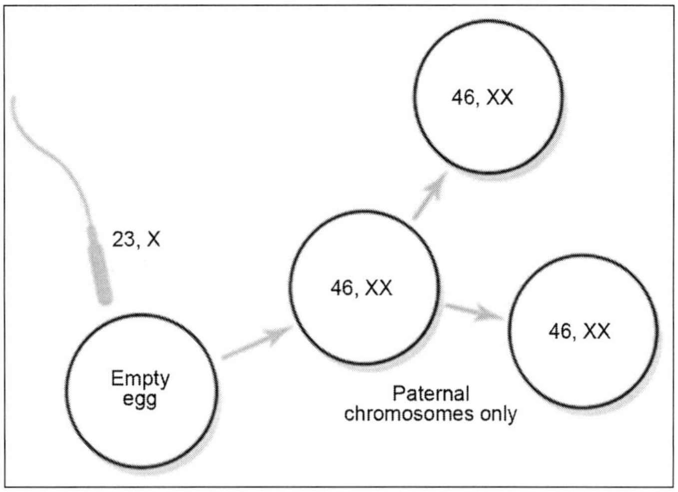

Figure 10.1: Origin of complete mole

Histologic Features

- Hydropic degeneration and marked edema of the villi **(hydropic villi)**
- Diffuse trophoblastic proliferation
- Absence of the villous blood vessels
- Absence of fetal tissue

Clinical Features

Symptoms

- **Vaginal bleeding**
  - **Most common presenting symptom (85%),** often presenting in first trimester of pregnancy
  - Molar tissue separating from decidua may disrupt maternal blood vessels leading to large volume of retained blood distending the endometrial cavity -> **anemia**
  - Patients may present with **passage of 'grape like' vesicular tissue** from the vagina (pathognomonic but occurs rarely classically described as white currant in red currant juice appearance)
- Additional classic symptoms that probably arise from stimulation by excessive hCG include:
  - **Hyperemesis gravidarum (8%)**
  - **Preeclampsia (25%)**
  - **Hyperthyroidism features (7%) (as Beta HCG simulates TSH). BL1> Abdominal pain may be present due to over-stretching of uterus, concealed hemorrhage or contractions**

Signs

- Uterine size may be **larger than expected for gestational age** (40%)

- **Uterus has a doughy consistency**
- **Absent fetal parts and fetal cardiac activity**
- **Theca lutein cysts** in the ovaries (50%)
- **Trophoblastic embolization (2%)**–patient may present with respiratory distress, chest pain, tachypnea, tachycardia during or after evacuation

Diagnosis

A **diagnosis of complete molar pregnancy** is suspected if:

- **hCG level is greater than100,000 mIU/mL**
- **Ultrasound reveals uterine cavity filled with small vesicles** instead of the expected gestational sac and fetus. **Characteristic 'snow storm appearance'**
- Pathologic correlation and cytogenetic analysis for DNA content confirms the diagnosis

Malignant Potential

- Complete molar pregnancies may result in malignant sequelae in about ***20% of cases. Risk of choriocarcinoma is 4%***

Extra edge

Theca lutein cyst:

- *Theca lutein cysts are commonly seen in Hydatiform mole*
- *Occur due to high circulating levels of hCG*
- *About 50% cases of complete mole have theca lutein cyts*
- *The cysts* ***regress spontaneously in 2-4 months after suction evacuation****. Hence, do not need any specific management*
- ***Complications :****Torsion, Infarction and Hemorrhage*

PARTIAL OR INCOMPLETE MOLE

- ***Origin:*** A partial mole occurs when two sperm fertilize a normal ovum. The resulting karyotype is 69, XXX, 69, XXY, or 69, XYY (Fig 10.2)

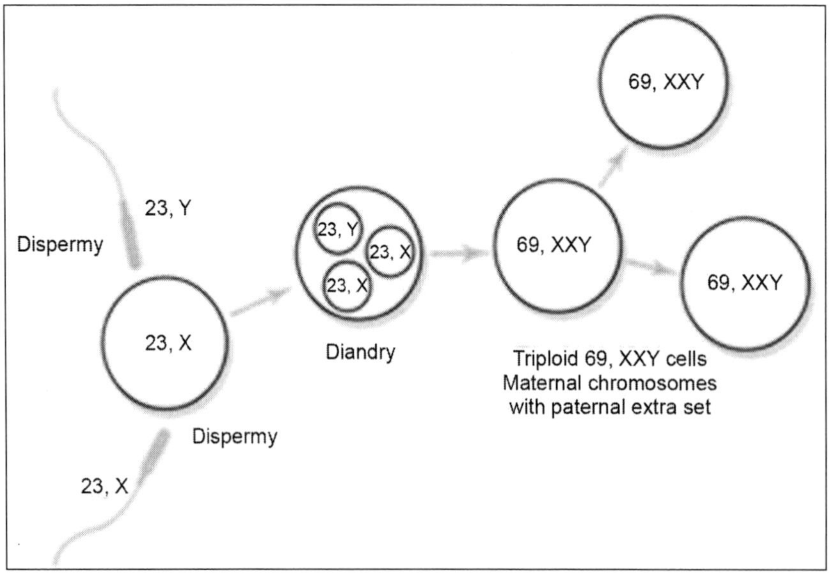

Figure 10.2: Origin of partial mole

Histologic Features

- Focal hydropic degeneration of villi
- Focal trophoblastic proliferation
- Identifiable **fetal tissue is present that is usually not viable and has features of a triploid gestation**

- Marked villous scalloping
- Prominent stromal trophoblastic inclusions

Clinical Features

- **Vaginal bleeding** is the most common presenting symptom in the first trimester, similar to complete mole
- Hyperemesis, preeclampsia, hyperthyroidism, and theca lutein cysts are rare features
- **hCG is generally not significantly elevated**
- **USG may show a fetus as well as hydropic villi and** may present as **missed abortion. Focal cystic spaces are seen within the placental tissue** are seen. The transverse to AP diameter of gestational sac is more than 3:2
- Pathologic correlation and cytogenetic analysis for DNA content confirm diagnosis
- Many spontaneous abortions may represent undiagnosed partial moles

Malignant Potential

- About 4% of partial moles progress to malignant disease. Risk of choriocarcinoma is less than 1%

Table 10.5: Comparison of complete and partial mole

Feature	Complete Mole	Partial Mole
Age	Greater risk at > 40 years	Not age related
Karyotype	90% XX, 10% XY	XXX or XXY (Triploid)
	All chromosomes paternally derived	1 chromosome set maternal origin; 2 chromosome sets paternal origin
Fetus	Absent	Present
hCG	Oftent > 100,000 mIU/mL	Rarely elevated above normal levels for pregnancy
Primary symptom	Bleeding	Rare
Secondary symptoms	Large uterine size for gestational age	Rare
	Hyperemesis	Rare
	Theca lutein cysts	Rare
	Preeclampsia	Rare
	Hyperthyroidism	Rare
Risk of persistent GTT	20%	4%

MANAGEMENT OF MOLAR PREGNANCY

Investigations

Laboratory tests

- Quantitative serum Beta hCG
- Complete blood count with platelets
- Blood grouping and typing
- Coagulation studies
- Baseline renal function test, liver function tests and thyroid function tests

Imaging studies

- Pelvic ultrasound
- Chest radiograph to evaluate for lung metastases

Treatment

- **Stabilize medical complications**-Blood pressure must be controlled (preeclampsia is common) and precautions should be taken to manage thyroid storm, if it occurs.
- **Dilatation and suction evacuation** of the uterus is the **preferred method of choice** for evacuating a molar pregnancy, independent of uterine size. Simultaneous ultrasound monitoring during the procedure is ideal

- **Steps of suction evacuation**
  - Packed cells kept ready for blood transfusion, if indicated
  - Regional/general anesthesia is administered
  - Large-bore needle for IV access is inserted
  - Cervix dilated to 10–12 mm with Hegar's dilators
  - Evacuation is done with suction cannula
  - Uterine curettage is done to ensure completion
  - Intravenous Oxytocin infusion 20 units should be given after the procedure to enhance uterine involution and minimize blood loss. Send material for histopathology
  - **Rh negative women** should be given Anti D injection following suction evacuation procedure, because if it is partial mole, there is expression of Rh factor in its fetal tissue. However, it may be with held if the diagnosis of complete mole is certain, as it does not contain fetal tissue
  - **Respiratory distress** resulting from **fluid overload, emboli of trophoblastic tissue, and thyroid storm may occur in about 2%** of cases in the perioperative period
  - **Theca lute in cysts** associated with molar gestation are not an indication for surgical intervention; resolves spontaneously as the hCG levels decreases following suction evacuation
  - **NOTE – Induction of labor and hysterotomy are not recommended**–increases maternal morbidity and the risk of post molar GTN

Role of Hysterectomy

- Hysterectomy is a treatment option for **women >40 years of age, who have completed their families. Ovaries are usually retained**
- **Also indicated in cases with uterine perforation, invasive mole uterine hemorrhage and sepsis BL 1> Advantage of hysterectomy - it averts or reduces risk of embolization**

Note

- *There is a concern that uterine contractions may force the trophoblastic tissues into the venous sinuses and cause embolization. Therefore,* ***oxytocin infusion should be started only after the evacuation is begun and prostaglandins for cervical ripening must be avoided***
- ***Hysterectomy eliminates the possibility of invasive mole and reduces risk of GTN. Metastatic gestational trophoblastic neoplasia can still occur even after hysterectomy; hence, follow-up is mandatory***

Risk of Gestational Trophoblastic Neoplasia (GTN) Following Evacuation of Molar Pregnancy

- **Risk of developing GTN** after evacuation is **20% for a complete mole and 4% for a partial mole**
- **About 15% develop locally invasive disease and 4–5% develop metastatic disease**
- **High Risk factors for development of GTN**
  - Uterus larger than period of gestation
  - Pretreatment hCG greater than 100,000 mIU/mL
  - Theca lutein cysts greater than 6 cm
  - Age more than 40 years
  - Women with previous history of molar pregnancy

Role of Prophylactic Chemotherapy

- Chemotherapy after evacuation of complete mole has been **tried in high-risk women who are not compliant with follow up for beta hCG surveillance and it has been shown to reduce the incidence of GTN**
- Both **Methotrexate and Actinomycin D** may be used as a single dose
- However, use of **prophylactic chemotherapy is controversial and is not routinely offered due to the risks of increased drug resistance and toxic side effects. This practice is not currently recommended by ACOG 2014**

- It is only used **in countries with limited resources to reliably monitor / follow up patients after evacuation**
- It may have a role in women with multiple **high-risk factors for developing GTN**

Postmolar Follow Up

- **Hyperthyroidism and hypertension, if present, usually regress after evacuation of mole**
- Theca lutein cysts regress spontaneously in 2–4 months
- Serum β-**hCG serves as a sensitive marker for surveillance** after evacuation of mole
- The earlier recommendation was to monitor quantitative serum HCG levels
  - Weekly till 3 consecutive values are normal (<5 mIU/mL)
  - Monthly for 6 consecutive months
- But it has been found that after a single normal level of β-hCG, progression to GTN is unlikely. Therefore, current recommendation is that **surveillance can be discontinued when a single value of β-hCG is undetectable or<2 mIU/mL**
- Average time for HCG to come back to normal is **9 weeks for complete mole and 7 week for partial mole**

Contraception

- If pregnancy occurs during follow-up, the associated increase in β-hCG can interfere with detection of GTN. Hence, contraception is advised during the follow up period
- **Intrauterine devices can cause irregular bleeding** and increases risk of uterine perforation if an invasive mole is present. Hence, **IUCDs are not recommended**
- **Combined oral contraceptive pills or depot medroxyprogesterone acetate (DMPA) is recommended of contraception during post molar follow up**
- Injectable medroxyprogesterone acetate is particularly useful when poor compliance is anticipated

DIAGNOSIS OF GTN FOLLOWING HYDATIDIFORM MOLE

- Most cases of GTN occur during postmolar surveillance; hence, certain criteria are used for diagnosis

Criteria for the diagnosis of Postmolar GTN/ Persistent GTD (FIGO 2000)
• Plateau of hCG lasting for four measurements, over a period of 3 weeks or longer, that is, days 1, 7, 14, 21
• Rise of hCG>10% on three consecutive weekly measurements, over a period of 2 weeks or longer, that is, days 1, 7, 14
• Persistence of detectable levels of hCG for >6 months
• Histological diagnosis of choriocarcinoma

Extra Edge

Quiescent Gestational Trophoblastic Disease

- *In few women, low levels (<200 mIU/mL) of hCG persist for several months after evacuation of mole, indicative of a small active focus of syncytiotrophoblast cells*
- *About 10% of these cases will develop active GTN; therefore, close follow-up is essential*
- *Quiescent GTN is however not an indication for chemotherapy*
- ***Hyperglycosylated hCG (hCG-H),*** *a variant of β-hCG, may be used to differentiate between* ***quiescent and active GTN***
- ***Hyperglycosylated hCG (hCG-H)*** *is produced by the invasive cytotrophoblasts during implantation and in GTN. It is* ***more sensitive and specific for the diagnosis of GTN and a rising level indicates development of active disease***

Extra Edge

Molar Pregnancy with Coexisting Fetus

In a twin pregnancy, rarely, one can be a complete mole and the other a normal fetus. Complications associated with this condition include:

- *Spontaneous abortion*
- *Chromosomal anomalies*
- *Pre-eclampsia*
- *Fetal growth restriction*

In the absence of complications and normal genetic and ultrasound findings, pregnancy can be continued.

GESTATIONAL TROPHOBLASTIC NEOPLASIA

INTRODUCTION

- **The locally invasive and metastatic subtypes of GTD are known as GTNs.** It includes
  - Invasive mole
  - Choriocarcinoma
  - PSTT
  - ETT
- **Majority of GTNs occur after a complete mole,** but GTN can occur after any gestation such as the following:
  - Molar pregnancy (50%)
  - Miscarriage
  - Tubal pregnancy
  - Normal term or preterm pregnancy
- **Invasive mole and choriocarcinoma are the GTN common;** PSTT and ETT are rare
- **Invasive mole and choriocarcinoma** are associated with **high levels of hCG; PSTT and ETT have low hCG levels**
- The diagnosis of GTN is often made on the basis of clinical presentation, elevated β-hCG and evidence of metastases on imaging. Hence, a definitive histological diagnosis of the type of GTN is not made in most cases
- **GTN require formal staging and respond favorably to chemotherapy**
- **The prognosis, preservation of fertility and successful subsequent pregnancy outcomes are good in most of the GTN**

Risk Factors

Risk factors for developing of GTN after hydatidiform mole includes:

- Uterus larger than period of gestation
- Pretreatment hCG greater than 100,000 mIU/mL
- Theca lutein cysts greater than 6 cm
- Age more than 40 years
- Women with previous history of molar pregnancy

INVASIVE MOLE

- Invasive mole is the **most common GTN**
- It is locally invasive but can metastasize in 5% of cases
- Invasive mole always develops after a complete or partial mole. BL1> The other name for invasive mole is chorioadenoma desterens

Clinical Features

- Vaginal bleeding
- Uterus size larger than POG
- Elevated serum β-hCG

Pathology

- Hydropic villi are present. The proliferating cytotrophoblasts and syncytiotrophoblasts invade the myometrium and serosa, parametrium and vaginal wall. Usually cells are monomorphic.
- **Presence of villi with trophoblasts extending into the myometrium** is the characteristic feature of invasive mole

Complications

- Uterine perforation
- Intraperitoneal hemorrhage
- Profuse vaginal bleeding
- Sepsis

CHORIOCARCINOMA

- This is the second common GTN after invasive mole
- It constitutes about 30–40% of GTN cases
- Choriocarcinoma can develop after term pregnancies, molar pregnancies, abortions or ectopic pregnancies
- **GTN that develops after a term pregnancy is often choriocarcinoma**
- Choriocarcinomais an aggressive tumor-locally invasive and metastasizes rapidly

Pathology

Macroscopic appearance: Choriocarcinoma appears as highly vascular, dark red or blackish mass with hemorrhage. The growth can be seen **extending into the myometrium**

Microscopic Appearance

- The tumor is composed of sheets **of anaplastic cytotrophoblasts and syncytiotrophoblasts and is seen extending into the myometrium**
- There is **extensive necrosis and hemorrhage** and is **characterized by the absence of chorionic villi**
- The metastatic lesions are hemorrhagic, dark red or black and well circumscribed

Pattern of Spread

- **Early hematogenous spread** is characteristic of choriocarcinoma (Table 10.6)

Table 10.6: Hematogenous spread in choriocarcinoma

	Frequency (%)
Lung	80
Vagina	30
Pelvis	20
Liver	10
Central nervous system	10
Other	
Spleen	<5
Kidney	<5
Gastrointestinal tract	<5

Lung Metastasis

- **Most common site of** metastasis
- Patient presents with respiratory symptoms like dyspnea, hemoptysis, chest pain
- **On X-ray it may produce the following four patterns:**
  - An alveolar **snow storm pattern**
  - Discrete rounded densities or **canon ball appearance**
  - Pleural effusion
  - An embolic pattern caused by pulmonary arterial occlusion

Vaginal Metastasis

- Second most common site of metastasis
- Occurs **as suburethral nodules or in fornices**
- Appears as **purple hemorrhagic projections**–highly vascular and bleed on touch

Metastasis to other pelvic organs, liver and brain also occurs through the hematogenous route

PLACENTAL SITE TROPHOBLASTIC TUMOR

- This is a rare tumor that develops from **extravillous, intermediate trophoblasts**
- **It is locally invasive but can metastasize**
- Serum **hCG levels are low**
- **Identification of high proportion of free b-hCG (>30%) is considered diagnostic**
- **Human placental lactogen (hPL) is another tumor marker that may be elevated**
- PSTT occurs more often following normal pregnancy or abortion
- Histology–**Intermediate cell hyperplasia; no villi**
- It has high potential for metastasis
- **Does not respond to chemotherapy**
- **Treatment of choice is hysterectomy**

EPITHELIOID TROPHOBLASTIC TUMOR

- This is a very rare tumor that **arises from intermediate trophoblasts, but is histologically distinct from PSTT**
- Histology–**no villi;** cells are smaller and display less nuclear pleomorphism; **Epithelioid trophoblastic tumor grows in a nodular fashion** (Intermediate trophoblast nodules surrounded by Extrachorionic membrane) rather than the infiltrative pattern of PSTT. **'Geographic' necrosis** is often present
- **Serum hCG levels are low** and diagnosis is usually late
- The diagnosis is usually **confirmed by endometrial biopsy**
- It is locally invasive but can metastasize
- Patients may present with metastasis and may be chemoresistance to multiagent therapy, leading to poor prognosis
- Hysterectomy is the primary treatment of choice

STAGING OF GESTATIONAL TROPHOBLASTIC NEOPLASIA

GTN Staging recommended by the International Federation of Obstetrics and Gynecology (FIGO, 2000) – Table 10.7; Figure 10.3

Table 10.7: Staging of Gestational Trophoblastic Neoplasia

Stage I	Disease confined to the uterus; persistent elevation of serum β-hCG
Stage II	GTN extends outside of the uterus but is limited to the genital structures (adnexa, vagina, broad ligament)
Stage III	GTN extends to the lungs, with or without known genital tract involvement
Stage IV	All other metastatic sites (brain,liver)

FIGO, International Federation of Obstetrics and Gynecology: GTN, gestational trophoblastic neoplasia; hCG, human chorionic gonadotrophin

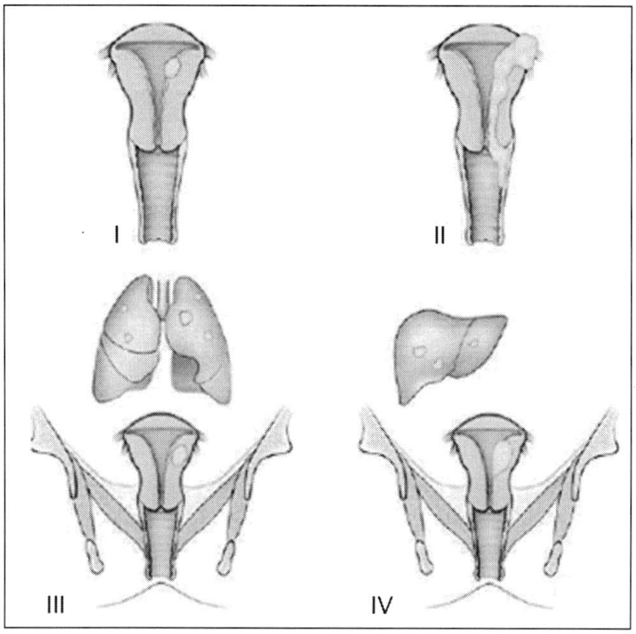

Figure 10.3: Staging of Gestational Trophoblastic Neoplasia

RISK FACTOR SCORING FOR GTN

- The risk factor prognostic scoring system was developed by the World Health Organization (WHO) and has been modified by FIGO and is currently recommended for risk scoring (Table 10.8)

Table 10.8: Risk Factor Scoring for GTN

	Score			
	0	1	2	4
Age (years)	<40	≥40	–	–
Antecedent pregnancy	Mole	Abortion	Term	–
Interval months from index pregnancy	<4	4-6	7-12	≥13
Pretreatment serum β-hCG (mlU/mL)	$<10^3$	10^3–$<10^4$	10^4–$<10^5$	$\geq 10^5$
Largest tumor size (including uterus)		3–<5 cm	≥ 5cm	
Sites of metastases	Lung	Spleen, kidney	Gastrointestinal	Liver, brain
Number of metastases	–	1-4	5-8	>8
Previous failed chemotherapy	–	–	1 drug	≥2 drugs
hCG, human chorionic gonadotroph				

- **A score of 0–6 is low-risk disease and can be managed by monotherapy**
- **A score of ≥7 is high-risk disease and requires combination chemotherapy**

COMBINATION OF FIGO STAGING AND RISK FACTOR SCORING FOR GTN

- **The combination of FIGO staging and risk factor scoring is currently used for management of GTN**
- Women with stage I usually have a low-risk score and most women in stage IV have a high-risk score. Therefore, combined scoring is most useful in stages II and III
- The stage is represented by Roman numeral (I–IV), followed by a colon and the risk score in Arabic numerals (e.g. FIGO stage III: 10)

CLINICAL FEATURES

- GTN that develops during follow-up after evacuation of hydatidiform mole is usually **diagnosed when serum β-hCG levels do not normalize as expected.** The criteria for diagnosis of post molar GTN has been mentioned earlier
- GTN can be metastatic or non metastatic
- Women who develop post molar GTN may present with **irregular vaginal bleeding or amenorrhea, enlarged uterus, persistent theca lutein cysts or vaginal nodules**
- When GTN develops following abortion or normal pregnancy, symptoms depend on the stage of the disease

Clinical Features of Non-metastatic Disease

- Disease confined to the uterus can be asymptomatic
- Vaginal bleeding
- Amenorrhea
- Uterine enlargement
- Persistent theca lutein cysts (due to persistently elevated hCG)
- Intraperitoneal bleeding (due to uterine perforation)
- Purulent vaginal discharge (due to sepsis)

Clinical Features of Metastatic Disease

- Can be asymptomatic
- Symptoms and signs of metastatic disease depend on the site of metastasis (Table 10.9)

Table 10.9 Clinical features of metastatic disease

Site of metastasis	Clinical features
Lung metastasis	• **Most common site of metastasis (80%)** • May present with cough, hemoptysis and secondary pulmonary hypertension
Vaginal metastasis	• Second most common site of metastasis (30%) • Most common site –**Suburethral nodule** • Nodules are very vascular and bleed profusely, if biopsied
Liver metastasis	• Occurs late, more common in GTN following term pregnancy • May present with jaundice, epigastric pain • Hepatic lesions can stretch the liver capsule and cause capsular rupture resulting in intraperitoneal bleeding
Brain metastasis	• Causes convulsions and focal neurological deficits depending on the location

NOTE-Liver and brain metastases are usually associated with lung and pelvic metastasis

Diagnostic Evaluation

The patient should be evaluated by history, clinical examination and investigations to determine the following:

- Extent of the disease
- Stage of the disease
- Risk factor scoring
- Presence or absence of metastases

History and Physical examination in a case of GTN

History in GTN	Physical examination in GTN
• Age • Symptoms • Duration of symptoms • Interval from antecedent pregnancy • Antecedent pregnancy – Mole – Miscarriage – Term pregnancy – Ectopic gestation • Prior treatment – Evacuation of mole – Hysterectomy – Chemotherapy o Single agent o Combination	• General examination – Pallor • Respiratory system – Respiratory rate – Rales on auscultation • Central nervous system – Level of consciousness – Focal neurological deficits • Abdominal examination – Hepatomegaly, tenderness – Uterine enlargement – Intraperitoneal bleeding o Guarding o Ragidity • Speculum examination – Suburethral/vaginal nodules – Bleeding • Bimanual examination – Uterine size – Theca lutein cysts

INVESTIGATIONS

Serum β-hCG

- When GTN is suspected, estimation of serum β-hCG is the first step in diagnostic evaluation
- Serum β-hCG levels are very high in choriocarcinoma
- Pretreatment value is of prognostic significance and should be documented

Imaging

- Imaging helps in diagnosis of the uterine lesion and metastases (Table 10.10)

Table 10.10: Imaging modality in evaluation of GTN

Imaging modality	Helps in detection of the following:
Ultrasonography of abdomen and pelvis	Uterine lesion Theca lutein cyst Hepatic metastasis
Chest X-ray	Diagnosis and number of pulmonary metastases Should be done in all cases of GTN
Computed tomography (CT) thorax	Pulmonary micrometastasis
CT abdomen	Hepatic and intra-abdominal lesions
Magnetic resonance imaging (MRI) or CT brain (done if pulmonary metastasis is present)	Brain metastasis
Positron emission tomography (PET)	Useful when MRI/CT does not reveal metastasis but β-hCG is elevated

NOTE-Metastatic lesions are very friable, and biopsy to confirm diagnosis is not recommended. *In the setting of appropriate clinical history and elevated hCG, lesions visualized on radiographic studies are treated presumptively*

Pretreatment investigations

All women with GTN need chemotherapy. Pretreatment investigations includes the following:

- Complete blood count
- Liver and renal functions
- Baseline serum β-hCG level must be documented

MANAGEMENT OF GTN

- **Chemotherapy is the mainstay of management of GTN**
- Women with **low-risk GTN by the risk scoring system are treated with single-agent chemotherapy**
- Women with **high-risk GTN are treated with multiagent therapy**
- Hysterectomy is warranted in some situations in the management of GTN

Indications for Hysterectomy

Hysterectomy followed by adjuvant single-agent chemotherapy is considered as the first choice in following cases:

Indications for hysterectomy
• Women with low-risk GTN who do not desire fertility
• Perforating mole with Intraperitoneal haemorrhage
• Uncontrolled vaginal bleeding
• Chemoresistant disease confined to the uterus
• Placental site trophoblastic tumor
• Epitheloid trophoblastic tumor

MANAGEMENT OF LOW-RISK GTN

Criteria for Low-risk Disease

Low-risk disease includes women with a WHO risk score of 1–6. It includes:

- Almost all women with stage I disease
- Women with stage II/III with WHO score 1–6

Management

- Hysterectomy should be considered in older women who do not desire fertility, followed by chemotherapy
- Treatment of **low-risk disease is by single-agent chemotherapy**
- **Methotrexate and Actinomycin D** are the commonly used chemotherapeutic agents
- Serum β-hCG should be monitored weekly, until three consecutive values are normal
- If hCG levels plateau or rise (no response to therapy), switch to alternative drugs–If methotrexate resistant, switch to Actinomycin D; If Actinomycin resistant, switch to methotrexate
- Other drugs that have been used are oral etoposide and 5-fluorouracil
- **Contraception should be continued for 12 months**
- Response to therapy is usually good, fertility is preserved and cure rate is 100%

Methotrexate

- Methotrexate is the **drug of choice for GTN**
- **MOA:** Methotrexate is a **folic acid antagonist,** that acts on the rapidly dividing cells. It acts by **inhibiting the enzyme folic acid reductase,** required for folic acid metabolism (Folic acid is required for the synthesis of thymidine and purine, which are essential for DNA and RNA synthesis)

- **Folinic acid rescue**–Folinic acid, which has the same action as folic acid, is not inhibited by methotrexate. Folinic acid is administered alternating with methotrexate to prevent toxicity when the drug is used in high doses
- **Both intramuscular (IM) and intravenous methotrexate regimens are** proved to be effective in the management of GTN
- **Dosage and administration** of methotrexate regimens are as follows (Table 10.11)

Table 10.11: Dosage and administration of methotrexate regimens

Dose	Frequency	Route of administration
30-50 mg/m^2	Weekly	IM
1 mg/kg, days 1, 3, 5, 7, alternating with 0.1 mg/kg, days 2, 4, 6, 8	Every 2 weeks	IM
0.4 mg/kg/day for 5 days	Alternate weeks	IM
100 mg/m^2	Every 2 weeks	IV infusion
IM, intramuscular; IV, intravenous		

- **Adverse effects**–mucositis, diarrhea, stomatitis, nausea, alopecia, bone marrow suppression, Hepatotoxicity
- **Complete blood count and Liver function tests** should be monitored during treatment with high-dose regimens. Methotrexate should be **with held, if the liver enzymes are elevated or the total leucocyte count and platelet count decreases**
- Remission rate is 80%
- Response rates are similar with all the regimens. The 8-day methotrexate with folinic acid rescue regimen and the weekly IM dosing are the frequently used regimens .

Actinomycin D

- **Second-line drug of choice** used in the treatment of GTN
- **Efficacy is similar to that of methotrexate but toxicity is higher**
- It is usually used when there is no response to methotrexate
- Dosage and route of administration are as follows:
  - Dosage
    - 9-13 μg/kg/day IV × 5 days every 2 weeks
    - 1.25 mg/m^2 IV bolus every 2 weeks
- Adverse effects–Alopecia, nausea, nephrotoxicity

MANAGEMENT OF HIGH-RISK GTN

Criteria for High-risk Disease

High-risk GTN includes patients with risk score of 7 or more. It includes:

- Women with stage IV disease
- Women with stage II/III disease with WHO score ≥7

Management

- High-risk GTN require aggressive therapy with multiagent chemotherapy (Table 10.12)
- **The multidrug regimen consists of Etoposide, Methotrexate, Actinomycin D, Cyclophosphamide and Vincristine (Oncovin) with Folinic Acid Rescue (EMA-CO / BAGSHAW regimen)**
- Each course is given for **over 8 days and next course started on day 15** (every 2 weeks)

Table 10.12: Multiagent chemotherapy for high risk GTN

Day	Drug	Dosage
1	Etoposide	100 mg/m^2 IV over 30 minutes
	Methotrexate	100 mg/m^2 IV bolus followed by 200 mg/m^2 IV over 12 hours
	Actinomycin D	0.5 mg IV bolus
2	Etoposide	100 mg/m^2 IV over 30 minutes
	Actinomycin D	0.5 mg IV bolus
	Folinic acid	15 mg oral Q12H for four doses
3	Cyclophosphamide	600 mg/m^2 IV
	Vincristine	1.0 mg/m^2 IV

GTN, gestational trophoblastic neoplasia; IV, intravenous

- Monitor serum Beta-hCG weekly till three consecutive values are normal; then, monthly Beta-hCG till 12 consecutive nondetectable levels
- Monitoring response by serum β-hCG:
  - Response: >10% decline in β-hCG
  - Plateau: ± 10% change in β-hCG
  - Resistance: <10% rise in β-hCG
- Switch to alternative regime if resistant to therapy-Alternative regimen is modification of the EMA-CO regimen by substituting with Etoposide and Cisplatin on day 8 **(EMA-EP)**
- **Adverse effects** of Multiagent chemotherapy - alopecia, stomatitis, gastrointestinal mucositis and myelosuppression
- **Management of chemoresistant metastases**–Surgery, Radiation and Selective arterial embolization
- Remission rate with **EMA-CO is 75-80%**
- The regimen is well tolerated and **fertility rate following treatment is good**
- **Surveillance and contraception should be continued for 24 months since late recurrences can occur**
- For those patients with liver metastases, brain metastases, or a very high-risk score, other more intensive chemotherapy regimen, may yield a better response and outcome, such as follows:

Salvage therapies
• EP-EMA (etoposide, cisplatin, etoposide, methotrexate and actinomycin-D)
• TP/TE (paclitaxel, cisplatin/paclitaxel, etoposide)
• MBE (methotrexate, bleomycin, etoposide)
• VIP or ICE (etoposide, ifosfamide, and cisplatin or carboplatin)
• BEP (bleomycin, etoposide, cisplatin)
• FA (5-fluorouracil, actionmycin-D)
• FAEV (floxuridine, actionmycin-D, etoposide, vincristine)
• High-dose chemotherapy with autologous bone marrow or stem cell transplant
• Immunotherapy with pembrolizumab

MANAGEMENT OF METASTASES

Patients with metastatic disease may require surgical intervention to remove chemoresistant disease or to control hemorrhage (Table 10.13)

Table 10.13: Management of metastases

Site	Intervention	Indication
Vagina	• Packing • Wide local excision • Local radiation • Arterial embolization (commonly performed in hypogastric embolization)	Profuse bleeding

Contd.

Contd.

Lung	Pulmonary wedge resection	Chemoresistant disease
Liver	Intra-arterial chemotherapy	Chemoresistant disease
	Partial hepatic resection	
	Arterial embolization	
Brain	Whole brain irradiation (intrathecal methotrexate can avert hemorrhage and can cause shrinkage of tumor if craniotomy is planned)	Chemoresistant disease

MANAGEMENT OF PLACENTAL SITE TROPHOBLASTIC TUMOR (PSTT) AND EPITHELOID TROPHOBLASTIC TUMOR (ETT)

- PSTT and ETT **do not respond well to chemotherapy**
- **Hysterectomy** is the recommended treatment
- In advanced stages, EP-EMA or TE/TP can be considered
- Interval from antecedent pregnancy of more than 48 months seems to be the most significant adverse prognostic factor
- Prognosis in metastatic disease is poor

Summary of the treatment Protocol for GTN

Stage I

Low-risk GTN : Single-agent chemotherapy

High risk : Combination therapy

Failure : Hysterectomy

Stages II and III

Low risk : Single agent till family is completed, then hysterectomy

High risk : Combination therapy; hysterectomy to reduce tumor mass

Resistant : Hysterectomy

Stage IV

Combination chemotherapy
Surgery (Hepatic resection, craniotomy)
Radiation (For cerebral metastasis)

Survival Rate

GTN has an **overall good prognosis** following therapy (Table 10.14)

Table 10.14: Survival rate in GTN

GTN	Survival rate
Low-risk disease	100%
High-risk disease	80-90%
Brain metastasis	50–60%

MANAGEMENT OF FUTURE PREGNANCIES FOLLOWING GTD

- **Contraception should be advised for all women during** the follow up period after treatment of molar pregnancy and GTN
- There is **1–2% risk of having a repeat molar pregnancy** in future conceptions following a molar pregnancy. Hence, ultrasonography should be performed in the first trimester to confirm a viable pregnancy
- An **hCG measurement should be obtained 6 weeks** after completion of any future pregnancy to exclude occult trophoblastic disease
- **Outcome of pregnancies after chemotherapy for GTN is found to be normal**

RECENT UPDATES

- *Recent evidence indicates that some patients with* ***recurrent CHM have diploid biparental CHM (BiCHM)*** *rather than the typical androgenetic CHM (AnCHM). In these cases, the molar phenotype is due to an* ***autosomal recessive condition,*** *familial recurrent HM (FRHM) that predisposes women to recurrent pregnancy loss, most usually CHM*
- *Mutations in two genes have now been associated with recurrent molar pregnancy:* **NLRP7** ***and*** **KHDC3L.** Reason for familial repetitive mole-missense mutation in NLRP7 gene located in chromosome 19
- *While women with recurrent* ***AnCHM are likely to have normal live births*** *in subsequent pregnancies and benefit from conventional in vitro fertilisation, women with* ***FRHM are unlikely to achieve a normal pregnancy*** *except through ovum donation from an unaffected individual*

Immunohistochemical staining and molecular genotypingin molar pregnancy

- ***Histopathologic evaluation of the tissue obtained can be enhanced by immunohistochemical staining and by molecular genotyping***
- ***p57KIP2 is a nuclear protein*** *whose gene is paternally imprinted and* ***maternally expressed and is produced only in tissues containing a maternal allele***
- *As complete moles contain only paternal genes,* ***p57KIP2 protein is absent in complete moles,*** *and tissues do not pick up this stain*
- *In contrast, this* ***nuclear protein is strongly expressed in normal placentas, spontaneous pregnancy losses with hydropic degeneration, and partial moles***
- *To* ***differentiatea partial mole from a nonmolar hydropic abortus (both express p57), molecular genotyping*** *can be used*
- ***Molecular genotyping determines the parental source of polymorphic alleles.*** *It can distinguish among a diploid diandric genome (complete mole), a triploid diandric-monogenic genome (partial mole), or biparental diploidy (nonmolar abortus)*
- *Genotyping can also be useful in the identification of BiCHM, associated with FRHM, since most are pathologically indistinguishable from typical AnCHM*
- *Unfortunately, there are no histological or immune histochemical features that reliably predict which patients will subsequently develop persistent GTD (pGTD)/GTN, and hence all HMs require hCG surveillance. BL1> Recently cytokeratin 20 is identified as biological marker which can distinguish between physiological and pathological trophoblastic tissue.*

GTD IMMUNO HISTOCHEMISTRY MARKERS

- *P63- myoepithelial layer*
- *CD10-endometrial stromal differentiation*
- *Perivascular epithelioid cells-melanocytic and smooth muscle markers.*
- *P57 immunostaining –positive in partial mole (maternal chromosome)*
- *Hsd3b1- specific trophoblastic tissue marker*
- *Cytotrophoblasts-positive for CD 10 and cytokeratin,negative for HCG, HPL*
- *Syncytiotrophoblasts-HCG, PLAP positive*
- *Placental site nodule-intermediate trophoblasts with CK18, plap, HCG, HPL positive, Ki 67 index low <10%*
- *Choriocarcinoma – b-HCG strong positive, CK 18, inhibin positive, high Ki 67 index, HPL –weak positive*
- *Placental site trophoblastic tumour-positive for HPL, mel- cam (cd 146), mucin 4 and CD10, ki67 index high, weak positive for b- HCG*
- *Epiththelioid trophoblastic tumour-p63 positive, Hsd3b1, e-cadherin, cyclin E positive*
- *Hyperglycosylated HCG (HCG-h) – more in active gestational trophoblastic diseases than quiescent GTN.*

CHAPTER 11

PRINCIPLES OF RADIOTHERAPY IN GYNECOLOGIC CANCERS

INTRODUCTION

- Radiotherapy and chemotherapy are the important modalities of cancer therapy apart from surgery
- They may have the following roles in treatment of cancers:
  - **Curative role** when used as a primary therapy (e.g. radiotherapy in carcinoma cervix and chemotherapy in gestational trophoblastic neoplasia)
  - **Adjuvant role** when multidisciplinary approach is used for treatment of some cancers to improve survival outcome
  - **Palliation role** in advanced cancers with in capacitating symptoms. Palliative radiotherapy aims to achieve symptomatic relief, when cure may not be achieved. It may have little or no impact on the survival outcome of the patient

Biological Effects of Radiation (Radiobiology)

Modes of action of Radiotherapy (Fig 11.1):

- **Direct action:** When the radiation is absorbed, it causes damage to cell DNA directly. This is the predominant mechanism of action of particulate radiation (neutrons)
- **Indirect action:** When the radiation interacts with other substances (H2O) in the cell, it produces free radicals (OH–) which in turn damage the cell DNA

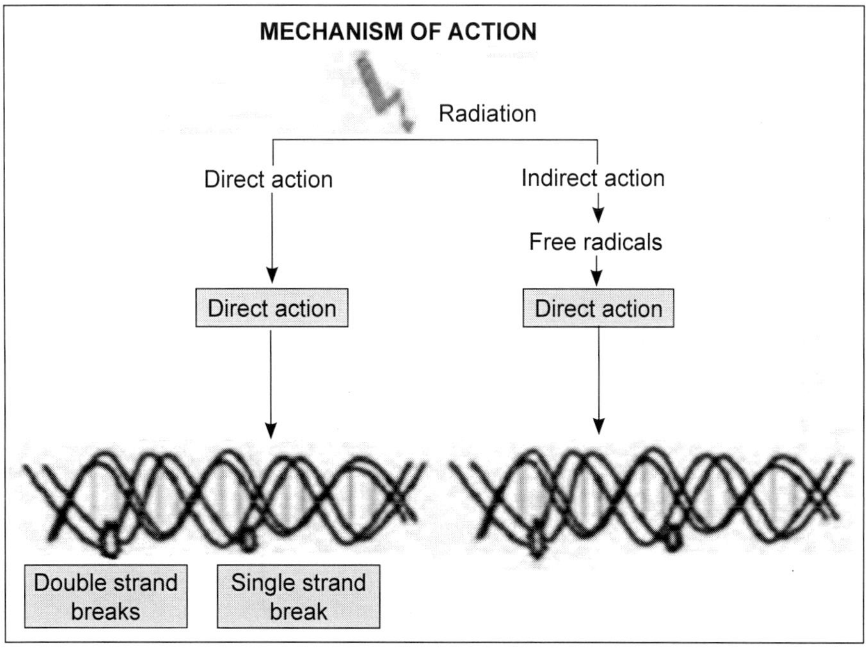

Figure 11.1: Mechanism of action of radiotherapy

Compton effect (Fig 11.2)

- Radiation while passing through tissues **produces fast electrons by dislodging** the orbital electrons -> This fast electron ionizes molecules along its path leading to production of **free hydrogen atoms, free hydroxyl radicals and hydrogen**

peroxide (H2O2) -> The ionized molecules react with proteins, enzymes and nucleic acids resulting in **structural and functional alteration of a cell**

- The target for radiation injury is cell DNA, leading to limited cell mitosis and cell death
- Ionizing radiation damages nuclear and plasma membranes and produces cytoplasmic vacuolation and fragmentation
- The effect of ionizing radiation is common for both the normal and neoplastic tissues encountered in the radiation path
- **Complications of RT are mainly due to interaction with the normal tissues**
- Lethal effect of radiation leads to cell death. When the radiation effect is sub lethal, cell DNA may undergo repair and the cell survives

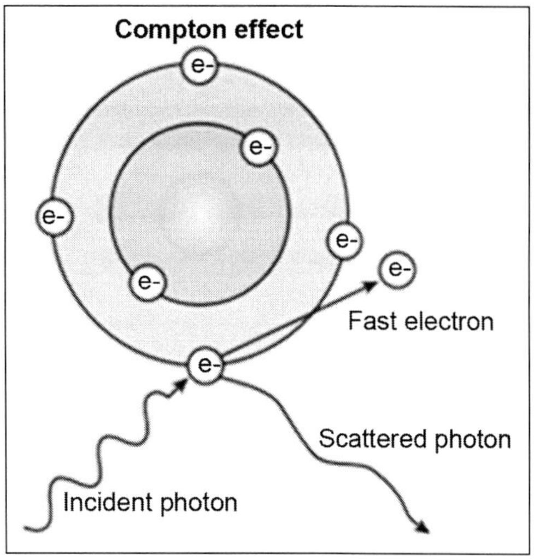

Figure 11.2: Crompton effect

Effect of Radiation on Tissues

It depends upon the **total dose of** radiation, **time duration** over which radiotherapy is administered and the **radio sensitivity** of the particular cell types

Effect of RT on tissues may be as follows:

- **Apoptosis or programmed cell death**–Loss of mature functional cells by apoptosis usually occurs within 24 hours of radiation
- **Loss of cellular reproductive capacity**
- **Gene mutation**

Four 'R's of Radiobiology

These are related to the influence of dose, time, and fractionation on the cellular response to radiation

- **Repair**–Fractionated irradiation permits greater recovery of sublethal injury during treatment. Therefore, **a higher total dose of radiation is required to achieve a given biologic effect when the total dose is divided into smaller fractions.** Broader the shoulder of the survival curve, the greater is the increase in dose required to achieve the same level of cell death as achieved by single dose
- **Repopulation**–Repopulation refers to the **cell proliferation that occurs during the delivery of radiation**
- **Redistribution**–Cells are usually **most sensitive to radiation in late G2 phase and during mitosis and are most resistant in the mid-to late S phase and early G1 phase**
- **Reoxygenation–Sensitivity of fully oxygenated cells to ionizing radiation** is approximately **three times** that of cells irradiated under **anoxic conditions**

Concept of Therapeutic Ratio (Figure 11.3)

- Concept of the therapeutic ratio for radiotherapy, **compares the radiation dose-response curves for tumor control and side effects in normal tissue**
- **Optimal tumor control curve lies to the left of the normal tissue curve**
- For every incremental increase in total dose required to control the tumor, there is a corresponding increase in likelihood of normal tissue side effects due to treatment
- **Magnitude of the difference between effective tumor cell kill and the likelihood of treatment related side effects corresponds to the therapeutic ratio**

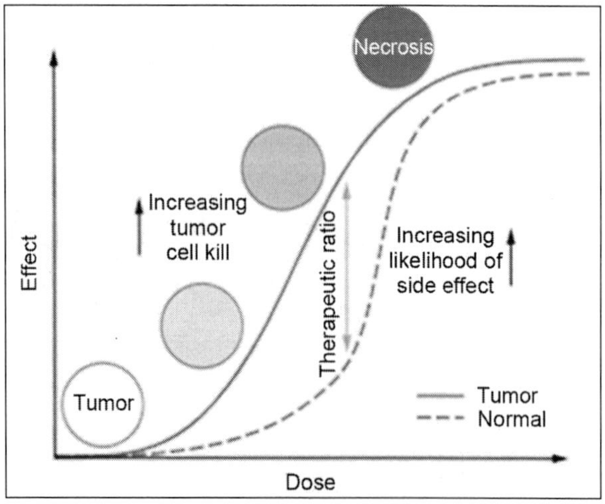

Figure 11.3: Therapeutic ratio for radiotherapy

TYPES OF IONIZING RADIATION USED FOR THERAPY

- Ionizing radiation may be electromagnetic (non particulate) or particulate radiation (Figure 11.4):

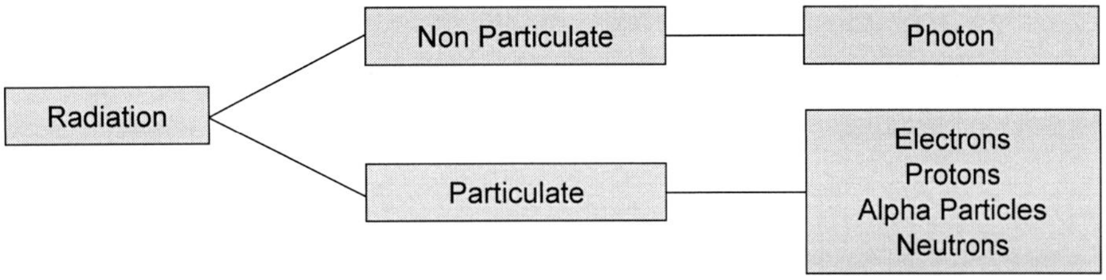

Figure 11.4: Types of ionizing radiation

Electromagnetic Radiation

- It consists of quanta of energy and wavelength (photon radiation)
- It is of two types–**X-rays and gamma rays that are collectively called photons**
- When photons interact with matter (tissue), **the following effects are observed**
  - Photoelectric effect
  - Compton scattering
  - Pair production.
- In human radiation therapy, **Compton scattering is the major interaction of photons with tissues**
- **X-rays and gamma rays have shorter wavelength and high frequency**
- **X-rays and gamma rays** possess considerable **power of tissue penetration** depending on the **photon energy and the density of the matter through which they pass**
- **Photons** have suitable tissue penetration property and can be used for **deep seated cancers**
- External photon beam radiation is usually derived from a **linear accelerator**

Radioactive Nuclei Particles

- **Isotopes** are atoms of an element with same number of protons but different number of neutrons at its nuclear core
- **Isotopes may be stable or unstable. Unstable isotopes try to attain stability by ejection of particles.** This process produces **ionizing radiation with emission of alpha and beta particles and gamma rays**
- Radioactive sources used for therapeutic purpose include **Radium 226, Cesium 137, Gold 198, Iodine 125, Cobalt 60, Iridium 192.** These give off **alpha and beta particles and gamma rays**
- **Radioactive substances** are **encapsulated** to **absorb alpha and beta particles, leaving gamma rays to attain therapeutic purpose**
- Half-lives of common radioactive isotopes are given in Table 11.1

Table 11.1 Half-lives of common radioactive isotopes

Radionuclide	Half-Life (Days)
Gold-198	2.7
Phosphorus-32	14.3
Iodine-125	60
Iridium-192	74.4
Cobalt-60	5.3
Caesium-137	30
Radium-226	1620

Particulate Radiation

- This consists of **atomic sub particles such as electrons, protons and neutrons**
- **Only electrons (β-rays) are used in radiotherapy**
- **High energy electron beams** are produced by **linear accelerators**

- Electrons lose energy rapidly as they travel in tissues and has limited tissue penetration
- **Transcervical electron irradiation** is used for **control of hemorrhage** in cervical carcinoma

Recent advances

High linear energy transfer

- X-rays and γ-rays are less effective against hypoxic cells compared to oxygenated cells
- **Fast neutrons or negative π mesons (pions) are very effective against hypoxic cells.** These have **high biologic effectiveness and low dependence on oxygen**
- **Cyclotron and D-T generators generate fast neutron beam for radiotherapy, emitted with an energy of 14-16 Mev**
- **Negative π mesons (pions)** with **energy of 40 -70 Mev** have a tissue penetration of about **6-13 cm**

RADIATION THERAPY FOR TREATMENT OF CANCERS

Radiotherapy Techniques

Radiation therapy may be administered as:

- **Brachytherapy**–The source of radiation is placed within, or close to the tumor
- **Teletherapy (External Beam Radiotherapy)–**Radiation is produced from a source external to the patient

BRACHYTHERAPY

- It gives a very high dose of radiation, where the source of radiation is placed within, or close to the tumor
- Damage to normal tissues is less, as there is rapid fall off of radiation around the source **(inverse square law)**
- The application may be **Intracavitary, Interstitial or Surface (skin)**

Brachytherapy techniques

Intracavitary brachytherapy

- It consist of **hollow stem (intrauterine tandem),** which is placed within the uterine cavity and devices designed for vaginal placements, **termed vaginal ovoids or colpostats**
- Most common radioactive source for **intra-cavitary RT in carcinoma cervix** is **Iridium-192**

Interstitial brachytherapy

- It consists of placement of radioactive sources (needles, wires or seeds) **within the tissues.** Normal tissues are spared from radiation injury
- **Most commonly used to treat prostate cancer**
- Permanent seed implants (Iodine-125, Au-198) can be inserted using a specialized **seed inserter** to treat early stages of **vaginal carcinoma**
- **Interstitial brachytherapy** can be used to **treat tumor beds.** Temporary **Teflon catheter implants** can be placed intraoperatively and subsequently loaded with radioactive sources (usually Ir-192)
- **Temporary transperineal template-guided interstitial needle implants** are used to treat **vaginal and some cervical tumors.** Needles are after loaded with Ir-192 for treatment of apical vaginal lesions. Laparoscopy/laparotomy guidance may facilitate needle placement. This can also be used to treat **pelvic/aortic lymph nodal recurrence after irradiation**
- **Temporary transperineal free hand implants are particularly useful for treating urethral and vaginal tumors**

Instillation of Radioisotopes into Peritoneal Cavity (Intraperitoneal instillation)

- This is a mode of local therapy employed in **early ovarian cancers**
- Radioactive isotopes of either gold or phosphorus, linked to carrier colloids, are commonly used in ovarian cancer

- These can give radiation to a depth of 4-8 mm. Small volume tumor in the peritoneal or pleural cavity can be treated with radioisotopes solution.
- Most common radioactive substance for **intraperitoneal instillation is Phosphorus-32**
- Radioactive phosphorus (P- 32) **emits pure β-rays and has got longer half-life (14.3 days) and deeper penetration (8 mm) power** compared to radioactive **gold (Au -198)**

After loading technique

- It is a modern technique of brachytherapy to prevent radiation complications to the medical and nursing personnel handling the case.
- **Procedure**
  - A mock insertion of applicators is performed and X-ray is taken to note their exact position
  - Later, live radioactive sources are introduced by remote control in the identical manner. **Remote control systems allow complete protection of staff from radiation exposure**
- Remote after loading system uses **Selectron (Cs -137) or high dose Selectron (Co-60)**

Low dose rate (LDR) and High dose rate (HDR) system of Brachytherapy

- Brachytherapy can be either **low dose rate (LDR) or high dose rate (HDR) system**
- **LDR system** requires **hospital admission** and **delivers dose at 50-100 cGy/hour**
- **HDR systems** are commonly done on **outpatient basis** and **delivers dose at 100 cGy/minute**

Advantages of brachytherapy

- Delivers localized high radiation dose to a small tumor volume with high local control
- Radiation dose to the surrounding normal tissues is less, as there is sharp fall-off, according to inverse square law

Disadvantages

- Usually unsuitable for large tumors, unless used following EBRT and/or chemotherapy
- Risks of radiation exposure to medical and nursing personnel due to gamma rays

EXTERNAL BEAM RADIOTHERAPY (EBRT)

- **EBRT or teletherapy** is the **treatment with beams of ionizing radiation produced from a source external to the patient**
- EBRT is designed to **deliver a uniform radiation dose to the tumor volume without 'hot' (excess dose) or 'cold' (under dose) spots**
- **Accurate tumor localization and volume measurement are essential**
- **Superficial tumors** may be treated with **X-rays of low energy in the range of 80-300KV**
- **Deep-seated tumors** are treated using **mega-voltage photons**
- EBRT is used to **treat large volumes of tumor (tumor, lymph nodes, parametrium)**
- **Greater the tumor volume, higher the radiation dose required**
- **Cobalt-60 and Cesium-137** are the common teletherapy sources for EBRT

NEWER TECHNIQUES OF RADIOTHERAPY

Three-dimensional conformal radiation therapy (3D CRT)

- **3D CRT uses imaging modalities such as CT, MRI and PET scanning**
- 3D conformal therapy can shape the beam to conform to the target, so as to maximize dose to the tumor and minimize dose to normal tissues

Intensity modulated radiation therapy (IMRT)

- IMRT uses computers to perform thousands of iterations of planning in order to maximize the tumor dose and minimize dose to normal tissue

Advantages of 3D CRT and IMRT

- 3D CRT and IMRT use small collimator "leaves" to vary the beam intensity, that allows irregular shapes (tumor tissue) to be treated and has the benefit of reduced radiation dose to normal tissues
- **Tomotherapy and cone-beam CT** allow more precise localization of beam and verification of dose delivered

Stereotactic radiotherapy

- This is similar to IMRT and 3D CRT that allows high dose delivery of external radiation to precise locations in the body
- Stereotactic radiation uses a **modification of linear accelerator**

Cyber knife

- Radiation is delivered from a robotic arm and targets the radiation at any body part, from any direction using fiducial markers as guidance

Gamma-Knife radiation

- This utilizes cobalt and delivers **gamma radiation** to precise location in the brain, for treatment of **brain tumors,** with the intent of delivering an ablative dose of radiation in one treatment session

MEASUREMENT OF RADIATION (Table 11.2)

- **Radiation absorption dose (Gray)** is the unit used to measure the amount of energy absorbed per unit mass of tissue
- **One gray (Gy)** is equivalent to **1 Joule/kg which is equivalent to 100 rads**
- **One centigray (cGy)is equivalent to one rad**
- The amount of radiation the patient receives is calculated by **dosimetry**
- Primary tumor should receive high dose. Homogeneous irradiation of tissues is desirable
- Brachytherapy and teletherapy should be combined to provide adequate irradiation to the primary tumor, as well as to the pelvic lymph nodes and parametrium

Table 11.2: Measurement units of radiation

Quantity	SI Unit (Special Name)	Non-SI Unit	Conversion Factor
Exposure	C kg^{-1}	roentgen (R)	1 C kg^{-1} ≈ 3,876 R
Absorbed dose, kerma	J kg^{-1} (gray [Gy])	rad	1 Gy = 100 rad
Dose equivalent	J kg^{-1} (sievert [Sv])	rem	1 Sv = 100 rem
Activity	s^{-1} (becquerel [Bq])	curie	1 Bq = 2.7 × 10^{-11} Ci

RADIATION DOSE

- ***Inverse square law:*** Dose of radiation at a particular point varies inversely proportional to the square of the distance from the source of radiation
- According to the **"inverse square law"** there is reduction of radiation dose at a distance from the brachytherapy source. This helps in **protection of normal tissues**
- A planning computer calculates the field sizes, the dose from each field and the angles of the treatment machine while delivering EBRT
- High energy machines such as the **Linear accelerators** that deliver X-rays of 4-8 Mev, spares the skin and deliver more radiation below the skin surface
- Treatment is carried out in a protected room. During the treatment period, the patient is supervised using a television camera
- Safety precautions of radiation are maintained

RADIOCURABILITY AND RADIOSENSITIVITY

Radiocurability–It is the **elimination of tumor at the primary or metastatic site due to direct effect of radiation**

Radiosensitivity–It refers to the **response of tumor to irradiation.** Radiosensitivity is measured in terms of loss of cellular proliferative capacity due to the DNA damage. Accumulation of sublethal injury following repeat radiation leads ultimately to DNA damage and cell death

Radiosensitivity depends on the following factors (Table 11.3)

Table 11.3: Factors Influencing Radiosensitivity

Factor	*Effect*
Tissue hypoxia	Hypoxic cells are more resistant to radiation compared to toxic cells; higher the hypoxic fraction of cells, the lesser is the radiation response
Proportion of mitotic (clonogenic) cells	Clonogenic cells are more radiosensitive
Cell cycle	**Mitotic cells (M phase) and G2 cells are more radiosensitive** compared to late S-phase cells
Tumor specificity	**Certain tumors (dysgerminomas) are more radiosensitive** than the others
Tumor volume	Smaller the tumor volume→lesser the hypoxic cells→less the radiation dose ->better the radiation response
Photon wavelength	**Lesser the photon wavelength** more is the penetrating power and energy of ionizing radiation

- **Supervoltage and megavoltage radiation (Co60, Cs137, Ra226, betatron, linear accelerator) have the following advantages:**
  - Higher energy of radiation
  - Less skin injury
  - Less lateral scattering
  - More tissue penetration at a greater depth-suitable for the deep seated tumors such as carcinomas of the cervix and endometrium)

RADIOSENSITIZERS AND RADIOPROTECTORS

Radiosensitizers: Agents that potentiate the radiation effect

Radiation Protectors: Agents that decrease toxicity of radiation on normal tissues

Examples of radiosensitizers and Radioprotectors are given in Table 11.4

Table 11.4: Examples of Radiosensitizers and Radioprotectors

Radiosensitizers	**Radioprotectors**
Metronidazole, Misonidazole	Amifostine
Hyperbaric oxygen	Pentoxyphyline
Cisplatin	II-1
5 FU	GM-CSF
Gemcitabine hydroxyurea	

HYPOXIC CELL SENSITIZERS

- ***Oxygen enhancement ratio (OER)***–It is defined as the ratio of radiation dose required for a given level of cell kill under hypoxic condition, compared with the dose needed in air
- Compared to well-oxygenated cells, **hypoxic cells require about three times the radiation dose,** to obtain the same proportion of cell kill
- Hypoxic cell can be sensitized to ionizing radiation by different agents in order to improve the **Oxygen Enhancement Ratio (OER)**

Agents used for treatment of radioresistance of hypoxic cells

- Hyperbaric oxygen or carbogen breathing
- Packed cell transfusion or use of growth factors
- Pharmacologic agents that act as **hypoxic cell sensitizers** improve response of hypoxic cells to radiation **(e.g., misonidazole)** or agents that selectively kill potentially radioresistant hypoxic cells (e.g., **tirapazamine**)
- High linear-energy-transfer radiation

FRACTIONATION

Definition: It is the division of the total dose of external beam radiotherapy into small daily doses

Principle: This is based on the ability of the cells to accumulate and repair the sublethal injury. Tumor tissue takes longer time to recover from radiation damage compared to normal tissue. Fractionation allows normal tissue (intestinal mucosa, bone marrow) to repair sublethal injury (sparing effect). However, it results in accumulation of sublethal damage and ultimate loss of reproductive capacity in tumor tissue. **Thus it preferentially spares normal tissue from damage**

- **External beam radiotherapy is usually fractionated** and is given once daily for five times a week. A dose of **180-220 cGy per fraction** is used.
- The types of fractionation are mentioned in Table 11.5

Table 11.5: Types of fractionation

Types of fractionation	Characteristics	Rationale	Results
Hyperfractionation	Total dose: Same Dose per fraction: Reduce Number of fractions: Increased Overall time: Same	Reduce dose per fraction reduces late effects Higher total dose increase tumor kill	Local control: Better Acute toxicity: Higher Late toxicity: Less
Accelerated fractionation	Total dose: Reduced Dose per fraction: Reduced/same Number of fractions: Same Overall time: Reduced	Reduced time reduces tumor repopulation Reduce dose per fraction reduces late effects	Local control: Better Acute toxicity: Higher Late toxicity: Less
Hypofractionation	Dose per fraction: Increased Number of fractions: Reduced Overall time: Reduced	Reduced time Repopulation reduced	Local control: Less Acute toxicity: Less Late toxicity: Higher

RADIATION DOSE AND ORGAN TOLERANCE (Table 11.6)

Table 11.6: Radiation Dose and Organ Tolerance

Organ	Tolerance dose (cGy)
Bone marrow	2,000
Spinal cord	5,000
Femoral head	5,000
Stomach	4,500
Bowel	5,000
Rectum	5,000
Ureter	7,500–8,000
Bladder	6,500
Ovary	600-1,000
Uterus	10,000-20,000
Cervix	9,000
Vagina	9,000–10,000
Vulva	2,000–3,000

INTERACTION BETWEEN DRUGS AND RADIATION (Table 11.7)

Table 11.7: Interaction between Drugs and Radiation

Effect	Explanation
Spatial Cooperation (Independent Action)	Spatial cooperation is the situation in which **drugs and radiation act independently with different targets** and mechanisms of action so that **total effect of combination is equal to that of each agent separately** For example, a site that is protected from chemotherapy (e.g., the brain) may be treated with radiation to prevent recurrence. Chemotherapy drugs may be used to destroy microscopic distant disease, while radiation is used to destroy local tumor
Additivity	Additivity is the situation in which **the two agents act on the same target to cause damage** that is **equal to the sum of their individual toxic effects**
Supra-additivity	When there is supra-additivity, a **drug potentiates the effect of radiation, causing a greater response** than that would be expected from simple additivity
Subadditivity	With subadditivity, amount of **cell death that results from the use of the two agents is less** than that expected from simple additivity

RADIATION DOSE PRESCRIPTION

- It should include the following:
  - **The total dose**
  - **Number of fractions**
  - **Dose and time for each fraction**
- **Example:** 40Gy in 20 fractions given five times weekly for 4 weeks at the rate of 2Gy per fraction
- **Intraoperative radiation** at the time of staging laparotomy is possible. Large fraction RT of 1500-2500 cGy can be delivered directly to selected areas such as biopsy proven periaortic node irradiation

RADIATION REACTIONS (Table 11.8)

Table 11.8: Radiation reactions

Early
• Anorexia, nausea, vomiting, lassitude or fever
• Diarrhea (radiation enteritis)
• Leukopenia, thrombocytopenia, anemia– (treated with hematinics, blood transfusion, G–CSF)
• Intestinal reaction such as enteritis, colitis, proctitis
• Cystitis, pyelitis, hematuria
Late (due to vasculitis and fibrosis)
• Atrophic changes of vulval skin and vaginal stricture-minimized with megavoltage therapy
• Radiation fibrosis–treated with Steroid enemas, antidiarrheal agents
• Pathological fracture due to osteoporosis
• Intestinal stricture, bleeding per rectum, perforation, obstruction
• Malabsorption syndrome with megaloblastic anemia–treated with folic acid
• Proctosigmoiditis
• Vesicovaginal *or* rectovaginal fistula(usually occurs 1-2 years following primary therapy)
• Radiation damage to ovaries and menopausal symptoms

Contraindications to Radiotherapy

- Severe anemia
- Poor general health
- Sepsis

- Pregnancy
- Fibroid uterus
- Tubo-ovarian mass
- Uterovaginal prolapse
- Presence of genital fistulae

Table 11.9: Advantages and Disadvantages of Preoperative and Postoperative Radiation

Advantages		Disadvantages	
Preoperative radiation			
1.	Surgically undisturbed tumor bed. Intact vascularity (good oxygenation)	1.	Precludes accurate pretreatment staging of the disease
2.	May facilitate surgical dissection, allowing a lesser procedure by shrinking the tumor	2.	May be considered unnecessary in cases with high chances of cure with surgery alone
3.	May decrease the likelihood of risk of implantation or dissemination of viable tumor cells during surgical handling of tissues	3.	Interferes with tissue healing
		4.	Combined therapy increases the morbidity
Postoperative radiation			
1.	Accurate surgical staging	1.	Surgery may alter the kinetics of tumor proliferation
2.	Extent of loco-regional disease accurately defined	2.	Surgery often disturbs tumor vascularity causing hypoxia
3.	Choice of omitting or selective use of radiation in some patients		

RADIOTHERAPY FOR CANCERS IN GYNECOLOGY

RT FOR CARCINOMA CERVIX

Indications

- It is a primary treatment modality that can be used for all stages of cancer cervix
- Postoperative RT is indicated in high- and intermediate risk cases as follows:
  - Positive margins
  - Positive lymph nodes
  - Microscopic parametrial involvement
  - Large tumor size
  - Lymphovascular space involvement (LVSI)
  - Cervical stromal invasion
- In case of recurrence following surgery, RT can be given
- Hemostatic RT can be given to control brisk hemorrhage
- **In early stages:** Brachytherapy is given first followed by EBRT
- **In advanced stages:** EBRT is given first to shrink the primary tumor and make the insertion of intracavitary source feasible, followed by brachytherapy

Intracavitary Brachytherapy

- Treatment is specified using variation of the Manchester system, **which uses two primary reference points (Fig 11.4):**
- **Point A**–A point 2 cm lateral and 2 cm superior to external os in plane of implant
- **Point B**–A point 3 cm lateral to point A
- **Total dose to point A** (from external beam and LDR intracavitary therapy) that is adequate to achieve central disease control is usually between **75 Gy (for small stage IB1 cancer) and 90 Gy (for bulky or locally advanced disease)**
- **Prescribed dose to point B is 45 to 65 Gy** depending on extent of parametrial and sidewall involvement

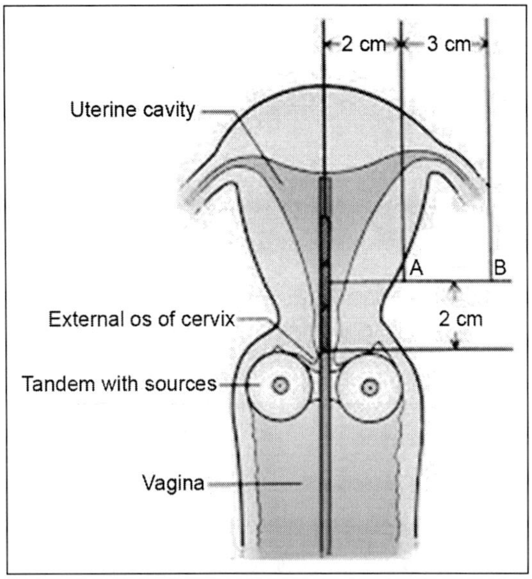

Figure 11.4: Reference points for radiotherapy in cancer cervix

External beam Radio therapy

- Typical external beam fields are designed to include the primary tumor, paracervical tissues, iliac and presacral lymph nodes, all with 1.5 to 2–cm margins
- The field borders are mentioned in Table 11.10

Table 11.10: Field borders in External Beam Radiotherapy

Superior border	Between L4 and L5 to include the common iliac nodes
Inferior border	At the inferior margin of obturator foramen to include the obturator nodes
Lateral borders	One cm lateral to the margins of the bony pelvis

RADIOTHERAPY IN EPITHELIAL OVARIAN CANCERS

- Chemotherapy has replaced radiotherapy for the management of early and advanced disease ovarian tumors
- RT may be used in the following cases who fail to respond to chemotherapy
  - Metastatic deposits over the peritoneal surfaces
  - Lymph node metastasis
  - Palliation for painful pelvic or bone recurrences

Moving strip technique

- Major limitation of the use of completely abdominal irradiation is radiosensitivity of normal tissues in the upper abdomen (e.g., kidney, liver, bowel, and spinal cord), which prevents delivery of more than 22 to 30 Gy to the whole abdomen. **This dose is inadequate to control areas of gross or even extensive microscopic disease**
- **Moving strip technique** is now used to irradiate whole of abdomen
- Presence of **residual disease** following debulking procedures in ovarian carcinoma is treated with this technique

Procedure of Moving strip technique

- Whole abdomen is divided into contiguous strips of 2.5 cm wide area. Each strip is irradiated from front and back over 2 days and the field is gradually moved up
- **Cobalt–60 machine** is generally used and a total tumor dose of 2600 to 2800 cGy is delivered
- Pelvic boost of 2000 to3000 cGy is given in addition
- **Kidneys and right lobe of liver are shielded** with lead to reduce the RT to these organs
- Bulky residual disease (> 2 cm) is not suitable for radiotherapy

ENDOMETRIAL CANCER

- **As adjuvant therapy following surgery:**
  - **Radiation therapy remains the standard adjuvant treatment modality following surgico-pathological staging** for most patients as there is risk for recurrence
  - **Post operative RT is required in all stages except endometrial Ca. Stage IA, Grades 1 and 2**
  - Currently, **intravaginal brachytherapy and external beam pelvic RT with/ without an extended field RT is commonly employed as post op adjuvant therapy**
  - Chemotherapy is recently supported as an **adjuvant treatment for patients with stage III and IV endometrial carcinoma**
- **Serous and clear cell ovarian cancers** have high propensity for upper abdominal relapse. **Whole abdomen RT along with systemic chemotherapy is required in these cases**
- **Preoperative RT followed by surgery**–indicated in patients who are unsuitable for extensive surgery (obese, elderly, medical problems)
- RT is preferred for patients with **inoperable stage** III endometrial carcinoma
- As palliative treatment of massive pelvic or metastatic disease
- **Curative treatment for patients with isolated vaginal or pelvic recurrence,** usually using combination of external beam and intracavitary or interstitial radiation therapy

VULVAL CANCER

Possible benefits of radiotherapy in the treatment of vulvar cancer include the following:

- Reduces risk of regional recurrence and improved survival in patients with inguinal node metastases
- Reduces risk of vulvar recurrence in patients with positive surgical margins
- Avoidance of exenterative surgery in patients with disease involving the anus or urethra

VAGINAL CANCER

- Most patients with **invasive vaginal cancers are treated with radiotherapy**
- The cure rates are similar to those achieved with radiation therapy for cervical cancer

CHORIOCARCINOMA

- Choriocarcinoma **responds extremely well to chemotherapy** which has replaced surgery and radiotherapy in young women.
- Radiotherapy is applicable in distal metastasis in few cases

RECENT ADVANCES

Recent technological developments for patients receiving EBRT include:

- *Intensity-modulated radiation therapy (IMRT)*
- *Volumetric modulated arc therapy (VMAT)*
- *Advantages - helps to offer greater precision to the target volume and simultaneously aims to reduce the radiation dose to organs at risk (OAR)*

Technical developments in brachytherapy:

- *Image guided adapted brachytherapy (IGABT)-improves the quality and efficacy of radiation*
- *BL 2 - Multileaf collimators (MLC) allows radiation beam shaping, which has permitted OAR shielding*

Ongoing research - *use of new targeted agents such as poly (ADPribose) polymerase (PARP) inhibitors in combination with radiation, where there may be a synergistic effect*

CHAPTER 12

PRINCIPLES OF CHEMOTHERAPY IN GYNECOLOGIC CANCERS

INTRODUCTION

- Chemotherapy is part of multidisciplinary approach in management of gynecological cancers
- Traditional chemotherapy has reached a plateau in most cancers; the only new agent to have emerged in the past few years is **trabectedin,** the marine-derived compound
- The identification of molecular pathways that lead to aberrant cell signaling and tumorigenesis has led to identification of new targets and drugs, a step forward towards **'personalised medicine'**
- Most of the new developments in chemotherapy relate to ovarian cancer. However, new molecular targeted agents for cervical, endometrial, vulval and vaginal carcinomas and gynaecological sarcomas are under trial
- Chemotherapy has moved on from single-agent therapy with alkylating agents and antimetabolites to the use of combination chemotherapy regimens that include taxanes, platinums, anthracyclines etc
- **Ovarian cancer** often requires surgery, with postoperative platinum based adjuvant chemotherapy. In some cases, neoadjuvant chemotherapy and interval debulking may be offered. Recurrent ovarian cancers are usually treated with chemotherapy, and the drug choice is often influenced by the platinum free interval prior to recurrence
- **Endometrial cancer** is usually treated with surgery followed by post operative adjuvant radiotherapy. The role of adjuvant chemotherapy for endometrial cancer remains open to debate. Adjuvant chemotherapy is increasingly offered for high-risk cases with lymphovascular space invasion. Carboplatin and paclitaxel are the most effective drugs in adjuvant therapy and recurrent cases
- The standard of care for **locally advanced cervical cancer** is combined chemoradiation ie., concomitant chemotherapy with radiation therapy. Recent studies have shown that the addition of bevacizumab to cisplatin and paclitaxel leads to improved response rates in recurrent and metastatic cases
- Gynecological cancers often require multidisciplinary management, and entry into clinical trials should be strongly supported.

Recap of Cell Kinetics

Normal cells have inherent capacity to multiply, which is **controlled** by various internal and external factors. There is also a constant balanced cell loss.

Cancer cells undergo **uncontrolled** and **excessive proliferation compared to cell loss. Speed of cell division is the same as compared to normal cell**

Normal cells may be classified as mentioned in Table 12.1

Table 12.1: Classification of Normal Cells

Cell type	Description	Example
Proliferating cells	Undergo constant cell division	Bone marrow, intestinal mucosa, epidermis
Quiescent cells	Can proliferate under special conditions (injury), otherwise they are in quiescent phase	Liver, kidney
Static cells	Comprises relatively well-differentiated cells, that after initial proliferative activity in the embryonic and neonatal period, rarely undergo cell division.	Neurons, striated muscles

Cell cycle: There are **four phases** of cell cycle. These are **G1, S, G2 and M (Figure 12.1)**

- **Normal tissues have huge number of cells in the G0 phase (out of cycle phase),** in contrast to **tumor cells, where more cells are in the active phase of cell division**
- **Tumor cells in active phase of cell division are most sensitive to cytotoxic agents whereas cells in the G0 are relatively insensitive**
- Proper understanding of cell cycle has evolved synergistic combinations of drugs with better cancer killing potential and less side effects

Terminologies in relation to Cell Cycle are given in Table 12.2

Gap 1 (G_1) (Synthesis of enzymes and regulatory proteins)	Postmitotic	4–24 hours (variable)
DNA Synthesis (S) and Replication		10–20 hours
Gap 2 (G_2) RNA synthesis Protein synthesis	Premitotic	2–10 hours
Mitosis (M)		0.5–1 hour
G_0 Resting phase		Variable Period

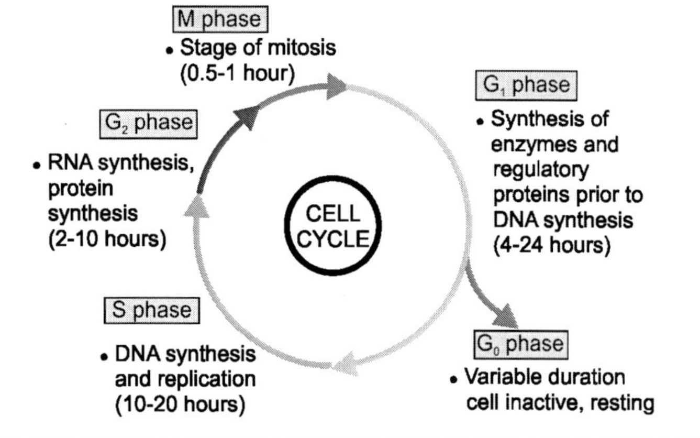

Figure 12.1: Cell cycle and cell generation time

Table 12.2: Various terminologies in relation to cell cycle

Term	Description
Cell cycle time	• It refers to the amount of time needed by a proliferating cell to progress through the cell cycle and produce a new daughter cell • Cell cycle time varies widely, but is relatively constant for a specific cell type
Doubling time	• Doubling time of a tumor is defined as the time taken by a tumor mass to double its size. Doubling time varies depending upon the specific type of tumor
Growth fraction	• It is the number of cells in the tumor mass that are actively involved in the phase of cell division • Tumor growth depends on growth fraction and cell death
Gompertzian growth	• It states that when a tumor volume increases in size, its mass doubling time becomes progressively longer.
Generation time	• It is the duration of the cycle from M phase to M phase (between two M phases). Tumor cells do not have faster generation time
Log kill hypothesis	• Antitumor agents kill a **constant fraction** of cells (rather than a constant number)with each course of therapy that is called **log kill hypothesis** • Intermittent courses of chemotherapy are found to destroy more tumor cells

CYTOTOXIC CHEMOTHERAPY

Uses of chemotherapy

- As a primary treatment of cancer–Complete remission of the tumor
- As an adjunct to surgery/radiotherapy–to prevent recurrence
- As neoadjuvant therapy for advanced disease following which additional treatment is planned
- As Palliation therapy–To alleviate the symptoms, so as to improve the quality of life

NOTE: The available chemotherapy agents damage both cancerous and normal tissues; however normal tissues recover from the insult, but cancerous tissues do not recover

Principles of Chemotherapy

- **Rapidly growing tumors are more amenable** to chemotherapy than slow growing tumors
- A **constant fraction of neoplastic cells are killed** with each dose of cytotoxic drug

- **Effect of chemotherapeutic drugs depends on:**
  - Tumor mass and growth rate
  - Sensitivity of resting phase cells
  - Immunocompetence of host cells
  - Type and dose schedule of the agent
- High dose **intermittent course of chemotherapy may result in high cell kill** and optimal destruction of the tumor (dose intensity)
- **Combination agent chemotherapy is superior** to single agent therapy for the treatment of most malignancies
- **Combination drugs** should have **synergistic effect, different mechanism of action and different spectrum of toxicity** in order to enhance the tumor cell kill and minimize drug resistance
- Prior to starting chemotherapy, **pre-treatment evaluation** should be done. Drug dose is adjusted according to the tolerance of the patient.

Classification of Chemotherapeutic Drugs Based on Cell Cycle Specificity (Table 12.3)

- **Cell cycle specific agents** act only on **proliferating cells**
- **Cell cycle non-specific agents** destroy both **resting and proliferating cells**

Table 12.3: Classification of Chemotherapeutic Drugs Based on their Cell Cycle Specificity

Cell Cycle	**Non-specific**	Cyclophosphamide, Cisplatin, Carboplatin
Cell Cycle	**Specific:** On G_1	Actinomycin D
	On S phase	Methotrexate, 5 FU, Doxorubicin
	On G_2	Bleomycin, Etoposide
	On M phase	Vinblastine, Vincristine Taxanes
	G_0	Nitrosoureas

Classification of Chemotherapeutic Drugs Based on Structural Similarity and Mechanism of Action (Table 12.4)

Table 12.4: Classification of Chemotherapeutic Drugs Based on Structural Similarity and Mechanism of Action

Agents	Mechanism of action	Examples
Alkylating agents	• These are **cell cycle non-specific agents** • **They prevent cell division by cross-linking the DNA strands. They produce single and double stranded DNA break** • Cyclophosphamide in addition, inhibits DNA synthesis	• Cyclophosphamide (endoxan) • Ifosfamide • Melphalan • Thiotepa • **Platinum agents:** Cisplatin, carboplatin, oxaliplatin
Antimetabolites	Act by **inhibiting essential metabolic processes** that are required for synthesis of **purines, pyrimidines and nucleic acids**	• **Methotrexate–Folic acid antagonist,** prevents reduction of folic acid to folinic acid by inhibiting the enzyme dihydrofolate reductase • **5-Fluorouracil–Pyrimidine analogue,** blocks thymidine synthesis and prevents DNA replication • **6-Mercaptopurine–Purine analogue** • **Gemcitabine** (2', 2' – fluorodeoxycytabidine) is a new agent used in ovarian, breast and cervical carcinoma
Antibiotics	• These are **cell cycle non-specific agents** • They **prevent DNA replication,** causes single and double stranded DNA break	• Actinomycin D • Bleomycin • Doxorubicin • Mitomycin C

Contd.

Contd.

Plant Derivatives and Taxanes	**These are cell cycle specific agents** They act as **spindle poison and cause arrest of mitosis at metaphase** – **Taxanes**–disturb the normal assembly, disassembly and stabilization **of microtubules** – **Camptothecin analogs (topotecan and irinotecan)** inhibit **topoisomerase-1,** causing single stranded DNA breaks	• **Vincristine and vinblastin** (from plant Vinca rosea) • **Taxanes** (from the bark of pacific yew tree Taxus brevifolia) **-paclitaxel (taxol) and docetaxol (synthetic)** • **Topoisomerase-1** inhibitors-**topotecan and irinotecan** • **Etoposide**
Hormones	The drugs induce **regression of a hormone responsive tumor** and also increase anabolic processes	• **Progesterones**–hydroxyprogesterone caproate, medroxyprogesterone acetate, megestrol acetate • **Anti-estrogen–Tamoxifen** acts by competitive receptor binding, thus helpful in **estrogen dependent tumors**
Miscellaneous agent		• **Hexamethylamine**–acts like antimetabolite • **Hydroxyurea**–increases radiosensitivity of malignant tissue
Biological agents	• Act by improving the host immune defense	• Interferons, Müllerian inhibiting factor

Single Agent Versus Combination Chemotherapy

- Combined chemotherapeutic agents **attack different phases of cell cycle (synergistic effect) and hence reduces the tumor volume effectively**
- Combination chemotherapy (cell cycle specific and cell cycle non-specific) **enhances tumor cell kill compared to single drug therapy**
- **Drug dose and duration of therapy** cannot be increased with **single agent** chemotherapy because of **toxicity**
- **Emergence of drug resistance** is more with **single agent** therapy

Principles in selecting the combination of drugs

1.	The drugs used must be active as single agents against the particular tumor
2.	The drugs should have different mechanisms of action to minimize emergence of drug resistance
3.	The combination of drugs should have additive or preferably synergistic effects
4.	The drugs chosen should have a different spectrum of toxicity so that they can be used for maximum cell kill at (or near) full doses
5.	The drugs chosen should be administered intermittently so that cell kill is enhanced and prolonged myelosuppression is minimized

Pretreatment Evaluation Prior to Chemotherapy

NOTE:

- Chemotherapeutic agents **are highly toxic to the erythropoietic system** such as bone marrow
- The drugs are **mostly metabolized in the liver and excreted through kidneys**
- The patients are also **immuno compromised** and any source of infection should be treated

Pretreatment evaluation includes the following (Table 12.5)

Table 12.5: Pretreatment evaluation

Evaluation	Comment
Hematological	Complete hemogram and platelet count (> 100,000/cu.mm)
Serum electrolytes	
Renal function tests	Blood urea, Serum creatinine and creatinine clearance (especially when cisplatin is used)
Liver function tests	Total proteins, liver enzymes, Sr. bilirubin
Cardiac function	Baseline ECG and ventricular ejection fraction when cardiotoxic drug **(doxorubicin)** is used
Pulmonary function tests	When **bleomycin** is used

Calculation of Drug Dose

- The dose of a chemotherapeutic agent is usually **calculated as square meter of body surface area (BSA). Normogram** is used for calculating body surface area of adults

Advantages of using BSA for calculation of drug dose:

- It provides a **better measure of potential toxicity than body weight**
- **The body surface area closely reflects cardiac output and blood flow**
- There is **minimal change in body surface area** during entire course of therapy compared to bodyweight

Route of administration

- **Oral:** Alkylating drugs such as Cyclophosphamide, Chlorambucil and Melphalan are mainly administered orally
- **Parenteral:** Intravenous administration at interval of 1-4 weeks allows recovery of bone marrow and of normal cells
- **Intraperitoneal:** Drug penetration will be only few cells depth. Systemic / Parenteral administration is more effective

Treatment principles while administering systemic chemotherapy

- Drugs used in combination should not be mixed together
- The infusion set should be flushed with normal saline between the administration of each drug
- To avoid sclerosis of the vein, the drugs should be washed through with normal saline
- Extravasation should be avoided
- Antiemetics should be given before start of chemotherapy

ASSESSMENT OF RESPONSE TO CHEMOTHERAPY

- History and physical examination
- Assessment by imaging studies–CT or MRI
- Measurement of specific tumor markers (i.e. CA125 for epithelial ovarian cancer, β-hCG for GTN)
- Detection of hyper metabolic state by PET scan

NOTE

- *All cases undergoing chemotherapy should be monitored for evidences of regression of the disease by changes in clinical, biophysical and biochemical markers*
- *Hematological profile must be checked at regular intervals*
- *Minor complications like nausea, vomiting, alopecia, glossitis should not preclude full treatment protocol*
- *The benefits should be weighed against toxic effects. Explaining the situation clearly helps in patient compliance and improves ultimate result*

Response evaluation criteria in solid tumors (Table 12.6)

Table 12.6: Response evaluation criteria in solid tumors

Response	**Definition**
CR (complete response)	Disappearance of all target lesions
PR (partial response)	30% decrease in greatest diameter of tumor
PD (progressive disease)	20% increase in greatest diameter of tumor
SD (stable disease)	Small change that do not meet the above criteria.

Mechanisms of Chemotherapy Drug Resistance

- Decrease in cellular drug uptake
- Increase in repair of DNA
- Increase in levels of target enzyme to make the cell immune to the drug
- Increase in drug degradation
- Spontaneous tumor cell mutations

ROLE OF CHEMOTHERAPY IN GYNECOLOGICAL CANCERS (Table 12.7)

Table12.7: Role of chemotherapy in Gynecological cancers

Type of neoplasm	Indication	Chemotherapy used
Squamous cell carcinoma of cervix	• Adjuvant chemotherapy in combination with radiation • Neoadjuvant chemotherapy • Palliation in recurrences	Cisplatin is commonly used. Various other drugs are tried • Bleomycin/vincristine/Doxorubicin/ vinblastine / 5- Flurouracil • Mitomycin, hydroxyurea–to increase radiosensitivity
Squamous cell carcinoma of **vulva** and **vagina**	In advanced stages and in recurrence as palliation	• Bleomycin
Endometrial carcinoma	In advanced stages and in recurrences as palliation	Progestational agents, Ifosfamide, Doxorubicin, Cisplatin, Tamoxifen, Leuprolide
Endometrial sarcoma	As an alternative to radiotherapy	Doxorubicin and Cyclophosphamide, VAC regimen, Progresterone, Ifosfamide
Fallopian tube carcinoma	Advanced stages	Doxorubicin/Melphalan/Cyclophosphamide
Ovarian tumors Epithelial carcinoma	• Stage IA: Used as a routine following surgery to improve outcome • Advanced stage • Palliative chemotherapy	Single or multiple drug therapy: Cisplatin or carboplatin (less toxic), taxol, melphalan, thiotepa, chlorambucil, hexamethyl melamine, cyclophosphamide and adriamycin/(CAP or CP), gemcitabine Usually combination therapy: • Taxol and cisplatin/carboplatin • Adriamycin and cyclophosphamide • Adriamycin, cyclophosphamide and cisplatin
Sex cord stromal tumor • Granulosa cell tumor	Not very sensitive to chemotherapy /RT Used in metastatic disease and recurrence	• Vincristine + Adriamycin + Cyclophosphamide **(VAC)** • Bleomycin + Etoposite + Cisplatin **(BEP)**
Germ cell tumor • Dysgerminoma • Endodermal sinus cell tumor, Embryonal carcinoma • Choriocarcinoma • Malignant immature teratoma, Polyembryoma	Usually used as adjuvant therapy following surgery	Combination agents: VAC therapy/BEP therapy/VBP therapy Combination therapy in recurrent cases • POMB–ACE-Vincristine (oncovin), Methotrexate, Bleomycin, Cisplatin, Etoposide, Actinomycin D, Cyclophosphamide
Hydatidiform mole	As a prophylactic therapy in selected cases	• Methotrexate and Actinomycin D are commonly used
GTN	Mainstay in the management of GTN-nonmetastatic and metastic GTN	• Single agent therapy with Methotrexate or Actinomycin used in low risk disease • Combination therapy (EMACO regimen) in high risk cases
Chemotherapy for intraperitoneal small volume residual disease (<1-2 cm) and/or malignant effusions		Intraperitoneal instillation of cisplatin

Toxicity of Chemotherapeutic Agents (Tables 12.8)

Drug toxicity depends on the type of drug used, method of administration, dosage and general condition of the patient

Table 12.8: Toxicity of chemotherapeutic agents and their management

Tissue or organ affected	Toxic effects and drugs	Management
Gastrointestinal	Nausea, vomiting, oral ulceration, stomatitis, necrotizing enterocolitis, diarrhea (cisplatin, methotrexate, paclitaxel, docetaxel, etoposide)	Antiemetics used for emetogenic chemotherapy • Dexamethasone 20 mg IV • Ondansetron 8 mg IV every 4 hours 2-3 doses • Metoclopramide 80-120 mg IV every 3-4 hours
Hair roots	Alopecia (paclitaxel, cyclophosphamide)	Generally reversible
Hematological (bone-marrow)	Anemia, granulocytopenia, thrombocytopenia. The danger level: Hb percent < 8 gm%, leukocyte count < 3,000/cumm and platelet count < 20,000/cumm (paclitaxel, etoposide, carboplatin)	Blood transfusion, platelet transfusion, drug dose may be modified. Granulocyte Colony-stimulating factor (G-CSF) and granulocyte macrophase colony-stimulating factor (GM-CSF) have been used (250 μg/M^2, subcutaneously) for myelostimulation
Skin	Dermatitis, pigmentation (bleomycin), extravasation of drug, skin necrosis (actinomycin D, doxorubicin)	For extravasation and skin necrosis–removal of intravenous line, local infiltration of corticosteroids, ice pack therapy
Cardiac	Cardiomyopathy, arrhythmias, endocardial fibrosis (doxorubicin, cyclophosphamide), toxic myocarditis (Paclitaxel)	Discontinuation of drug, drug and dose modification, cardiologist consultation
Liver	Hepatitis, elevated transaminases and bilirubin (Methotrexate)	Discontinuation of drug, drug and dose modification
Lungs	Fibrosis (Bleomycin, alkylating agents, doxorubicin)	Pulmonary function tests; stop therapy; steroids may be helpful
Nervous system	Neurotoxicity, ototoxicity, peripheral neuropathy (Cisplatin, Ifosfamide)	Vitamin B complex, pyridoxine therapy, drug and dose modification
Urinary system	Renal failure, azotemia (Cisplatin), hemorrhagic cystitis (Cyclophosphamide, Ifosfamide), red urine (doxorubicin)	Prehydration and mannitol induced diuresis before therapy, avoid simultaneous use of nephrotoxic drugs (aminoglycosides). **Mesna** is used for hemorrhagic cystitis caused by cyclophosphamide or ifosfamide
Immune system	Supression of cellular and humoral immunity, loss of host defense mechanism	Usually reversible
Metabolic	Hyperkalemia, hyperuricemia, hypocalcemia–due to rapid tumor lysis Hyponatremia–due to inappropriate ADH secretion	Estimation of serum electrolytes and appropriate correction
Surgical wound	Delayed healing	
Gonads	Infertility, amenorrhea, premature ovarian failure	Patient counseling
Embryo	Teratogenic effects, congenital malformation	Patient counseling to assess risk benefit
Secondary malignancies	Due to mutagenic effects-leukemia (melphalan)	

NOTE:

- ***Nausea and vomiting are the most common side effects*** *due to stimulation of chemoreceptor trigger zone, which secretes neurotransmitters (serotonin, dopamine and histamine) to activate the vomiting center*
- ***Chemotherapy induced nausea and vomiting are more common (risk >90%) with Cisplatin, Dacarbazine, Doxorubicin and Ifosfamide. Ondansetron (5 HT3 receptor antagonist), dexamethasone and metoclopramide*** *are commonly used for treatment*
- ***Chemotherapy agents commonly causing peripheral neuropathy are Cisplatin, Oxaplatin, carboplatin, Paclitaxel, Docetaxel, Vincristine, Altretamine. Agents commonly used for chemotherapy-induced peripheral neuropathy pain include Duloxetine, Gabapentin, Lidocaine patch, Opioids, Pregabalin, Tramadol and Tricyclic antidepressants***

Table 12.9: Impact of pre-existing/physiological conditions on cancer chemotherapy		
Physiologic condition	**Causation**	**Impact and examples**
Renal insufficiency	Obstruction, chronic kidney disease, hypovolemia, hypotension, on steroidals, nephrotoxins (aminoglycosides, cisplatin)	Decreased clearance of methotrexate, carboplatin and other agents
Hepatobiliary dysfunction	Biliary obstruction, hepatitis, cirrhosis	Decreased clearance of doxorubicin, mitoxantrone, vincristine, vinblastine, etoposide, paclitaxel, docetaxel
	Gilbert's syndrome, impaired glucuronidation and polymorphisms	Increased exposure to SN-38 (active metabolite of irinotecan)
	Decreased microsomal activity	Impaired activation of cyclophosphamide and ifosfamide
Reduced protein binding	Carrier displacement (sulfonamide, salicylates, phenytoin)	Increased toxicity, higher free drug levels (methotrexate)
	Reduced carrier proteins (malnutrition)	Increased toxicity, higher free drug levels (cisplatin, paclitaxel, docetaxel, etoposide, SN-38)
Altered intestinal absorption	Oral antibiotics (neomycin)	Decreased absorption of methotrexate
	High-fat meal	Increase bioavailability of lapatinib
		Decrease bioavailability of capecitabine
	Grapefruit (intestinal CYP3A4 inhibition)	Increased bioavailability (Cyclosporine, erythromycin, benzodiazepines)
Decreased metabolism	Caused by allopurinol	Delayed clearance of 6-mercaptopurine
	Dihydropyrimidine dehydrogenase (DPD) deficiency	Lethal toxicity from 5-fluorouracil
Cholinesterase inhibition	Caused by cyclophosphamide	Decreased clearance of succinylcholine
Monoamine oxidase inhibition	Caused by procarbazine	Neurotoxicity and seizures (tricyclic antidepressants and phenothiazines)
MDR-1 competition	Associated with natural products and other substrates, including verapamil, cyclosporine tamoxifen	Decreased efflux and increased toxicity from natural products (doxorubicin, vincristine, paclitaxel, docetaxel)
CYP2C9 Inhibition	Caused by capecitabine	Increased AUC of warfarin
CYP3A4 Induction	Caused by glucocortiocoids, barbiturates, rifampin	Increased activation of cyclophosphamide
Substrate Inhibition	Caused by ketoconazole, itraconazole, fluconazole, erythromycin	Decreased metabolism of substrates (potentially significant)
Substrate competition	Caused by cyclophosphamide, ifofamide, paclitaxel, docetaxel, etoposide, vincristine, vinblastine, tamoxifen, gefitinib	Decreased metabolism of other substrates (usually not clinically significant)

Extra Edge

Table 12.10: Grading of chemotherapy induced diarrhea					
	Grade 1	**Grade 2**	**Grade 3**	**Grade 4**	**Grade 5**
Diarrhea	Increase of < 4 stools per day over baseline; mild increase in ostomy output compared to baseline	Increase of 4-6 stools per day over baseline; moderate increase in ostomy output compared to baseline	Increase of > 6 stools per day over baseline; incontinence; severe increase in ostomy output compared to baseline; limiting self-care activities of daily living (ADL)	Life-threatening consequence; urgent intervention indicated	Death

Table 12.11: Grading of chemotherapy induced peripheral neuropathy					
	Grade 1	**Grade 2**	**Grade 3**	**Grade 4**	**Grade 5**
Paresthesia	Mild symptoms	Moderate symptoms: limiting instrumental ADL	Severe symptoms: limiting self-care ADL	–	–

Contd.

Contd.

Peripheral neuropathy	Asymptomatic; observation; intervention not indicated	Moderate symptoms; limiting instrumental ADL	Severe symptoms; limiting self-care ADL; assistive device indicated	Life-threatening consequences; urgent intervention indicated	Death

Table 12.12: Types of hypersensitivity reaction of platinums and their characteristics

Type of hypersensitivity reactions	Antigen	Mediated by	Mechanism	Involved in platinum hypersensitivity	Symptoms related
I	Soluble antigen	IgE	Mast cell and basophil degranulation	Carboplatin, cisplatin, oxaliplatin (most)	Early onset symptoms; itching, chest pain, rash, anaphylactic reactions
II	Cell-or matrix associated antigen	IgG, IgM	Phagocyte and NK-cell activation	Oxaliplatin	Hemolysis, thrombocytopenia
III	Soluble antigen	IgG	Immune complex, phagocyte and NK-cell activation, complement fixation	Oxaliplatin	Chronic urticaria, joint pain, proteinuria
IV	Soluble or cell-associated antigen	T-cell	Macrophage and eosinophil activation, cytotoxicity	Carboplatin, cisplatin	Delayed reactions, hours or even days after infusion

Table 12.13: Grading of hypersensitivity reactions

	Grade				
	1	2	3	4	5
Hypersensitivity (allergic reaction)	Transient flushing or rash, drug fever (38.0°C), intervention not indicated	Intervention or infusion interruption indicated: responds promptly to symptomatic treatment (e.g., antihistamines, NSAIDS, narcotics): prophylactic medications indicated for $\leq$ 24 hours	Prolonged (e.g., not rapidly responsive to symptomatic mediation and/or brief interruption of infusion); recurrence of symptoms following initial improvement; hospitalization indicated for clinical sequelae (e.g., renal impairment, pulmonary infiltrates)	Life-threatening consequences, urgent intervention indicated	Death
Acute infusion reactions (Cytokine release syndrome)	Mild reaction; infusion interruption not indicated; intervention not indicated	Therapy or infusion interruption indicated and responds promptly to symptomatic treatment (e.g., antihistamines, NSAIDS, narcotics IV fluids); prophylactic medication indicated for $\leq$24 hours	Prolonged (e.g., not rapidly responsive to symptomatic medication and/or brief interruption of symptoms following initial improvement; hospitalization indicated for clinical sequelae (e.g., renal impairment, pulmonary infiltrates)	Life-threatening consequences; pressor or ventilator support indicated	Death

Table 12.14: Common Terminology Criteria for Adverse Events (CTCAE) grading of myelosuppression

Element	Grade			
	1	2	3	4
Leukocytes (per mm^3)	LLN to 3,000	<3,000 to 2,000	<2,000 to 1,000	<1,000
Granulocytes (per mm3)	LLN to 1,500	<1,500 to 1,000	<1,000 to 500	<500
Hemoglobin (g/dl)	LLN to 10.0	<10.0 to 8.0	<8.0 to 6.5	<6.5
Platelets (per mm^3)	LLN to 75,000	<75,000 to 50,000	<50,000 to 25,000	<25,000

Representative drug dose medications for hematologic toxicity

Category (Timing)	Parameters	CTCAE (Grade)	Dose or Schedule
Granulocytes (day of therapy)	>1,500/mm^3	0,1	Full doses of all drugs
	<1,500/mm^3	2,3,4	Delay until recovered. If delay < 7 days, reduce doses by one level or add G-CSF. If delay > 14 days, reduce doses by one level and add G-CSF
Platelets (day of therapy)	WNL	0	Full doses of all drugs
	< LLN to 75,000/mm^3	1	Delay until recovered
	<75,000/mm^3	2, 3, 4	Delay until recovered. If delay > 7 days, reduce doses by one level
Granulocytes (cycle nadir)	>1,000/mm^3	0, 1, 2	Full doses of all drugs
	<500/mm^3 for ≥ 7 days	4	Reduce doses by one level. If already reduced, add G-CSF for future cycles
	< 1,000/mm^3 with fever	3, 4	Add G-CSF for current episode, reduce doses by one level for future cycle. If already reduced, add G-CSF for future cycles
Platelets (cycle nadir)	≥ 50,000/mm^3	3	Full dose of all drugs
	< 50,000/mm^3 with bleed	3, 4	Reduce doses by one level
	< 25,000/mm^3	4	Reduce doses by one level

LLN – Lower limit of normal; G-CSF –Granulocyte colony stimulating factor

Table 12.15: Assessment scale to determine patient's prognosis

Score	Karnofsky performance status scale
100	Normal, no complaints; no evidence of disease
90	Able to carry on normal activity, minor signs or symptoms of disease
80	Normal activity with efforts, some signs or symptoms of disease
70	Cares for self but unable to carry on normal activity or do active work
60	Requires considerable assistance but is able to care for most personal needs
50	Requires considerable assistance and frequent medical care
40	Disabled; requires special care and assistance
30	Severely disabled; hospitalization indicated, although death not imminent
20	Very sick; hospitalization necessary; active support treatment necessary
10	Moribund; fatal process progressing rapidly
0	Dead
Grade	**Gynecologic Oncology Group of performance status scale**
1	Fully active, able to carry on all predisease performance without restriction
2	Restricted in physically strenuous activity but ambulatory and able to carry out work of a light or sedentary nature (e.g., light house work, office work)
3	Capable of only limited self-care, confined to bed or chair >50% of waking hours
4	Completely disabled; cannot carry on any self-care totally confined to bed or chair
5	Dead

Note

***Karnofsky Performance Scale**–It is an assessment tool for functional impairment. It can be used to compare effectiveness of different therapies and to assess the prognosis in individual patients. In most serious illnesses, the lower the **Karnofsky** score, the worse the likelihood of survival*

SUMMARY OF THE COMMON CHEMOTHERAPEUTIC AGENTS, ROUTE OF THERAPY, TOXICITY AND CANCERS Table 12.16

Table 12.16: Chemotherapy agents used in treatment of gynecological cancers

Drug	Route of administration	Common toxicities	Used in
Cyclophosphamide	PO, IV	Myelosuppression cystitis + bladder fibrosis, alopecia, hepatitis	Breast, ovarian cancer, soft tissue sarcomas
Chlorambucil	PO	Myelosuppression, nausea dermatitis, hepatotoxicity	Ovarian cancer
Melphalan	PO	Myelosuppression, nausea and vomiting (rare), second malignancies	Ovarian, breast cancer
Cisplatin	IV	Nephrotoxicity, tinnitus and hearing loss, nausea and vomiting, myelosuppression, peripheral neuropathy	Ovarian carcinoma, cervical, endometrial cancer
Carboplatin	IV	Less neuropathy, ototoxicity and nephrotoxicity than cisplatin; more hematopoietic toxicity, especially thr; ombocytopenia, than cisplatin	Ovarian carcinomas, endometrial and cervical cancer
Dacarbazine	IV	Myelosuppression, nausea and vomiting, flu-like syndrome, hepatotoxicity	Uterine sarcoma soft tissue sarcoma

Antitumor antibiotic used for gynecologic cancer

Drug	Route of administration	Common toxicities	Used in
Actinomycin D (dactinomycin)	IV	Nausea and vomiting, skin necrosis, mucosal ulceration myelosuppression	Germ cell ovarian tumors, choriocarcinoma, soft tissue sarcoma
Blecomycin	IV, IM	Fever, dermatologic reactions, pulmonary toxicity, anaphylactic reactions	Germ cell ovarian tumor
Doxorubicin (Adriamycin)	IV	Myelosuppression, alopecia, cardiotoxicity, nausea and vomiting, mucosal ulceration	Ovarian, breast, endometrial cancer
Liposomal doxorubicin	IV	Palmar-plantar erythrodysesthesia, myelosuppression stomatitis	Ovarian and endometrial cancer

Antimetabolitics used for gynecologic cancer

Drug	Route of administration	Common toxicities	Used in
5 - Fluorouracil (flucecuncil 5FU)	IV	Myelosuppression, nausea and vomiting anorexia, alopecia	Breast, cervical cancer
Methotrexate	PO, IV, II	Mucosal ulceration, myelsuppression, hepatototoxicity, allergic pneumonitis with intrathecal: Meningeal irritation	Choriocarcinoma, breast cancer
Gemcitabine	IV	Myeosuppression, fever	Ovarian, breast cancer leiomyosarcoma

Contd.

Contd.

Plant alkaloids			
Drug	**Route of administration**	**Common toxicities**	**Used in**
Vincristine (Oncovin)	IV	Neurotoxicity myelosuppression, cranial nerve palsies, gastrointestinal	Ovarian germ cell tumors, sarcomas, cervical cancer
Vinblastine	IV	Myelosuppression, alopecia, nausea and vomiting, neurotoxicity	Ovarian germ cell tumors
Epipodophyllotoxin (etoposide)	IV/PO	Myelosuppression, alopecia	Ovarian germ cell tumors, choriocarcinoma, Ovarian cancer
Paclitacel	IV	Myelosuppression, alopecia, allergic reactions, cardiac arrhythmias	Ovarian, breast cancer
Vinorelbine	IV	Myelosuppression, constipation, peripheral neuropathy	Ovarian, breast cancer
Docetaxel	IV	Myelosuppression, alopecia, hypersensitivity reactions, peripheral edema	Breast, ovarian cancer

Topoisomerase 1 Inhibitors			
Drug	**Route of administration**	**Common toxicities**	**Used in**
Topotecan	IV	Myelosuppression	Ovarian cancer
Trinotecan	IV	Myelosuppression, diarrhea	Cervical, ovarian cancer

Anti-angiogenesis agents			
Drug	**Route of administration**	**Common toxicities**	**Used in**
Bevacizumab	IV	Hypertension, proteinuria, bowel per-formation	Breast, ovarian and cervical cancer
VEGF Trap (Aflibercept)	IV	Hypertension, proteinuria, fatigue	Colon cancer

Other agents			
Drug	**Route**	**Toxicities**	**Used in**
Progesterones: 17–α-Hydroxy progesteronecaproate	IM	Hepatic dysfunction , Alopecia	Carcinoma endometrium
Medroxyprogesterone acetate	Oral		
Megestrol acetate	Oral		
Anti-estrogen: Tamoxifen	Oral	Hot flushes, pruritus vulvae, vaginal bleeding	Carcinoma Breast Carcinoma Endometrium
Hydroxyurea	Oral	Bone marrow depression, megaloblastic anemia, stomatitis, alopecia, diarrhea	Carcinoma cervix (with radio-therapy).

CHAPTER 13

TARGETED THERAPY FOR GYNECOLOGICAL CANCERS

INTRODUCTION

- **Targeted therapy** is a new medical treatment for cancer that inhibits the growth of cancer cells by interfering with specific molecules needed for their pathway of carcinogenesis and progression (different from traditional cytotoxic chemotherapy)
- **Recent advances** in molecular biology of cancer have led to the development of **targeted agents such as monoclonal antibodies and small-molecule compounds that** target the signaling pathways of cancer cells and vasculature in tumor tissues
- In addition, novel **immunotherapy using immune checkpoint inhibitors such as anti-PD-1 antibody** for modulation of local immunity have also been developed

DRUGS FOR TARGETED THERAPY (Table 13.1)

One of the earliest and most extensively used molecular Targeted drugs is tamoxifen, a selective estrogen receptor (ER) modulator that competitively antagonizes ER in breast tissue–widely used to prevent recurrence of ER–positive breast cancer

New drugs for targeted therapy are divided into two categories

- **Monoclonal antibodies** that do not penetrate the cell membrane but bind with the ligands and receptors of the specific growth factors
- **Low molecular organic compounds** that can enter the cytoplasm and act on targets such as tyrosine kinases, PI3K/AKT/mTOR pathways and DNA repair mechanisms

Table 13.1: New Drugs for Targeted Therapy and Their Mechanism of Action

Drug	MOA	Indication
Monoclonal antibodies targeting ligands and receptors		
Trastuzumab	Human epidermal growth factor-2 (HER2/neu) is over expressed in about 15–20% of early stage breast cancers and is associated with poor prognosis Trastuzumab is a Humanized monoclonal antibody that selectively binds to the HER2 receptors	Metastatic breast cancer expressing HER2 receptors
Cetuximab	Epidermal growth factor receptor (EGFR blocker)	Treatment of head and neck cancer, colorectal cancer
Bevacizumab	Anti-VEGF monoclonal antibody-inhibit the signaling pathways of angiogenesis	• Cancer of the colon, lung, breast, kidney, and brain • It is an important targeted drug for ovarian and cervical cancers
Tyrosine kinase inhibitors		
Imatinib mesylate	• Philadelphia chromosome seen in CML is related to BCR-ABL tyrosine kinase over expression • Imatinib inhibits the activated BCR-ABL tyrosine kinase and suppresses the growth of Philadelphia chromosome-positive CML	Chronic myeloid leukemia

Contd.

Contd.

Gefitinib	EGFR tyrosine kinase inhibitor-prevents cell proliferation, stimulates apoptosis and increases levels of cyclin-dependent Kinase inhibitor p27, which leads to G1 cell cycle arrest	Treatment of advanced Non small cell lung cancer (NSLC)
Erlotinib	EGFR tyrosine kinase inhibitor	Treatment of metastatic NSLC
Lapatinib	Inhibits both EGFR and HER2	HER2-positive breast cancers refractory to trastuzumab
Phosphatidyl inositol 3-kinase(PI3K)/mTOR (mammalian target of rapamycin) pathway inhibitors • **PI3K signaling pathway mediates cell growth and proliferation** • **mTOR acts within the PI3K signaling pathway and is an important integrator of several targetable signaling cascades**		
Pictilisib	PI3K inhibitors	• Approved for astrocytoma, breast cancer, renal cell carcinoma • Studied for treatment of endometrial cancer and ovarian cancers with PTEN mutation
Temsirolimus, Everolimus	mTOR inhibitors	
Poly (ADP-ribose) polymerase (PARP) inhibitors–		
Olaparib, Rucaparib and Niraparib	Prevent DNA repair in the tumor cells and make them vulnerable to apoptosis	Approved for use in ovarian cancer

MOLECULAR–TARGETED DRUGS FOR GYNECOLOGICAL CANCERS

Numerous agents that target specific gynecologic cancer-related molecules have been tried, mainly for patients with advanced or recurrent disease

- **Anti-VEGF antibodies**–in treatment of **ovarian and cervical cancers**
- **PARP inhibitors**-in treatment of **ovarian cancer**

Anti-VEGF Antibodies–Bevacizumab

- VEGF plays an important role in angiogenesis. **Bevacizumab is an** anti-VEGF antibody, a recombinant humanized monoclonal immunoglobulin G antibody that binds to circulating VEGF and prevents it from binding to its receptors
- Clinical benefits reported in patients with colorectal cancer and breast cancer and ovarian cancer
- **Adverse events**–hypertension, proteinuria, and serious gastrointestinal toxicities such as perforation and fistula
- Phase II trials that evaluated bevacizumab as monotherapy for ovarian cancer yielded favorable results with response rates of 16–21%
- Phase III trials that evaluated paclitaxel and carboplatin chemotherapy plus bevacizumab resulted in significantly longer progression-free survival than chemotherapy alone
- **AURELIA study for platinum-resistant recurrent ovarian cancer**
  - Significant improvement in progression-free survival but not in overall survival was observed in the chemotherapy plus bevacizumab group
  - The benefit of bevacizumab in quality of life was consistent in patients with ascites
- **OCEANS study for platinum-sensitive recurrent ovarian cancer**
  - Significantly, longer progression-free survival but no difference in overall survival was observed in chemotherapy with bevacizumab group
- Following these studies, bevacizumab has been approved for ovarian cancer patients in both primary and recurrent settings
- A phase III clinical trial in patients with metastatic, persistent, or recurrent cervical cancer disease showed overall survival improvement by addition of bevacizumab to chemotherapy

PARP Inhibitors

- *BRCA1* and *BRCA2* are tumor suppressor genes involved in repair when double-strand DNA breaks occur in normal cells; BRCA1/2 germline mutations account for 5–10% of breast cancers and 15% of ovarian cancers

- **Poly (ADP-ribose) polymerase (PARP)** is a key enzyme involved in repair of DNA single-strand breaks using the base excision repair pathway
- PARP inhibitors in tumors with BRCA1/2 mutations prevent DNA repair in tumor cells and make them vulnerable to apoptosis referred to as "synthetic lethality"
- PARP inhibitors have emerged as one of the key targeted therapies in the management of ovarian cancer
- The evolution of clinical trials of PARP inhibitors in ovarian cancer has led to a progression from its use only in patients with BRCA germline mutations to patients with platinum-sensitive recurrent ovarian cancer
- **NOVA, SOLO and ARIEL trials**–showed significant improvement in the progression-free survival after recurrence
- PARP inhibitors that have been approved for use in ovarian cancer are **Olaparib, Rucaparib and Niraparib**
- Major advantages–availability of oral formulations and have good tolerance

IMMUNOTHERAPY

It is defined as administration of agents that can modulate, induce, modify and alter inflammatory and immune responses in the body

Facts that have led to the idea that host immune response can prevent tumor growth

- Immune suppressed patients are more likely to develop malignant disease
- Therapy with monoclonal antibodies is found to destroy tumor cells, which is due to antibody dependent cellular cytotoxicity
- Natural killer (NK) cells and lymphokine-activated killer (LAK) cells together with IL-2 TNF, IFN can cause tumor cell destruction (adoptive immunotherapy)

Principles of Immunotherapy

- Tumor mass must be reduced to a minimum by surgery, chemotherapy or radiation prior to immunotherapy
- Single agent therapy is often ineffective. Immunotherapeutic approach should be a combined therapy
- Immunotherapy is more effective against tumors that are highly antigenic

Immune response leading to rejection of tumor can occur when the following conditions are fulfilled

- Biological response modifiers are in direct contact with tumors
- Tumor bulk is minimal
- Blood supply is good
- Monoclonal antibodies should be conjugated with agents (chemotherapy drugs, interferon) for precise delivery to tumor cells

Tumor Associated Antigens

- **HER-2/Neu:** Transmembrane protein of the HER-2 family amplified in 20–30% **ovarian cancers and breast cancer**
- **Folate-Binding Protein (FBP):** FBP functions as a transmembrane transporter of folate expressed in **ovarian cancers**
- **MUC-1:** High molecular weight glycoprotein expressed on membranes of epithelial cancer cells including ovary, breast and gastrointestinal malignancies
- **CEA:** Over-expressed in more than **50% of ovarian mucinous carcinomas**
- **p53:** Tumor suppressor gene p53 mutated in 30–50% of ovarian cancers
- **Sialyl–Tn:** Common in **mucinous tumors** and is extremely immunogenic

Types of Immunotherapy

- **Approaches to augment the immune response to tumor include the following:**
  - **Active immunotherapy**–to induce host immune response
  - **Passive immunotherapy**–immunologically active substances are directly transferred to the host

Active immunotherapy for ovarian cancer:
  - CD4+ T cells that target MUC1
  - Vaccination with p53 peptide, HER2-derived peptide, and WT-1 peptide
- **Passive immunotherapy**
  - **Anti CA–125 antibody, Oregovomab, Abagovomab in advanced Ovarian tumors**
- **Yttrium- 90 monoclonal antibody-binds specifically to polymorphic epithelial mucin (PEM), an antigen expressed in more than 90% ovarian cancers**
- **Trifunctional antibody Catumaxomab (EPCAM X anti-CD33)** has been evaluated in patients with malignant ascites

Novel Immuno Therapy for Gynecologic Cancers

- Clinical trials using Immunotherapy as immune checkpoint inhibitors has demonstrated efficacy in a subset of patients with recurrent ovarian cancer
- **Cervical cancer**–phase III trials with therapeutic vaccine targeting **HPV oncoproteins E6 and E7** are under evaluation
- Cancer cells frequently express either CTLA-4 or PD-L1 which reduce the immune attack by T cells. Immunotherapy using anti-CTLA antibodies or PD-L1/PD-1 antibodies is a novel targeted therapy against the immune checkpoint signals
  - **Anti-CTLA-4 antibodies-Ipilimumab, Tremelimumab**
  - **Anti-PD-1 antibodies-Nivolumab, Pembrolizumab**
  - **Anti-PD-L1 antibodies-Atezolizumab, Durvalumab, Avelumab**
- **Nivolumaband avelumab- tried for recurrent ovarian cancer**
- **Pembrolizumab**–tried for **advanced cervical cancer**
- **Adverse effects** of immune checkpoint inhibitors–colitis, endocrinopathies and pneumonitis
- **Topical IFN-α** has been used in persistent **atypia and dysplasia**
- **Paternal leucocyte immunization** used in **choriocarcinoma with pulmonary metastasis**

IMMUNOTOXINS

Immunotoxins are molecules that bind to surface antigens (which internalize) and kill cells by catalytic inhibition of protein synthesis within the cell cytosol

Examples of immunotoxins include:

- Ricin A
- Pseudomonal exotoxin
- Salmonella endotoxin
- Methotrexate
- Adriamycin

RECENT UPDATES

Recent and ongoing clinical trials using targeted therapeutics for high-grade serous carcinomas (Table 13.2)

Table 13.2: Recent and ongoing clinical trials using targeted therapeutics

Class	Agent	Target(s)
Anti-angiogenics		
	Bevacizumab[a]	*VEGF*
	Cabozantinib	*c-met, VEGFR2, RET, AXL*
	Cediranib	*VEGFR 2/3/4, c-kit*
	Fosbretabulin	*Endothelial microtubules*
	Trebananib	*Angiopoietin-1/2*

Contd.

Contd.

PARP inhibitors		
	Olaparib	*PARP*
	Niraparib	*PARP*
	Veliparib	*PARP*
	Rucaparib	*PARP*
	Pazopanib	*PARP*
	Cabozantinib	*PARP*
Immunologics		
	EGEN-001	*IL-12*
	Nivolumab	*PD-1*
	Ruxolitinib	*JAK1, JAK2*
	VTX-2337	*TLR8*
Pathway inhibitors		
	Temsirolimus	*MTOR*

Poly-ribose polymerase (PARP)IL-12, interleukin-12; JAK, Janus Kinase; MTOR, mammalian target of rapamycin; PD-1, programmed death 1; PFS, progression-free survival; TLR8, Toll-like receptor 8; VEGF, vascular endothelial growth factor; VEGFR2, vascular endothelial growth factor receptor 2

CHAPTER 14

TUMOR MARKERS IN GYNECOLOGIC CANCERS

INTRODUCTION

A tumor marker is a substance that is selectively produced by the neoplastic tissue and released into the blood where from it can be detected

An Ideal tumor marker should fulfill the following criteria

- It should be specific. It should be produced only by the tumor cells
- Its measurement should be sensitive enough to detect microscopic or subclinical disease
- Tumor markers are used to monitor the response of therapy. Ideally the tumor marker level should represent the tumor volume correctly. Progressive rise in marker value indicates ineffective chemotherapy
- The assay should be inexpensive and acceptable
- The tumor marker should indicate the presence as well the site of tumor origin
- **Tumor markers can be classified as follows:**
  - Tumor derived markers which originate from neoplastic cells themselves
  - Tumor associated markers that include various enzymes and proteins produced by cells of uninvolved organs or tissue infiltration by metastasis

TUMOR MARKERS IN OVARIAN TUMORS

- **The best tumor marker for epithelial ovarian tumors is CA–125**
- **CA-125 (carcinoma antigen 125) also known as mucin 16 or MUC 16** is a protein that is **encoded by the MUC16 gene** in humans. MUC16 is a member of the mucin family **glycoproteins**
- The reference range for CA -125 is **0-35 U/ml**
- **Apparently healthy pre-menopausal women can have levels of about 100 U/mL during menstruation**
- **Apparently healthy postmenopausal women can have levels< 20 U/mL**
- Although elevated CA 125 levels are found in about 80% of cases with epithelial ovarian cancers, **higher levels are found in only 50% of patients with FIGO Stage I disease (early stage ovarian cancer)**
- **Lack of sensitivity for early disease limits the use of CA 125 for diagnosis of early stage epithelial ovarian cancers**
- In addition to menstruation and first trimester of pregnancy, CA 125 levels can be elevated in multiple benign diseases as mentioned in Table 14.1
- **CA 125 can also be elevated in adenocarcinomas other than of ovarian tumors**

Table 14.1: Benign diseases and Non ovarian cancers which can have elevated CA 125 levels	
Benign diseases giving rise to elevated CA 125 levels	**Non ovarian malignancies giving rise to elevated CA 125 levels**
Endometriosis Benign ovarian tumors Acute salpingitis Uterine myoma Cirrhosis Cirrhosis with ascites Chronic active hepatitis	Endometrial Cervical Breast Colorectal Pancreas
Acute pancreatitis Chronic pancreatitis Renal failure	Lung Liver Gastric Biliary tract

Tumor Marker Application in Epithelial Ovarian Cancers	
Screening	• As a screening test, the main problem with CA 125 are: – Lack of sensitivity for early stage disease (only 50% patients with Stage I have elevated levels) – Lack of specificity (elevated in other adenocarcinomas and several benign conditions) • Due to these limitations, CA 125 is not currently recommended for general population screening for detection of sporadic form of disease • CA 125 in combination with TVS may have a role in early detection of ovarian cancer in women with hereditary ovarian cancer syndrome
Diagnosis	• Diagnosis of ovarian cancer is usually carried out by surgery followed by histopathology • Pre operative serum levels of CA 125, especially in post menopausal women may be useful in the differentiating of benign and malignant ovarian masses
Prognosis	• The traditional prognostic factors for ovarian cancer include tumor stage, grade, histological type and size of residual tumor after primary debulking (cytoreductive surgery) • Studies have shown that CA 125 levels is one of the strongest indicators of disease outcome; prolonged half-life of CA 125 or less than 7 fold decrease in CA 125 levels during the early months of treatment has been shown to predict poor outcome
Monitoring	• The most important application of CA 125 is in the monitoring of patients with epithelial ovarian cancers • Serial CA 125 levels can pre clinically detect recurrent disease earlier and more cost effectively than radiological procedures

Tumor Markers in Ovarian Germ Cell Tumors

- **AFP and hCG** are the main markers for ovarian germ cell tumors and the particular tumor marker expressed depends on the state of differentiation of the tumor and the histological tumor

Table 14.2: Tumor markers in ovarian cancers	
Tumor markers in ovarian tumors	
Ovarian tumor	**Tumor marker**
Dysgerminoma	Placental alkaline phosphatase, LDH
Yolk sac tumor (endodermal sinus tumor)	AFP and alpha-1 antitrypsin
Embryonal cell carcinoma	hCG and AFP
Polyembryoma	hCG and AFP
Choriocarcinoma	hCG
Teratoma	hCG
Nonmucinous malignant epithelial tumor	CA 125
Mucinous ovarian tumor	Carcinoembryonic antigen (CEA), CA 19-9
AFP, alpha fetoprotein, hCG, human chorionic gonadotropin, LDH, lactic acid dehydrogenase; Inhibin is used in granulosa cell tumors	

TUMOR MARKER IN CANCER CERVIX

- **Squamous cell carcinoma antigen (SCCA)** is the **tumor marker of choice for squamous cell carcinoma of cervix**
- SCCA is a 48 kDa protein with strong homology to a family of protease inhibitors known as serpins
- **Sensitivity of SCCA for carcinoma of cervix varies from less than 30% for stage I disease to over 90% for Stage IV disease**
- SCCA can be elevated in other squamous cell cancers (lung, head and neck, vagina) and in benign diseases of the skin (psoriasis, eczema), lung (sarcoidosis), liver and kidney

Tumor Marker Applicationin Cancer Cervix	
Screening	Screening asymptomatic women for cervical cancer with PAP smear helps in detection of pre invasive lesions of the cervix Serum tumor markers currently have no role in screening for cervical cancer
Diagnosis	The diagnosis of cervical cancer is based on histopathology SCCA lacks sensitivity and specificity and hence contribute little to the diagnosis of early stage disease Pre treatment levels of SCCA in squamous cell cancers may be an independent predictor of lymph node metastasis
Prognosis	Few studies have shown that high pre treatment levels of SCCA have been found to be an independent predictor of poor outcome in patients with squamous cell cancers In adenocarcinoma of cervix, CA 125 was found to be a prognostic indicator
Monitoring	Potential applications of SCCA in the follow up of patients with diagnosed SCC of cervix include • Early detection of recurrent disease • Monitoring of neoadjuvant chemotherapy • Monitoring treatment of recurrent disease In the follow up of cervical cancer, the overall correlation between clinical course of disease and variation in SCCA levels is usually greater than 80%. However, a clinical value in monitoring patients with SCCA has not been shown

TUMOR MARKER IN ENDOMETRIAL CANCER

Tumor Markers in Endometrial Cancers	
Screening	No existing marker has the sensitivity and specificity to screen for early endometrial cancer
Diagnosis	Endometrial cancer is diagnosed based on the histological examination of tissue obtained at curettage As CA 125 is elevated in only a minority of patients with low stage disease, it contributes little to early diagnosis
Monitoring	For monitoring patients with endometrial cancer, CA- 125 is the best available marker Elevated levels are found in 60% cases with recurrent endometrial cancers As with SCCA in cancer cervix, there is no evidence that follow up with serial CA 125 levels improves patient outcome The role of CA 125 in monitoring patients with uterine serous carcinoma is of questionable value

RECENT ADVANCES

Potential tumor markers for epithelial ovarian tumors under research include the following:

- *Complementary markers include CA 15-3, OVX1, CA 72-4 and cytokeratin 8 and 18 markers*
- *Further studies are required to establish how these markers can contribute to the diagnosis and management of patients with ovarian cancers*
- *Prognostic indicators–Kallikrein 8, Mesothelin, CYFRA 21-1, M-CSF, TATI, VEGF, CASA, Tetranectin*
- *Differentiation of adnexal masses–Osteopontin, TPS, CA-15-3, CA-72-4, CA-19-9, TATI, GAT, free serum DNA methylation, free glycans, IL-7, TNF a receptors*
- *Monitoring response to therapy–CASA*
- *Monitoring disease recurrence–HE4 BL1> hTERT - human telomerase reverse transcriptase has a beneficial role in carcinoma cervix.*

CHAPTER 15

GYNECOLOGICAL CANCERS DURING PREGNANCY

INTRODUCTION

- Cancers during pregnancy is infrequent, with an incidence of about 1 in 1000 pregnancies
- Cancers during pregnancy can pose several challenges to healthcare professionals due to lack of clinical consensus as there is lack of major cohort studies and randomized controlled trials
- Current recommendations state that pregnancy should be preserved whenever feasible, alongside providing accurate information to the mother and consideration of her wishes regarding continuation or termination of pregnancy
- **Pregnancy is not known to cause any deleterious effect on the prognosis of cervical and ovarian cancer** and pregnant women with these conditions are known to have **similar outcomes as nonpregnant women**
- Common tumors presenting during pregnancy **are breast cancer, cervical cancer, lymphomas, leukemia and ovarian cancers**
- The most **common gynecological cancers** diagnosed in pregnancy are **cervical and ovarian cancers**
- **Endometrial cancer** in young women is generally an **incidental diagnosis made during endometrial curettage following abortion or delivery**
- **Vulvar or vaginal cancers in pregnancy** and young women are rare
- **Diagnosis of cancer during pregnancy may be delayed for the following reasons**
  - Many symptoms of malignancy are similar to the symptoms of pregnancy, including nausea/vomiting, breast changes, abdominal pain, anemia and fatigue
  - Breast changes and the pregnant uterus may make physical examination difficult
  - Owing to its rarity, cancer during pregnancy might not be considered in the differential diagnosis
  - The sensitivity and specificity of tumor markers may be low during pregnancy-CA 15-3 used in breast cancer, CA 125 used in epithelial ovarian cancer, and alpha-fetoprotein used in germ cell tumors are physiologically elevated in pregnancy
  - Alteration of commonly used laboratory values may complicate the diagnosis of malignancy-Hemoglobin and hematocrit values are typically lower, whereas alkaline phosphatase and lactate dehydrogenase are typically higher in pregnancy

Ethical Issues

- A decision may often be needed to prolong or terminate the pregnancy, in order to optimize maternal therapy and hence the clinician needs to adopt a sensitive approach
- The patient should be well informed of the available treatment options, their complications and implications to the pregnancy and the fetus

IMAGING IN PREGNANCY

The following issues need to be taken into account when choosing the appropriate imaging technique in pregnancy:

- Safety of the fetus
- Viability of the fetus
- Risk of metastasis

- Radiation exposure above 100 mGy is associated with fetal malformation and childhood cancer in the newborn

- X-rays if needed, to be taken with proper abdominal shielding
- Mammogram images are difficult to interpret owing to physiological hypervascularity and density of the breast tissue
- CT scan is best avoided during pregnancy because of the unacceptable cumulative radiation and contrast doses
- Positron-emission tomography (PET) scan in pregnancy is debatable owing to the risk of radiation exposure to the fetus
- Ultrasound as a tool for diagnosis and staging is noninvasive and helps to perform guided biopsies of the breast and lymph nodes
- MRI scan is safe in all trimesters of pregnancy. It is the imaging technique of choice for diagnosis and staging of cancers during pregnancy
- Histopathology of tissues provides definitive diagnosis of tumor type and grading. The pathologist should be informed of the pregnancy status of the patient, to avoid incorrect interpretation resulting from pregnancy-associated tissue changes

CANCER CERVIX IN PREGNANCY

- Cervical cancer is the **most common gynecological malignancy associated with pregnancy**
- Cervical cancers in pregnancy generally present as Stage I disease at diagnosis
- **Vaginal bleeding is the usual presenting symptom**
- Women with suspicious cervical lesion in pregnancy should be subjected to cytology and colposcopic examination. Patients with a visible cervical lesion should have a directed biopsy
- Cervical cytology during pregnancy frequently cause concern, as, the presence of decidual cells may be mistaken for atypia
- Colposcopy can be challenging during pregnancy owing to increased vascularity and increase in genital edema
- Punch biopsy during pregnancy can lead to profuse bleeding due to increased vascularity
- Staging of cervical cancer is based on clinical examination
- CT scan carries a risk of radiation exposure to the fetus and is not recommended in pregnancy
- MRI for assessment of local and regional spread is safe in pregnancy
- **The safety and complications of procedures used** for diagnosis and treatment of cancer cervix in pregnant women are listed in Table 15.1

Table 15.1: Safety and complications of procedures in cervical cancer in pregnancy

	Procedure	Safety/complications
Diagnostic procedures	Colposcopy	Safe
	Cervical biopsy	Bleeding tends to be more
	Endocervical curettage	Rupture of membranes
	Conization	Increased risk of abortion, preterm labor
Imaging modalities	Ultrasonography, MRI	Safe
	CT scan	Fetal radiation
Treatment modalities	Surgery	Bleeding tends to be more
	Chemotherapy	Abortion, congenital malformation, fetal death
	Radiotherapy	Abortion, fetal death

Management of premalignant disease and cervical cancer during pregnancy (Table 15.2)

- **Management of preinvasive disease (CIN 1 to CIN 3)** can be deferred until 6–8 weeks after delivery. However, it is recommended that a colposcopy is performed in each trimester to assess lesion size and disease progress
- Principle factors considered in the **management of cervical cancers in pregnancy:**
  - Stage of the disease
  - Gestational age
  - Histological subtype
- **Immediate definitive treatment,** regardless of gestational age, is appropriate for invasive cancer in the following settings:
  - Documented lymph node metastases

- Progression of disease during the pregnancy
- Patient's choice to terminate pregnancy

- **With early-stage disease (up to small volume stage IB1 (2 cm)) and in the absence of any nodal disease, the current trend is continuation of pregnancy, following treatment with** large loop excision of the transformation zone **(LLETZ), conization or radical trachelectomy and consideration of pelvic lymphadenectomy to assess disease spread**
- **Cesarean section is preferred,** as vaginal delivery is associated with an increased risk of spread of the tumor
- Cases of **Stage IA1, IA2, and IB1 cervical cancers** should be managed on an individual basis; the key factors in determining treatment are tumor type and size
- **Stage IA1 tumors can be managed by LLETZ or cold-knife conization alone**
- **LLETZ or cold-knife conization should be undertaken early in pregnancy**
- Conization is best done between 12 and 20 weeks of pregnancy. The term "coin biopsy" is used in pregnancy to highlight that the incision should not be deep enough to cause damage to the fetal membranes
- **As pregnancy progresses, conization** is associated with risks such as bleeding, pregnancy loss, premature delivery or premature rupture of membranes
- **In stage IA2 and above, lymphadenectomy is performed,** to assess spread of the tumor and to gain prognostic information which helps in further management of the case
- **Laparoscopic pelvic lymphadenectomy** for assessment of pelvic node status is best performed before 20 weeks of pregnancy
- **Histopathological evaluation of nodes can be difficult to interpret** due to decidual changes in pelvic nodes, which can mimic nodal metastases
- Postoperative chemoradiation is usually advised, if lymph nodes are positive
- **Stage IB1 tumors (up to 2 cm)may be managed with radical trachelectomy in the first trimester, thereby preserving pregnancy.** Obstetric outcome is poor and hence radical trachelectomy is not recommended during pregnancy
- In **Stage IB1 cervical cancer diagnosed in advanced pregnancy,** once fetal is viable, delivery should be by caesarean section, immediately followed by radical hysterectomy and pelvic lymphadenectomy
- **Stage IB1 tumors (>2 cm) may be treated with neoadjuvant chemotherapy (NACT) with or without pelvic lymphadenectomy**
- **Chemotherapy is relatively safe in the second trimester,** although there is risk of preterm labor, premature rupture of membranes and fetal growth restriction. NACT stabilizes the tumor until fetal maturity is achieved so that cesarean delivery and radical hysterectomy can be performed
- In **advanced cervical cancer > stage IB1,** prognosis is not good and the standard management is with **chemoradiation. Pregnancy termination and treatment as in nonpregnant women is advocated**
  - **In early gestation (less than 12 weeks), spontaneous abortion occurs after pelvic radiation**
  - **In second trimester cases, hysterotomy followed by definitive chemoradiation is preferred**
  - **If the fetus has attained viability,** deliver the fetus to enable treatment to be started
- The prognosis of squamous cell carcinoma, adenocarcinoma or adenosquamous carcinomas are similar as in nonpregnant women
- **Postpartum follow-up** is the same as for nonpregnant women

Table 15.2: Management of cervical cancer during pregnancy

Stage	Management during pregnancy
Stage IA1	Pregnancy can be followed till term and vaginal delivery can be allowed. Vaginal hysterectomy can be done, 6 weeks later
Stage IA2	Continue pregnancy till fetal maturity. Do cesarean section and modified radical hysterectomy with pelvic lymph node dissection (PLND)
Stage IB1	Do not delay treatment for more than 4 weeks to attain fetal maturity. Do classical cesarean section and radical hysterectomy with PLND
Stage II-IV	If the fetus is viable, deliver by classical cesarean section followed by radiotherapy immediately

Management of pregnant women previously treated for cervical cancer

- These women might have had either a LLETZ or cone biopsy or trachelectomy for treatment of the lesion
- Women previously treated with **trachelectomy** are at increased risk of **preterm rupture of membranes, chorioamnionitis, mid-trimester loss and preterm delivery**
- Patient should be counseled about the need for delivery by **cesarean section**

OVARIAN AND FALLOPIAN TUBE CANCERS IN PREGNANCY

- Ovarian cancer is the **second most frequent gynecological malignancy** occurring in pregnancy, next to cancer cervix (the most common benign ovarian tumor associated with pregnancy is Dermoid cyst)
- **The common ovarian malignancies in pregnancy are: borderline ovarian tumors, germ cell tumors, sex cord-stromal tumors and epithelial tumors**
- **The most common symptom is abdominal or pelvic pain**
- Preoperative ultrasound may be helpful in differentiating benign from malignant ovarian tumors
- **MRI** of the abdomen and pelvis should be used to characterize ovarian masses and the extent of disease **(CT scan is not recommended in pregnancy)**
- The tumor marker **CA125 is not very reliable during pregnancy, particularly in the first trimester,** with concentrations reported being more than 65 IU/ml
- **Definitive diagnosis** can be made only on removal of the adnexal mass, inspection of the abdominal cavity and biopsy of any suspicious lesions, with necessary cytological analysis

Management of ovarian tumors in pregnancy

- **Surgery for asymptomatic masses should be undertaken only when the mass has obvious malignant features** by assessment of risk malignancy index. If the risk of malignancy is high, surgical staging is done
- When suspicion of malignancy is low, expectant management can be adopted
- Surgery is indicated in cases with risk of **ovarian torsion or rupture**
- Surgery should **ideally be performed between 12 and 27 weeks of gestation**
- **Laparoscopic management can be recommended upto 20 weeks of gestation, if** the risk of malignancy is low

Management of borderline ovarian tumors in pregnancy

- Management is similar to that in nonpregnant women
- The recommendation is for **continuation of the pregnancy with the aim of having a normal delivery, irrespective of the time of diagnosis**
- These tumors have **good prognosis** and can be managed surgically in the postpartum period

Management of non-epithelial ovarian cancers in pregnancy

- Patients with **non-epithelial cancers** are **often symptomatic,** frequently due to large mass and are **usually at stage I when diagnosed** in pregnancy
- **Fertility-preserving surgery with a unilateral salpingo-oophorectomy is done,** generally without lymphadenectomy, unless suspicious lymph nodes are visualised during surgery
- **Alpha-fetoprotein is raised in pregnancy,** but the **levels with germ cell tumors are significantly higher than those found in normal pregnancies**
- In germ cell tumors, **BEP regime is considered highly toxic** because fetal growth restriction and neonatal complications are high. **Weekly paclitaxel and cisplatin is usually recommended**

Management of epithelial ovarian cancers in pregnancy

- **Management depends on the stage of the tumor**

- **With stage I,** treatment is similar to that of non-pregnant women. **Unilateral salpingo-oophorectomy** with surgical staging, preserving the uterus and contralateral ovary is usually performed. Pelvic and para-aortic lymphadenectomy should be performed, if suspicious nodes are identified
- With **stage II–IIIB** disease, surgical debulking should be done as soon as possible that involves hysterectomy and termination of the pregnancy
  - If she wishes to continue with the pregnancy, neoadjuvant chemotherapy should be offered until fetal maturity, with the aim to perform cytoreductive surgery following delivery
- With **advanced or unresectable disease (Stage IIIC–IV)** neoadjuvant chemotherapy and interval debulking surgery are offered; Prognosis is often poor.
- Paclitaxel/carboplatin-based chemotherapy can be given safely in the second and third trimester in epithelial ovarian cancer, stopped before 37 weeks to avoid myelosuppression in the neonate
- Bevacizumab is not recommended during pregnancy
- Vaginal delivery is ideal in early-stage ovarian cancer that has been treated surgically

Management of pregnant women previously treated for ovarian malignancy

- **CA-125 levels can be elevated in pregnancy**
- **CA-125 and MRI** scan should be performed only **if the woman has symptoms or there is strong clinical suspicion of recurrence**

FALLOPIAN TUBE CANCER IN PREGNANCY

- Very little is found in the literature about the management of fallopian tube cancer in pregnancy
- **Fallopian tube cancer are managed similar to epithelial ovarian cancers**
- More recently, an increasing number of cases that were thought to be ovarian malignancies have been diagnosed as **primary fallopian tube cancers**

ENDOMETRIAL CANCER IN PREGNANCY

- Endometrial carcinoma is rarely diagnosed in pregnancy, with most cases incidentally diagnosed in women who have undergone endometrial curettage for miscarriage or termination of pregnancy
- Increased incidence of **obesity** is linked to an increase in incidence of **endometrial carcinoma in a relatively younger age group.** This poses a challenge in young women who wish to preserve their fertility

Management of endometrial carcinoma in pregnancy

- The standard treatment for endometrial carcinoma remains total hysterectomy and bilateral salpingo-oophorectomy
- In young women, case series have been published on managing **atypical endometrial hyperplasia and cases of grade 1, stage IA endometrioid cancers confined to the endometrium with progestogen therapy, with surveillance hysteroscopy and achieving successful pregnancy outcomes**
- As the number of young women with endometrial hyperplasia who are managed conservatively with progestogens and surveillance hysteroscopy are on the rise, recommendations should be developed for management of these women during pregnancy

VULVAR CANCER IN PREGNANCY

- Vulvar cancer in pregnancy is very rare, with <5% of vulvar cancers arising in women <40 years of age
- Progression of vulvar carcinoma is not affected by pregnancy
- Majority of **women present with stage I disease and squamous cell carcinoma is the commonest type** in pregnancy

Management of vulvar cancers in pregnancy

- Once confirmed by biopsy, it should **be managed surgically, as in non pregnant women with vulvectomy and inguinal lymphadenectomy**
- Inguinal lymphadenectomy in women with early disease can be associated with high morbidity and **sentinel lymph node sampling may be a safe alternative** for these women

- If diagnosis is made at >= **36 weeks of gestation, it is recommended that surgery should be delayed until after delivery**

Management of pregnant women previously treated for vulvar cancers

- **Previously treated vulvar carcinoma is not a contraindication to pregnancy**
- In women previously managed with surgery alone, vaginal delivery can be considered. However, cases with removal of periurethral or perivaginal tissue are relative contraindications to vaginal delivery
- Patients **treated with radiotherapy in the past** are at an **increased risk of intrauterine growth restriction** because of potential impairment of the uterine vascular supply and radiation fibrosis affecting the myometrium. Therefore **increased fetal surveillance** is required

VAGINAL CANCER IN PREGNANCY

- Very few cases of vaginal cancers in pregnancy have been reported in the literature
- The commonest type is **squamous cell carcinoma**
- Diagnosis is confirmed by taking a biopsy from the lesion and subsequent staging with MRI is done

Management of vaginal cancers in pregnancy

- Treatment is planned on a case-to-case basis
- **In tumors arising from upper third of the vagina**
  - **Stage I tumors** should be managed by radical hysterectomy, upper vaginectomy and bilateral pelvic lymphadenectomy
  - In women presenting in their first and second trimester, a potential need to terminate the pregnancy must be discussed
  - In the third trimester, early delivery can be considered to allow treatment
  - **In cases more advanced than stage I, radiotherapy is the mainstay of treatment**
- In **tumors arising from lower two-thirds of the vagina,** surgery will not be of benefit and is **treated with radiotherapy**
  - The radiotherapy field is likely to involve the uterus and fetus, and is not compatible with fetal life
  - Consideration should be given for termination of the pregnancy in the first or early second trimester and for delaying treatment to achieve fetal viability in later gestations

CHEMOTHERAPY, RADIOTHERAPY AND SURGERY IN PREGNANCY

Radiotherapy

- Pelvic radiotherapy is not compatible with fetal life and should be avoided during pregnancy. Attempts are usually made to delay the treatment to attain fetal viability. If needed, delivery should be performed at a suitable gestation to maximize viability by cesarean section and the ovaries transposed at the time of cesarean section so that they are out of the radiotherapy field
- The fetal dose should not exceed **50–100 mGy**
- **Fetal risk with radiotherapy** include-Lethality, gross malformations, growth retardation, sterility, cataracts, other neuropathology and malignant disease
- In cases where pelvic radiotherapy is a necessity (cervical, vulvar and vaginal cancers), it can be administered in the third trimester with lead shielding to limit the radiation dose to the fetus. Careful monitoring of fetal growth is indicated during such treatment
- Scatter and leakage radiation are a concern even with proper shielding, although adequate shielding can minimize risks
- Shielding of the gravid uterus, especially in advanced pregnancy, can be difficult owing to the heavy materials used
- Radioactive isotopes should be avoided in pregnancy as they cross the placenta

Chemotherapy

- **Chemotherapy should be avoided in the first trimester because of an increased risk of congenital malformations and fetal toxicity**

- After the first trimester, most chemotherapeutic agents can be used with relative safety
- Transplacental transport of chemotherapeutic agents differs widely-agents such as **paclitaxel crosses the placenta at a low rate, anthracyclines at an intermediate rate and carboplatin at a high rate**
- Carboplatin can be administered after 12–14 weeks of pregnancy with little harm to the developing fetus
- **Trastuzumab is contraindicated in pregnancy** because of HER2 receptors on the kidneys of the fetus, resulting in oligohydramnios and fetal lung hypoplasia
- **Bevacizumab, a vascular endothelial growth factor, a monoclonal antibody,** used in the management of advanced ovarian cancer is **contraindicated in pregnancy** because of **teratogenic effects**
- **Antifolates, such as methotrexate, are contraindicated in pregnancy**
- The **risk of congenital malformation is linked directly to gestational age. At less than 12 weeks,** there is risk for abnormalities of the eyes, ears, and blood systems; the risk decreases significantly after complete organogenesis
- Chemotherapy may cause a significant reduction in maternal blood production, **leading to low platelet counts and risk of overwhelming infection**
- **Elective delivery should not be planned within three weeks after chemotherapy.** Hence, chemotherapy should not be administered after 37 weeks of pregnancy owing to risk of spontaneous onset of labor
- **Carboplatin, paclitaxel and cisplatin are all excreted in breast milk** and hence breast feeding should be avoided in women receiving such treatment
- Long-term follow-up of children born to mothers who received chemotherapy during pregnancy did not indicate an increased risk of congenital abnormalities or mental delay. However, the data should be interpreted with caution due to the small study population
- Potential risks include concern for **cardiac dysfunction in children exposed to anthracyclines** (commonly used for breast cancer treatment) during the fetal period

Surgery

- Cancer surgery in pregnancy may be indicated for diagnosis, treatment and staging
- Surgery may be delayed until fetal maturity
- Surgical procedures are best undertaken in the second trimester to prevent spontaneous abortion
- Surgery in the second trimester is technically less complicated than in third trimester owing to the size of the uterus
- When surgery is performed after 28 weeks, tocolytics should be administered to prevent premature labor and corticosteroids administered to enhance lung maturity. Handling of the uterus should be kept to a minimum
- Unilateral or bilateral oophorectomy can be carried out safely after the first trimester. Whenever possible, regional anesthesia is preferred over general anesthesia owing to the potential risk of aspiration
- A lateral tilt during surgery may help to prevent aortocaval compression
- Therapeutic surgery can be performed in any trimester
- Laparoscopy can be performed with relative safety upto 20 weeks of gestation. Recommendations for laparoscopy during pregnancy are as follows:

16-20 weeks of gestational age
Tilting table to left or right
Left upper quadrant or subxiphoid insertion (6 cm between point of entry and top of fundus)
Open Hasson technique preferable
Ultrasound guidance with elevation of abdominal wall if Veress technique is used
Intraabdominal pressure is maintained at 15 mm Hg
Trendelenburg position
Fetal monitoring as indicated

PLACENTAL AND FETAL TUMOR INVOLVEMENT

- Metastatic disease to the placenta and the fetus is rare. **The most likely tumors to metastasize to the placenta include melanomas and hematological malignancies**
- In cases where malignant spread is possible, the placenta should be submitted to histologic evaluation
- The fetus should be examined at birth and at regular intervals after birth for any signs of metastatic disease

CHAPTER 16

AN OVERVIEW OF BENIGN TUMORS

VULVA

Benign Tumors of Epithelial Origin

Condylomata Acuminata

- These are papillary/verrucous lesions caused by **HPV 6 and 11.** Transmitted sexually and are highly contagious
- **Always appear as multiple lesions** on any part of vulva and around the anus; **Most commonly on the posterior fourchette.**
- Immunosuppressed women (HIV or organ transplant recipients) are at increased risk of developing large condylomata

Treatment

- Control of epithelial viral expression can be accomplished with topical agents such as **trichloroacetic acid, podophyllin or topical 5-fluorouracil (5-FU). Cryotherapy, laser vaporization, and electro excision or desiccation are other methods of treatment**
- **Imiquimod is a Topical immune response modifier, used for treatment of condyloma acuminata**

Hidradenoma

- Hidradenomas are tumors of the **apocrine sweat glands**
- These are benign lesions, usually less than 1 cm in diameter, occur on the medial aspect of the labia majora
- The lesions are firm and freely mobile. Ulceration and pain may develop, if the lesion connects with the epithelial surface

Treatment-Surgical excision

Syringoma

- Syringomas are benign hamartomas of the **eccrine sweat glands.** Usually, multiple lesions are present, and they may occur at more than one site on the body
- The lesions are asymptomatic and no treatment is needed unless pain or pruritus develops

Acrochordon

- **Fibroepithelial polyps,** referred to as skin tags are common in the vulva. It has no malignant potential
- They are soft, flesh-colored, polypoid structures. Skin appendages and hair are not characteristic of acrochordon

Treatment–local excision of symptomatic lesions

Benign Pigmented Vulvar Lesions

Benign pigmented lesions are classified as **lentigines, vulvar melanosis and nevi**

- ***Lentigines***-small, well-circumscribed macules. Lentigines can occur as part of several syndromes that include atrial myxoma and other cardiac structural and conduction defects **(LAMB syndrome, LEOPARD syndrome).** No therapy is required
- ***Vulvar melanosis***–lesion that is larger than lentigo and has an irregular border. Vulvar melanosis and lentigines are part of a spectrum of pigmentation changes of the vulva. It is important to distinguish them from melanomas by taking biopsy

- *Vulvar nevi*–Nevi are classified as intradermal, junctional, and compound nevi. The **intradermal nevus arises within the dermis and junctional nevus arises from the basal epidermal layer.** The **compound nevus** has **characteristics of both intradermal and junctional nevi.** Histologic evaluation of the melanocytes for atypical architecture and cytologic changes distinguishes pigmented nevi from melanoma. Irritable or bleeding nevi should be excised

Tumors of Mesenchymal Origin

Leiomyoma–Leiomyomas are derived from **smooth muscle** component of the vulva. These include round ligament remnants, cutaneous smooth muscle tissues, erectile tissue and blood vessels. The tumors usually are smooth and most frequently occur in the **labia majora**. Treatment is **local excision**

Lipoma–They arise in vulvar fatty tissue and histologically, they are composed of mature fat cells with a thin capsule. Treatment is **local excision**

Fibroma–Fibromas occur as small exophytic projections composed of dense collagen fibers and fibroblasts; usually appear on the labia majora. They may become large and produce symptoms. Treatment consists of **local excision**

Neurofibroma–Neurofibromas are dermal tumors that appear as small, flesh-colored, pedunculated lesions on the labia that develop after puberty. Patients with **Von Recklinghausen's** disease may have vulvar neurofibromatosis as component. These lesions have **eosinophilic fibrils, usually exclusive of neural tissue.** Occasionally, they form a large symptomatic mass that requires excision; otherwise, no treatment is necessary

Vulvar Cysts

Sebaceous Cysts: These are usually located in the labia majora and are formed by accumulation of the sebaceous material due to occlusion of the ducts. If infected, treated with antibiotics and surgical drainage

Epidermoid Cyst (Implantation Dermoid): Cysts lined by stratified squamous epithelium that appear in perineum and posterior vaginal wall. Most cysts arise from small portions of perineal skin which become buried at the time of obstetrical injuries. Usually asymptomatic. Symptomatic cysts should be excised

Bartholin's cyst

- Formed when Bartholin's duct is blocked by inflammation or by inspissated secretion
- **Appears on inner side at the junction of anterior 2/3rd and posterior 1/3rd of labium majora**
- Small cyst remains asymptomatic
- As the cyst enlarges, it bulges across the vaginal introitus causing dyspareunia and mechanical discomfort and it may get infected
- Treatment–cyst excision or marsupialization

Bartholin's Abscess

- Most common organism–**Gonococcus**
- Presents with a painful vulval swelling and purulent discharge
- Requires drainage under anesthesia
- Pus should be sent for culture sensitivity and appropriate antibiotics should be administered

Cyst of the canal of Nuck–arises from persistent processus vaginalis, which accompanied the round ligament (normally gets obliterated prior to birth). It invariably occurs in the anterior part of the labia majora. Excision is required if cysts reaches symptomatic size

Granular Cell Tumor

- Granular cell tumors (granular cell myoblastomas) of the vulva range in size from 1-4 cm and lesions characteristically form firm nodules with poor encapsulation
- Usually located on the **labia majora**
- These asymptomatic, slowly growing **benign neoplasms arise from neural tissue,** and may occur in a deep or superficial location with respect to the epidermis. The tumor infiltrates the underlying tissue and may ulcerate if it reaches the epidermis

- Microscopically, the tumors are composed of large, eosinophilic, polygonal cells
- Treated by **wide local excision because of the infiltrative nature** of the tumor. Although benign, incomplete excision may lead **to recurrenc**e of the lesion

Vascular Tumors

Malformations of vascular and lymphatic tissue may occur on the vulva, that include **capillary hemangioma, cavernous hemangioma, angiokeratoma, lymphangioma, and Kaposi's sarcoma**

Hemangiomas–Both capillary and cavernous, are well-demarcated papules. They may be congenital or acquired, and usually are asymptomatic. Hemangiomas are usually managed expectantly, unless bleeding or other symptoms develop. Treatment methods **include excision, laser therapy, sclerosing agents or cryotherapy**

Angiokeratomas–Dark red to brown papules with an irregular verrucous surface. If the lesion becomes symptomatic, or if clinical suspicion of melanoma exists, an excisional biopsy should be performed

Lymphangiomas–These are similar to hemangiomas, but do not have red blood cells. Absence of a muscular layer around the vascular structures further distinguishes these lesions from hemangiomas. They present as multiple, white or gray, vascular nodules with epithelial thickening. The lesion is usually subdermal. Treatment is surgical excision, if symptomatic

Kaposi's sarcoma–This is a multifocal vascular tumor and is associated with acquired immunodeficiency syndrome (AIDS), rarely occurring on the vulva. The diagnosis should prompt further clinical study of the immune status of the patient. Smaller lesions can be excised. Larger lesions are managed with local radiation therapy or systemic chemotherapy

Endometriosis

- The common location of endometriosis in the vulva is in **healed episiotomy scars.** Clinically, patients report cyclic pain and dyspareunia. Histologically, endometrial glands and stroma with extensive hemosider in deposition are identified. Excision is the best method of treatment. Recurrences are common

Common Vulvar Dermatosis (Table 16.1)

Table 16.1: Clinical characteristics of common vulvar dermatosisare given in

Disorder	Lesion	Hallmarks
Lichen sclerosis	Atrophic thin, whitish epithelium with frequent perianal halo or "keyhole" distribution	"Cigarette paper" parchment-like skin, halo or loss of elasticity
Lichen planus	White lacy network (Wickham striae) with flat-topped lilac papules and plaques	Erosive vaginitis with demarcated edges
Lichen simplex chronicus	Lichenified, hyperplastic plaques of red to reddish brown	Symmetric with variable pigmentation
Psoriasis	Annular pink plaques with silvery scale that bleed if removed (Auspitz sign)	Elbows, knees, scalp also often affected
Dermatitis: Irritant, allergic, or atopic	Eczematous lesions with underlying erythema	Symmetric with extension into areas of irritant or allergen contact
Seborrheic	Pale red to yellowish pink plaques, with scaly crust	Other hair-bearing areas often affected-scalp and chest; also back and face

VAGINA

Benign or malignant neoplasms of the vagina are uncommon

Cystic Tumors

Gartner's Duct Cyst

- Gartner's duct cysts develop as a result of **incomplete regression of the mesonephric or Wolffian duct during fetal development.** In the male, these ducts form the epididymis
- The gartner's cysts may be multiple, located submucosally **along the lateral aspects of the upper vagina**

- Histologic evaluation reveals **non secretory, columnar** epithelium. If these cysts are small and asymptomatic, no treatment is indicated. Symptomatic cysts should be excised
- Vaginal adenosis should be excluded

Paramesonephric Duct Cyst

- These cysts may be found **anywhere in the vagina** and frequently contain mucus
- In contrast to Gartner's duct cysts, paramesonephric duct cysts are **lined with secretory epithelium resembling endocervix or fallopian tube, suggesting Müllerian origin**
- The diagnosis is established with an excisional biopsy, if the cyst is symptomatic
- Vaginal adenosis should be excluded

Inclusion Cyst

- Inclusion cysts of the vagina result from **mucosa trapped in the submucosal region by surgical procedures such as episiotomy, trauma during childbirth, colporrhaphy etc.**
- The cysts are lined **with squamous epithelium** and contain keratin and squamous debris
- Symptomatic cysts are treated by **excision**

Endometriotic Cyst

- These appears as **bluish bulge in posterior fornix.** It behaves similar to endometriotic cyst of the vulva
- It is treated with surgical excision

Solid Tumors

Leiomyoma

- Vaginal leiomyomas or fibromyomas are rare lesions, usually located in the anterior vaginal wall
- Proposed sites of origin include vaginal smooth muscle, local arterial musculature, or smooth muscle of the bladder or urethra
- Symptoms include vaginal discharge or bleeding, dyspareunia, or urinary retention
- The differential diagnosis of a midline anterior vaginal mass includes urethral diverticulum, fibroepithelial polyp, cystocele, Skene duct abscess, or vaginal malignancy
- Therapy involves excision, if symptomatic

Fibroepithelial Polyp

- Fibroepithelial polyps of the vagina are uncommon and usually asymptomatic
- They are usually small and may be multiple. In infants and young girls, sarcoma botryoides must be ruled out
- Histologically, the polyps are composed of a squamous epithelial surface with a fibrovascular stalk and edematous stroma
- Therapy involves excision of the polyp and stalk in symptomatic patient

Condyloma Acuminatum

- Condyloma acuminatum represents a clinical manifestation of human papillomavirus infection
- These lesions may be associated with condyloma lesions of the cervix and vulva or appear only as vaginal lesions
- Histologic evaluation confirms the diagnosis and rules out dysplasia
- Treatment–Topical therapy with Trichloro acetic acid. For large or multiple lesions, excision, cauterization, laser vaporization, or loop electrical excision (LEEP) may be required

Other Benign Tumors of Vagina

- Hemangiopericytoma, neurofibromas, granular cell myoblastoma, myxoma, rhabdomyoma, and benign cystic teratoma are other rare neoplasms of vagina
- Excisional biopsy is required to make the diagnosis

OTHER RELATED CONDITIONS

In Utero Diethyl Stilbesterol (DES) Exposure

- **Clear cell adenocarcinoma** of the vagina has been observed with in utero exposure to DES
- **Nonmalignant structural changes** of the cervix and vagina including **cocks comb, cervical collar, cervical hood, pseudopolyp, and hypoplastic cervix -described in 25–48% of in utero DES exposed women**
- **Vaginal adenosis** has been reported in 35–65% cases of in utero DES exposure. Adenosis is described as the retention of müllerian-derived glandular epithelium in the vagina after vaginal embryogenesis is completed
- The evaluation of the DES exposed women include careful palpation of the entire vagina, followed by careful colposcopic examination of the vagina. Cytologic samples are taken from the cervix and vagina. The entire vagina is stained with Lugol's solution and re-examined to search for any non staining areas. Biopsy is performed on any non staining areas and colposcopically detected columnar epithelium in the vagina
- Annual examination include cytologic evaluation and palpation of the cervix and vagina
- **Treatment:** Vaginal adenosis is observed, without any therapy (No intervention required)

Urethral Caruncle

- Urethral caruncles present as localized, red, friable lesions at the urethral meatus
- They are generally seen in the postmenopausal woman and are thought to result from a localized area of prolapse of the urethral mucosa with secondary inflammatory changes
- May present with pain, dysuria, and bleeding
- Small asymptomatic urethral caruncles may not require any treatment. Large and symptomatic lesions can be treated by **topical application of estrogen**
- To establish the diagnosis, biopsy may be performed under local anesthesia

CERVIX

Nabothian cysts

- Seen in majority of multiparous women
- Nabothian cyst arises when duct of gland becomes obstructed by injury, fibrosis or plug of epithelial debris
- **Cyst is lined by columnar cell epithelium.** Contains clear mucus. Treated as in chronic cervicitis

Endometriotic cysts

- Situated in portio vaginalis part of cervix
- Implantation of endometrium occurs during delivery or any gynecologic surgery. Lining epithelium shows endometrial glands and stroma
- Treatment is by destruction with cauterization and rarely by excision

Cervical Polyp

- Cervical polyps are the most common benign lesions of the cervix. Cervical polyps often occur in women over 20 years of age and are rare prior to menarche
- They appear as red, finger-like growths and may protrude out into the vagina
- Cervical polyps may be asymptomatic. Women with a cervical polyp may have abnormal vaginal bleeding or vaginal discharge
- Polyps that are large, bleeding or appear abnormal can be removed, usually during a pelvic examination

Cervical Fibroid

- Cervical fibroids arise in the muscle fibers of cervix. They are similar to uterine fibroids but less common
- The common symptoms are abnormal vaginal bleeding or urinary retention. The typical appearance is described a 'Lantern on Top of St. Mount's cathederal'
- Treatment is hysterectomy

Papilloma

Cervical papillomas are usually asymptomatic or can cause blood stained discharge. **Treatment is surgical removal**

Hemangioma

- Rare lesions; can with increase in growth during pregnancy. Usually asymptomatic; Can cause irregular bleeding
- Treatment is by local excision, diathermy, coagulation or laser

UTERUS

Endometrial polyps

- Endometrial polyps represent focal, accentuated benign hyperplastic processes within endometrial cavity
- **Can be associated with endometrial hyperplasia and carcinoma**
- Endometrial Polyps occur more frequently in perimenopausal women
- Associated with unopposed estrogen exposure
- **Most common presenting symptom is abnormal uterine bleeding (AUB)**
- Small polyps are often incidentally found as part of endometrial curettage done for evaluating AUB
- Large polyp may protrude through cervical canal and present with irregular bleeding and pain, as cervix becomes slowly dilated and effaced.

Surgical removal controls bleeding and prevent infection developing within the exposed endometrial surface

- Less than 5% polyps show malignant change. Polyps in postmenopausal women or women taking Tamoxifen are more likely to be associated with endometrial carcinoma than those found in reproductive-age group women

Placental polyp

- Placental polyp forms from ***retained placental tissue*** following abortion or normal delivery
- May present with secondary postpartum hemorrhage or intermittent vaginal bleeding
- **Hysteroscopy** serves both diagnostic and therapeutic purpose.
- Hysteroscopic removal of multiple polyps may be desirable to ensure complete removal

Fibroids/Leiomyoma

- Most common benign uterine tumor
- **Etiology:** Predominantly estrogen-dependent tumors, associated with obesity, early menarche, nulliparity, late menopause, infertility, chronic anovulation associated with PCOD

Classification

- **Subserous**
  - Project from the uterus into the peritoneal cavity
  - Sometimes pedunculated
  - Least likely to cause symptoms
- **Submucous (~ 5% of all fibroids)**
  - Project into the uterine cavity
  - Sometimes pedunculated
  - Most likely to cause symptoms
- **Intramural**
  - Most common
  - Usually multiple

- Most common type of fibroid–**Intramural fibroid**
- Most common **Extrauterine fibroid–Cervical fibroid**
- Most common **symptom of fibroid is menorrhagia**
- Fibroid to cause **maximum symptoms–Submucous fibroid**
- Most common fibroid to cause **urine retention–Cervical fibroid**
- Most common fibroid to cause **Pseudomeig's syndrome–Subserous fibroid**
- Most common fibroid to cause uterine **inversion–Fundal submucous fibroid**
- Most common fibroid to undergo **torsion–Subserous fibroid**
- Most common fibroid to cause **abortion–Submucous fibroid**
- Most common **degeneration in fibroid–Hyaline degeneration**
- Least common degeneration–**Sarcomatous degeneration**
- Most common fibroid to undergo **calcareous degeneration–Subserous fibroid**
- Most common fibroid to undergo **malignant change–Submucous fibroid**
- **Lantern on dome of St. Paul Cathedral–Cervical fibroid**
- Wandering or **parasitic fibroid–Subserous fibroid**

Complications of fibroid

- Torsion (common in subserous pedunculated fibroid)
- Hemorrhage into fibroid
- Infection (submucous fibroids are prone to infection and ulceration)
- Degeneration
- Uterine inversion can rarely occur in a submucous fibroid
- Malignant change (very rare)

Secondary changes in fibroid

- Atrophy–occurs during menopause
- Degeneration
  - Hyaline degeneration (most common)
  - Fatty degeneration
  - Cystic degeneration
  - Calcareous degeneration–seen in old women with long-standing fibroid (phosphates and carbonates are deposited along the course of the vessels and visualized in X-ray)
  - Red degeneration (common during pregnancy)
- Sarcomatous change
  - Incidence is 0.2%
  - Presents as sudden increase in size of fibroid, postmenopausal bleeding and tenderness on palpation
  - Absence of capsule and increased vascularity in USG

Red Degeneration of Fibroid
• **Etiology:** Probably vascular in origin
• ***Occurs mainly in pregnancy during second half and puerperium***
• May also occur in female >40 years of age with painful myomas
• **Symptoms:** Severe abdominal pain, constitutional upset and fever
• **Signs:** Patient is febrile with moderate leukocytosis and increased ESR
• **Treatment:** Conservative-with bed rest and analgesics until pain subsides

TREATMENT: Refer Flowchart 16.1: On Next Page

OVARY

Benign ovarian cysts can be classified as non-neoplastic cysts of the ovary and Benign ovarian neoplasms

Non-Neoplastic Cysts of Ovary (Functional cysts or Cystic Ovaries)

- Non-neoplastic cysts of ovary are very common and can occur from adolescence to perimenopausal age
- The term includes the following: **follicular cysts, corpus luteal cysts and theca lutein cysts**

Features of functional ovarian cysts

- Related to temporary hormonal disturbances
- Usually **not more than 5-8 cm in diameter**
- Unilocular
- Contain clear fluid except when hemorrhage occurs
- Usually asymptomatic
- Usually **regress spontaneously**

Flowchart 16.1: Management of uterine fibroids

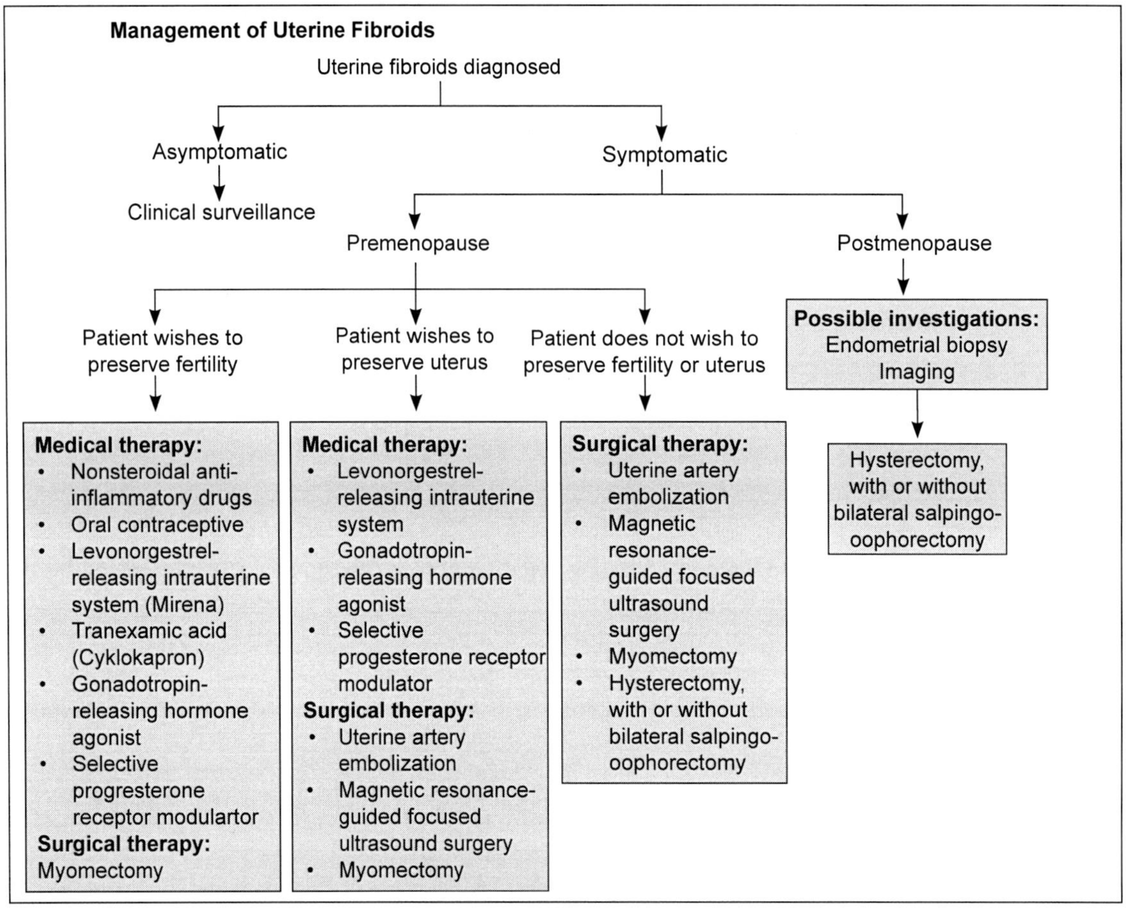

Follicular cysts

- **Most common functional cysts**
- Usually <5 cm size
- Can be single or multiple cysts
- Usually asymptomatic; can undergo torsion, hemorrhage, and rupture, and can present with symptoms of acute abdomen
- Disappear spontaneously within few weeks to few months

Theca lutein cysts

- Usually bilateral
- **Associated with excessive human chorionic gonadotropin (hCG) secretion** such as in gestational trophobastic tumors and cases with hCG and clomiphene therapy for infertility
- Usually regresses spontaneously following treatment of gestational trophoblastic tumors
- May present with local pain and tenderness

Corpus luteal cysts

- Usually occur due to **over activity of corpus luteum leading** to hemorrhage inside corpus luteum
- May present with amenorrhea
- May present similar to threatened abortion or the corpus luteal cyst may rupture leading to intraperitoneal hemorrhage, simulating a ruptured ectopic pregnancy
- **May be associated with pregnancy and can persist for about 12 weeks**
- Spontaneous regression usually occurs, unless complicated

Benign Ovarian Tumors (Table 16.2)

Table 16.2: Common benign ovarian tumors	
Epithelial cell tumors	Derived from mesothelial cells lining peritoneal cavity and ovary Examples: serous cystadenoma, mucinous cystadenoma, endometrioid tumor
Germ cell tumors	Derived from germ cells: may contain ectoderm, mesoderm, or endoderm Example: mature cystic teratoma (dermoid cyst)
Sex cord-stromal tumors	Derived from sex cords and stroma of developing gonad; often cause feminizing/virilizing effects, depending on type of cells present. Examples: granulosa-theca cell tumor, Sertoli-Leydig cell tumor

Serous Cystadenoma

- It arises from the totipotent surface epithelium of the ovary
- It accounts for 40% of ovarian tumors (most common ovarian tumor)
- It is bilateral in 40% of cases
- Risk of malignancy is 40% (serous cystadenocarcinoma)
- The cysts are not very large unlike mucinous cystadenoma
- The wall is smooth, shiny, and grayish white
- It may be uniloculated or multiloculated
- The content fluid is clear and rich in serum proteins.

Mucinous Cystadenoma

- It arises from the totipotent surface epithelium of the ovary
- It accounts for 20–25% of all ovarian tumors
- It is bilateral in 10% of cases
- Risk of malignancy is 10% (mucinous cystadeno carcinoma). It may enlarge to a huge size and is the largest benign ovarian tumor
- The wall is lobulated with whitish or bluish white hue
- The cyst is multiloculated and cut section shows **honey comb pattern**
- The contents are thick, viscid, and mucinous
- Rupture of the cyst can result in **pseudomyxoma peritonei**

Dermoid Cyst

- Dermoid cyst arises from germ cells of ovary
- It constitutes 95% of teratomas (most common teratoma)
- It accounts for 30–40% of ovarian tumors
- It is bilateral in 15–20% of cases
- Risk of **malignancy is 1–2%. Squamous cell carcinoma is the most common malignancy**
- It is the **most common ovarian tumor associated with pregnancy**
- **Torsion is the most common complication**
- The cyst is of moderate size and the capsule is smooth.
- It contains structures from all three germ layers. The content is predominantly sebaceous material and may contain hair, teeth, and bones

Ovarian Fibroma

- Solid benign ovarian tumor of connective tissue
- **Meigs syndrome**–association of **ovarian fibroma with ascites and pleural effusion**
- **Pseudo-Meigs syndrome:** When ascites and pleural effusion are seen in conditions other than ovarian fibroma such as **Brenner tumor and granulosa cell tumor, it is termed as Pseudo-Meigs syndrome**

MULTIPLE CHOICE QUESTIONS (MCQs)

GENERAL ONCOLOGY
(Genetics, Radiation, Chemotherapy & Molecular biology)

1. Apoptosis is characterized by all except: (NEET SS PATTERN 2017)

A. Condensation of chromatin
B. Nuclear and cytoplasmic blebbing
C. Cellular shrinkage
D. Autophagy

Ans: D

APOPTOSIS	NECROSIS
Membrane blebbing	Loss of membrane integrity-disruption
Cellular shrinkage	Swelling of cytoplasm and mitochondria
Apoptotic bodies-membrane bound vesicles	Complete cell lysis; no vesicles
Condensation of chromatin;DNA fragmentation	Nuclear disruption

2. First to show the signs of radiation damage among the following is:

A. Kidney
B. Muscle
C. Nerves
D. Small intestine

Ans: D

3. Bladder tolerates radiation of:

A. 45-50 Gy
B. 85-90 Gy
C. 100 Gy
D. 30 Gy

Ans: A

RADIATION TOLERANCE DOSES (DEVITA 10th e/d p.155)

ORGAN INVOLVED	TOLERABLE DOSE (Gy)
Bladder	40-50
Anus, Great vessels	30
Brachial plexus	60-66
Brain stem	55-60
Kidney	50
Spinal cord	50
Lung	45
Stomach, Esophagus, Heart	60
Small intestine	50
Colon	55
Rectum	60
Liver	50

4. **Log kill hypothesis implies all of following except:**

   A. Treatment will be effective if tumours are treated at level of micrometastases

   B. Chemotherapy works by first order kinetics and kills a constant fraction of cells rather than constant number of cells.

   C. It is basis for use of intermittent chemotherapy and rationale for use of combination chemotherapy

   D. It is not basis for use of adjuvant chemotherapy

   Ans: A

LOG KILL HYPOTHESIS/SKIPPER EXPONENTIAL TUMOUR GROWTH:

- Cytotoxic actions of anticancer drugs follow first-order kinetics.
- Destruction of cancer cells by chemotherapeutic agents follows first-order kinetics mean that a given dose of drug destroys a constant fraction or proportion of a cell population rather than a constant number of cells.
- They kill a fixed percentage of tumor cells, not a fixed number.
- Log-kill hypothesis also proposes that the magnitude of tumor cell kill by anticancer drugs is a logarithmic function.

GOMPERTZIAN MODEL OF TUMOUR GROWTH:

- A pattern of cell growth in tumors in which there is increased doubling time and decreased growth fraction as a function of time.

NORTON SIMON MODEL:

- Chemotherapy results in a rate of regression in tumor volume that is proportional to the rate of growth for an unperturbed tumor of that size.

GOLDIE COLDMAN MODEL:

- According to this hypothesis, even the smallest detectable cancers would contain at least one drug-resistant clone; therefore, the best chance of cure would be to use all effective chemotherapy drugs.

5. **TRASTUZUMAB (antibody against HER-2/neu gene) is active against which malignancy?**

   A. Breast Ca
   B. Cervical Ca
   C. Uterine Ca
   D. Ovarian Ca

   Ans: A

TRASTUZUMAB:

- Trastuzumab-HERCEPTIN→anti HER 2 antibody
- Indications: carcinoma breast (adjuvant/metastatic) and metastatic adenocarcinomas of stomach/GE junction that overexpress HER 2 protein.
- DOSE LIMITING SIDE EFFECT: Cardiomyopathy

6. **Dosage of carboplatin in treatment of ovarian cancer calculated by:**

   A. Dose (mg) : Target AUC * (GFR + 25)
   B. Dose (mg) : Target AUC + (GFR * 25)
   C. Dose (mg) : Target AUC * (GFR + 50)
   D. Dose (mg) : Target AUC * GFR

   Ans: A

CARBOPLATIN:

- Calvert formulaà Dose (mg) : Target AUC x (GFR + 25)
- Target AUC – area under curve;
- 4-6 for previously treated patients & 5-7 for previously untreated patients.

7. **Total radiation dose to point A & B in treatment of cervical cancer:**

A. 75-90 Gy ; 45-65 Gy
B. 45-65 Gy ; 75-90 Gy
C. 20-60 Gy ; 70-90 Gy
D. 30-60 Gy ; 70-90 Gy

Ans: A

RADIOTHERAPY IN CA CERVIX:

Point A	Point B
2 cm above & 2 cm lateral to external os	2 cm above & 5 cm lateral to external os
PARACERVICAL/PARAMETRIAL Nodes	OBTURATOR Nodes
70-80 Gy	60 Gy

8. **Each unit of packed RBCs should increase haematocrit in a 70 kg adult by:**

A. 1-2%
B. 3-4%
C. 5-6%
D. 7-8%

Ans: B

GUIDELINES FOR BLOOD TRANSFUSION:

- Accepted 3% increase in hematocrit to 1 "unit" of blood transfused is based on a calculation from total blood volume and hematocrit of blood transfused.
  - Approximately 300 +/- 25 mL
  - Hematocrit: 70 +/- 5%;
- **One unit of pRBCs should increase hemoglobin by approximately 1 gm/dl.**
- **One pRBC unit will raise the hematocrit of standard adult patient by 3%.**

9. **Cancer cachexia can be managed using combinations of following except:**

A. Parenteral nutrition
B. Enteral nutrition
C. Synthetic progestins
D. FFP

Ans: D

TREATMENT OF CACHEXIA:

- Provide small frequent feedings 6 times a day
- **Appetite stimulants:** Megestrol acetate, Dexamethasone, Metaclopramide, Antidepressants, Methylphenidate
- **Other measures:** Enteral & parenteral nutrition may be given in severe cachexia patients.

10. **All are alkylating agents except:**

A. Cyclophosphamide
B. Melphalan
C. Ifosfamide
D. Doxorubicin

Ans: D

DOXORUBICIN:

- Doxorubicin belongs to antitumour antibiotic group.

- Side effect is cardiomyopathy.
- Belongs to anthracycline group.

11. All are microtubule inhibitors except:

A. Paclitaxel
B. Vincristine
C. Ixabepilone
D. Topotecan

Ans: D

TOPOTECAN:

- Hycamtin-Ovarian cancer after failure of response to cisplatin therapy.
- Dose limiting side effect: **Myelosuppression.**

12. Only drug which is US-FDA approved for treatment of relapsed cervical cancer:

A. Paclitaxel
B. Irinotecan
C. Topotecan
D. Liposomal doxorubicin

Ans: C

LIST OF FDA APPROVED DRUGS:

Drug	Cancer
Alecensa (alectinib)	ALK +ve metastatic non-small cell lung cancer
Cotellic (cobimetinib)	BRAF, V600E/V600K +ve melanoma
Darzalex (daratumumab)	Multiple myeloma
Empliciti (elotuzumab)	Multiple myeloma after receiving prior therapies
Farydak (panobinostat)	Multiple myeloma
Ibrance (palbociclib)	ER +ve, HER 2 –ve breast cancer
Lenvima (levatinib)	Thyroid cancer
Lonsurf (trifluridine & tipiracil)	Metastatic colorectal cancer
Ninlaro (Ixazomib)	Multiple myeloma
Odomzo (sonidegib)	Locally advanced basal cell carcinoma
Onivyde (irinotecan liposomal)	Metastatic pancreatic cancer following gemcitabine based therapy
Opdivo (nivolumab)	Metastatic squamous non-small cell lung cancer
Portazza (necitumumab)	Metastatic squamous non-small cell lung cancer
Tagrisso (osimertinib)	EGFR T790M mutation +ve non-small cell lung cancer
Unituxin (dinutuximab)	High risk neuroblastoma
Varubi (rolapitant)	Delayed nausea and vomiting associated with chemotherapy
Yondelis ***(trabectedin)***	Liposarcoma/Leiomyosarcoma

13. Following are published clinical trials for solid cancers. Select incorrect one:

A. FUTURE trial-Endometrial cancer
B. AURELIA trial-Cervical cancer
C. OCEANS trial-Ovarian cancer
D. LACE trial-Cervical cancer

Ans: B

TRIALS OF ONCOLOGY:

TRIAL	CANCER	
FUTURE	Endometrial cancer	
AURELIA	Ovarian cancer (Recurrent)	Platinum resistant
OCEANS	Ovarian cancer (Recurrent)	Platinum sensitive
LACE	Cervical cancer	
AVAglio	Metastatic renal cell cancer	Bevacizumab + IFN alpha
FOLFIRI	Metastatic colorectal cancer	Aflibercept+5-FU+Irinotecan
VELOUR	Metastatic colorectal cancer	Aflibercept+5-FU+Irinotecan
DECISION	Differentiated thyroid cancer	RAI
COMPARZ	Metastatic RCC	Pazopinib & sunitinib
SUMMIT	Multiple myeloma	Bortezomib
CREST	Multiple myeloma	Bortezomib
VISTA	Multiple myeloma	Bortezomib+velcade+melphalan+ prednisolone
CORRECT	Metastatic colorectal cancer	Regorafenib

14. GOG-0218 and ICON7 studies assessed combination of following drugs except for:

A. Lipodoxorubicin
B. Bevacizumab
C. Carboplatin
D. Paclitaxel

Ans: A

GOG-0218 & ICON 7 TRIALS:

- Trials done for Advanced epithelial ovarian tumours
- Included drugs like Bevacizumab in combination with carboplatin and paclitaxel.

15. HPV all are true except:

A. Member of papovaviridae
B. DNA Virus
C. 31,33 are high risk types
D. Can infect fibroblasts

Ans: D

HUMAN PAPILLOMA VIRUS:

- HPV is a non-enveloped DNA virus with protein capsid.
- High affinity for lower ano-genital tract-cutaneous and mucosotropic.

LOW RISK TYPE	HIGH RISK TYPE
HPV 6 & 11	HPV 16,18,31,33,45,58
Causes genital warts and subclinical HPV infection	Causes high grade CIN progress to invasive cancer.

16. Optimal vaccine schedule for HPV vaccine:

A. 0, 2 , 6 months
B. 0, 1, 6 months
C. 0, 6 months
D. 0, 1 months

Ans: A & B

HPV VACCINE:

GARDASIL	CERVIRAX
Quadrivalent	Bivalent
HPV-6,11,16,18	HPV-16,18
0,2,6 months	0,1,6 months
Against Ca. cervix & genital warts	Against Ca. cervix
Intramuscular	Intramuscular

17. Following are matched correctly except:

A. **Age specific incidence rate:** It is the number of new cancers that occur over specified time among individuals of a particular age group divided by population in that same age group

B. **Age adjusted incidence rate:** It is obtained by summing weighted averages of incidence rates for each age stratum

C. Relative survival is defined as ratio of observed survival rate for patient group to survival rate for population with similar demographic characteristics

D. Prevalence is number of new cases of disease in population with in a specified time period

Ans: D

➢ Number of new cases of disease in population with in a specified time period is defined as incidence not prevalence.

18. Hereditary breast ovarian cancer associated with which genes:

A. BRCA 1, BRCA 2

B. HNPCC

C. TP53

D. VHL

Ans: A

HEREDITARY BREAST OVARIAN CANCER:

➢ Occurs due to mutation of BRCA 1 & BRCA 2.

➢ 0.125-0.20% of general population carry these mutations,

➢ Life time risk: 40% for BRCA 1, 20% for BRCA 2.

➢ **Average age of onset of ovarian cancer:**

- 49-53 yrs for BRCA 1.
- 55-58 yrs for BRCA 2.

➢ Most of them are epithelial and non-mucinous type(serous).

➢ Ovarian cancers with BRCA 1 & BRCA 2 have better prognosis compared to those without mutations-respond well to platinum compounds.

19. No role of radiation in management of which of the following gynecologic cancers:

A. Primary treatment of vulvar cancer

B. Primary treatment of cervical cancer

C. Curative treatment of cervical cancer metastases

D. Postsurgical adjunctive therapy of endometrial cancer

Ans: C

20. Which is not a particle radiation?

A. Photons
B Electrons
C Protons
D Helium ions

Ans: A

21. Radionuclides not used in brachytherapy include?

A. Cobalt
B. Cesium
C. Iridium
D. Phosphorus

Ans: D

22. Technique used to reduce risk of radiation induced ovarian failure during treatment in premenopausal women:

A. Omental sling
B. Ovarian transposition
C. Ovarian transplantation
D. All of the above

Ans: B

23. Not a criterion for diagnosing radiation-induced cancer?

A. Occurs with radiation doses exceeding 60 Gy
B. Located within previously irradiated region.
C. Pathology is different from original malignancy.
D. Diagnosed atleast few years after completion of therapy

Ans: A

RADIATION INDUCED MALIGNANCY:

Cahan's criteria is used to define a radiation-induced sarcoma. They are currently being used as the standard for demonstration of Radiation induced malignancy (RIM).

The modified Cahan's criteria for diagnosis of RIM are as follows:

(a) A RIM must have arisen in an irradiated field

(b) A sufficient latent period, preferably longer than 4 years, must have elapsed between the initial irradiation and the alleged induced malignancy

(c) The treated tumor and alleged induced tumor must have been biopsied. The two tumors must be of different histology

(d) The tissue in which the alleged induced tumor arose must have been normal (i.e., metabolically and genetically normal) prior to the radiation exposure.

24. Paclitaxel is:

A. Cell cycle non specific agent
B. Cell cycle specific agent that acts during M phase
C. Cell cycle specific agent that acts during G2 phase
D. Cell cycle specific agent that acts during G1 phase

Ans: B

PACLITAXEL:

- It is a cell cycle specific agent that acts during M phase.
- **Indications**: CA breast, ovary, lung, esophagus and AIDS related Kaposi's sarcoma
- **Toxicity:** Neutropenia, Hypersensitivity, peripheral neuropathy are dose limiting side effects. Alopecia- 90% total and sudden within 3 weeks of treatment.

25. Most sensitive to radiation therapy among the following is?

A. Glioma

B. Dysgerminoma

C. Osteosarcoma

D. Squamous carcinoma

Ans: B

ENDOMETRIAL CARCINOMA

26. Untreated atypical complex endometrial hyperplasia progresses to malignancy in:

A. 50%

B. 29%

C. 49%

D. 9%

Ans: B

ENDOMETRIAL HYPERPLASIA:

Type Of Hyperplasia	Progression To Cancer
Simple without atypia	1%
Complex without atypia	3%
Simple with atypia	8%
Complex with atypia	29-30%

27. Endometrial cancer which spreads in peritoneal cavity is:

A. Adenocarcinoma

B. Endometroid cancer

C. Sarcoma botyroides

D. Uterine papillary serous cancer

Ans: D

UTERINE PAPILLARY SEROUS CARCINOMA:

- Aggressive subtype of endometrial cancer typically arises in post-menopausal women.
- Has high propensity for early lymphatic and intraperitoneal spread.
- Does not develop from **endometrial hyperplasia** and is not hormone-sensitive.
- It arises in the setting of endometrial **atrophy** and is classified as a **type II endometrial cancer**

28. HNPCC is hereditary cancer caused by:

A. Mutation of RAS

B. Mutation of P 53

C. Inactivation of P 53

D. Inactivation of DNA mismatch repair gene

Ans: D

HNPCC- LYNCH SYNDROME-most repeated question**

- Accounts for 3% of all colorectal cancers and 15% in patients with family history of colorectal cancer.
- Right sided and proximal to splenic flexure. 5 to 10% of hereditary ovarian cancer.

TYPES:

- Type 1 – upto 100 polyps in right proximal colon, Mean age is 43 yrs.
- Type 2 – in addition involves extracolonic tumours involving stomach, small bowel, bile duct, renal pelvis, ureter, bladder, uterus, ovary, skin and pancreas
- **RISK FOR COLORECTAL CANCER IN HNPCC is 80%.**
- For endometrial cancer it is 50-60%. Rest of the cancers risk is 1-3%.
- Screening: colonoscopy should begin by 20-25yrs and should be repeated every 1-2yrs.Prophylactic hysterectomy and b/l salphingo-oophorectomy is option after child bearing.
- MUTATIONS involve hMSH2, hMLH1, hMSH6, hPMS2.
- Mutations of hMSH6 results in increased Endometrial cancer incidence.

29. Women with HNPCC is not true:

A. Increased risk of colon cancer
B. life time risk of endometrial risk is 50%
C. 50% will develop endometrial cancer before colon cancer
D. increased risk of breast cancer in 80%

Ans: D

RISKS:

CANCER	%	SCREENING
Colorectal cancer	80%	Colonoscopy every 2 yr beginning age 20 yr annually after 40 yr/10 yr younger than earliest case in family
Endometrial cancer	50%	Pelvic examination,transvaginal ultrasound,endometrial aspirate every 1-2 yr,beginning 25-35yrs age.
Upper urinary tract cancer	10%	USG and urinalysis every 1-2yr starting 30-35 yrs.
Gall bladder and biliary cancer	18%	-
CNS cancer	<5%	-
Small bowel cancer	<5%	-

30. Regarding endometrial cancer which is not true:

A. Type 1 is of endometroid pathology
B. Type 1 has bad prognosis
C. Type 2 seen in elderly
D. Type 2 has worst prognosis

Ans: B

TYPES OF ENDOMETRIAL CANCER:

- **Type 1:**
  - Women with obesity and hyperestrogenism.
  - Moderately differentiated with minimal invasion.
  - Good prognosis.
  - Alterations in PI3K and PTEN/AKT pathway.
- **Type 2:**
  - Elderly
  - Poorly differentiated with deep myometrial invasion.
  - Worst prognosis
  - Alterations in tumour suppressor genes P 53/P 16.

31. Medical management of endometrial cancer can be considered when following criteria are met:

A. Normal serum levels of cancer antigen (CA)-125

B. Disease confined to the endometrial cavity

C. No evidence of tumor invasion deeper than outer half of myometrium detected on pelvic MRI

D. Histology includes Endometrioid & Papillary serous carcinoma but not clear cell carcinoma

Ans: B

32. Risk factors for developing papillary serous uterine cancer include:

A. Obesity

B. Diabetes mellitus

C. African American race

D. Prior use of unopposed estrogens as naturopathic hormone replacement therapy

Ans: C

- ***Caucasian women have high risk of Endometroid cancer***
- ***African American race have poor prognosis- Because of high Type 2 E. cancers***

33. A 65-year-old retired school teacher presented to her gynecologist with a 3-month H/O vaginal bleeding. She is diabetic and hypertensive, has no children, and has been post-menopausal for 12 years. On examination, she has a diffusely enlarged uterus. Endometrial biopsy shows grade II endometrioid carcinoma. Next best step in management is:

A. Dilation and curettage

B. Total abdominal hysterectomy & bilateral salpingo-oophorectomy +/-adjuvant therapy

C. Chemotherapy

D. Pelvic radiation

Ans: B

34. Type II endometrial cancer has following characteristics except:

A. Older, non obese women

B. Pathology is serous cancer

C. Associated with PTEN mutation

D. May have been treated for breast cancer with tamoxifen

Ans: C

TYPES OF ENDOMETRIAL CANCER:

- **Type 1**–Women with **obesity** and hyperestrogenism-TAMOXIFEN

  Moderately differentiated with minimal invasion.

  Good prognosis.

  Alterations in PI3K and PTEN/AKT pathway.

- **Type 2–Elderly**.

  Poorly differentiated with deep myometrial invasion.

  Worst prognosis.

  Alterations in tumour suppressor genes P 53/P 16.

35. Unopposed estrogen is pathology for which type of endometrial cancer:

A. Type 1

B. Type 2

C. Both

D. None

Ans: A

- Hyperestrogenism is associated with type 1 endometrial tumours.

TYPES OF ENDOMETRIAL CANCER:

- **Type 1-**Women with **obesity** and hyperestrogenism-TAMOXIFEN

  Moderately differentiated with minimal invasion.

  Good prognosis.

  Alterations in PI3K and PTEN/AKT pathway.

- **Type 2- Elderly.**

  Poorly differentiated with deep myometrial invasion.

  Worst prognosis.

  Alterations in tumour suppressor genes P 53/P 16.

36. Following risk factors are common to both cancer endometrium and cancer ovary except:

A. Increase risk in nulliparous

B. Oral contraceptives and tubal ligation are protective

C. Risk decreases with increasing parity

D. Obesity

Ans: B

RISK FACTORS:

Carcinoma Endometrium	Carcinoma Ovary
Nulliparous	Nulliparous
Obesity, DM, HTN, PCOD	Obesity, PCOD
Late menopause/Early menarche, Atypical endometrial hyperplasia, H/O infertility/menstrual irregularity	Turner's syndrome, HNPCC, Hereditary breast ovarian syndrome
Tamoxifen / radiation therapy, Feminizing ovarian tumour	Ovulation inducing drugs, Exogenous estrogens

- ***OC pills and smoking are protective for carcinoma endometrium.***
- ***OC pills, pregnancy, breast feeding, multiparity, tubal ligation, hysterectomy are protective for carcinoma ovary.***

37. Malignant potential of complex endothelial hyperplasia without atypia:

A. <5%

B. 5-15%

C. 15-30%

D. >30%

Ans: A

ENDOMETRIAL HYPERPLASIA:

Type of Hyperplasia	Progression to Cancer
Simple without atypia	1%
Complex without atypia	3%
Simple with atypia	8%
Complex with atypia	29-30%

38. Percentage of women with postmenopausal bleeding who has endometrial hyperplasia:

A. 30%
B. 15%
C. 5%
D. 10%

Ans: D

POST MENOPAUSAL BLEEDING:

- Most common cause of post menopausal bleeding is Endometrial atrophy.
- Most common cause of post menopausal bleeding in india is CA CERVIX.

Cause of Bleeding	Percentage
Hormonal replacement therapy	15-25%
Endometrial atrophy	60-80%
Endometrial polyps	2-12%
Endometrial hyperplasia	5-10%
Endometrial cancer	10%

39. Choice of adjuvant treatment for endometrial carcinoma stage IA grade I:

A. Radiotherapy
B. Chemotherapy
C. Chemoradiotherapy
D. None

Ans: A

TREATMENT OF ENDOMETRIAL CANCER:

Stage	Grade	Treatment
I A	I & II	TAH + BSO (no adjuvant therapy needed
I A	III	TAH + BSO + ***Vaginal vault irradiation***
I B	I & II	TAH + BSO + ***Vaginal vault irradiation***
I B	III	TAH + BSO + ***Pelvic irradiation & Vaginal Brachytherapy***
II	***All grades***	***Modified radical hysterectomy + radiotherapy (pelvic + external fields)***
III	***Chemotherapy*** + Radiotherapy and weekly injection of medroxyprogesterone	
IV	Palliative chemotherapy ; Radiotherapy & hormonal t/t	

Treatment Recommendations for Early-Stage (FIGO 2009) Endometrioid Adenocarcinoma of the Uterus		
	Grade 1 or 2	**Grade 3**
IA	Observation[a]	Observation vs. IVRT
IB	IVRT	IMRT
II[b] (<50% cervical stromal invasion)	IVRT	IMRT vs. IVRT plus CT
II (<50% cervical stromal invasion)	IMRT	IMRT vs. IVRT plus CT

Ref: Devita 11th Edition

40. Endometrial hyperplasia is seen in:

A. Endodermal sinus tumour
B. Dysgerminoma
C. PCOD
D. Ca cervix

Ans: C

CAUSES OF ENDOMETRIAL HYPERPLASIA:

Simple	Complex
Due to increased estrogen	Unknown
PCOD; HRT; Follicular cysts of ovary; Granulose & theca cell tumours of ovary	PCOD; Glucose intolerance

41. Carcinoma endometrium that has involved vagina is staged as:

A. IIIB
B. IA
C. IIB
D. IVA

Ans: A

42. Which of the following doesn't increase risk of developing endometrial cancer?

A. Obesity
B. Tamoxifen
C. Cigarette smoking
D. Unopposed estrogen

Ans: C

43. What is the most common genetic syndrome associated with endometrial cancer?

A. Cowden syndrome
B. Li Fraumeni syndrome
C. Hereditary breast ovarian cancer syndrome
D. Hereditary nonpolyposis colorectal cancer syndrome

Ans: D

44. Which of the following methods does NOT reduce risk of endometrial cancer?

A. Bilateral tubal ligation
B. Copper intrauterine device
C. Combination oral contraceptives
D. Levonorgestrel-releasing intrauterine system

Ans: A

45. Which of the following is an appropriate treatment of 35 yr old woman with the diagnosis of complex endometrial hyperplasia without atypia?

A. Medroxyprogesterone acetate
B. Combination oral contraceptive pills
C. Levonorgestrel-releasing intrauterine system
D. All of the above

Ans: D

46. Which of the following subtypes is not a type II endometrial cancer?

A. Clear cell carcinoma
B. Papillary serous carcinoma
C. Endometrioid adenocarcinoma with squamous differentiation
D. None of the above

Ans: C

47. Most common method of spread of endometrioid adenocarcinoma is?

A. Lymphatic
B. Hematogenous
C. Direct extension
D. Intraperitoneal exfoliation

Ans: C

48. Which chemotherapeutic agent doesn't have definitive activity against endometrial cancer?

A. Cisplatin
B. Topotecan
C. Paclitaxel
D. Doxorubicin

Ans: B

49. Most important prognostic factor for a woman with endometrioid adenocarcinoma?

A. Age
B. Grade
C. Stage
D. Positive peritoneal washings

Ans: C

50. Histologic specimen demonstrates < 5 percent solid growth with severe nuclear atypia. What grade is assigned to this type of the uterine adenocarcinoma?

A. Grade 1
B. Grade 2
C. Grade 3
D. Not adenocarcinoma

Ans: B

51. An 80-year-old Woman is diagnosed with a grade 1 endometrioid adenocarcinoma of the uterus by office endometrial biopsy. She has a body mass index of 45 kg/m2, has uncontrolled type 2 diabetes mellitus, has had a prior right below-the-knee amputation, and is wheelchair bound, What is the most appropriate management?

A. Radiation
B. Tamoxifen
C. Vaginal hysterectomy
D. TAH & BSO

Ans: A

52. Most appropriate surgical approach to a 50 yr old woman with BMI of 35 kg/ml and preoperative diagnosis of complex atypical hyperplasia?

A. Transvaginal hysterectomy, bilateral salpingo-oophorectomy
B. Total abdominal hysterectomy, bilateral salpingo-oophorectomy, pelvic washings
C. Total laparoscopic hysterectomy, bilateral salpingo-oophorectomy, pelvic washings
D. Any of the above

Ans: C

53. Highest incidence of breast cancer is associated with which type of endometrial cancer?

A. Endometroid
B. Serous
C. Carcinosarcoma
D. Villoglandular

Ans: B

- Papillary serous–BRCA1 and BRCA 2 associated (Ovarian Cancers, 5-10%, Early spread through omentum–Omentectomy needed.
- Clear cell carcinoma– < 5%, Hobnail cells seen, Very aggressive, Older women–Omentectomy needed

54. Which of the following is not protective from endometrial cancer?

A. Progesterone therapy
B. Granulosa cell tumor
C. Exercise
D. Smoking

Ans: B

55. Which ovarian tumor causes risk of Endometrial cancer?

A. Serous cystadenoma
B. Mucinous cystadenoma
C. Granulosa cell tumor
D. Teratoma

Ans: C

ENDOMETRIAL SARCOMAS

56. A Patient has undergone an ultrasound at 20 weeks of gestation. She is diagnosed to have several fibroids in her uterus on USG. All of the following are complications that can occur during pregnancy except?

A. Fibroid necrosis and degeneration
B. Fetalmalpresentation
C. Progression to leiomyosarcoma
D. Preterm labor

Ans: C

- Uterine fibroids or myomas are benign smooth-muscle tumors of the uterus.
- Most women with fibroid are asymptomatic and do not require therapy.
- Uterine myomas are hormonally responsive and grow in response to estrogen exposure.
- Therefore, during pregnancy a woman with fibroids may have an increase in size of these fibroids to the point where they outgrow their blood supply (carneous/red degeneration).
- In pregnancy, uterine fibroids can also be associated with fetal malpresentation due to distortion of the endometrial cavity, antepartum hemorrhage, cervical dystocia, obstructed labor, postpartum atony due to inability of the uterine muscle to contract normally after delivery, and preterm labor.
- Uterine leiomyosarcomas are smooth muscle malignancies characterized by more than 5 mitoses per 10 HPF
- Uterine leiomyosarcomas typically occur in postmenopausal women with a rapidly enlarging uterus.

57. In leiomyoma of uterus, least likely change to occur is:

A. Red degeneration
B. Sarcomatous change
C. Calcifications
D. Hyaline generation

Ans: B

Various degenerative changes which occur in fibroid:

- Hyaline degeneration is the most common (65%). The central part is the common site.
- Fatty changes are rare and are found at/or after menopause.
- Calcification/calcific degeneration (10%) usually occurs in postmenopausal subserosal fibroids. When whole of tumor is converted to a calcified mass it is called 'womb stone.'
- Red degeneration presents almost exclusively in pregnancy with acute pain, fever and localized tenderness. It is due to aseptic inflammation and thrombosis. It is usually managed conservatively.
- **Sarcomatous degeneration is the least common.** Exact risk of sarcomatous change is probably **less than 0.1%.**

58. SARCOMA BOTYROIDES is mostly seen in:

A. Neonates
B. Children <2 yrs
C. Adults
D. Post menopausal

Ans: B

SARCOMA BOTYROIDES/EMBRYONAL RHABDOMYOSARCOMA:

- Special type of mixed mesodermal tumor arising from cervix, vagina & uterus.
- Children <6 yrs are frequently affected. Can be seen in adults
- ***Sarcoma botryoides*** *usually presents as an asymptomatic mass and may first be observed by the parents when bathing the child.*
- On vaginal examination, pinkish grape like polypoidal soft growth arising from cervix & fills whole vagina
- **Diagnosis**-HPE
- **Treatment**-intravenous Vincristine, Doxorubicin, Cyclophosphamide (VAC) Every 2 wks for 6 months

59. Which of the following was previously termed malignant mixed mullerian tumor?

A. Adenosarcoma
B. Carcinosarcoma
C. Leiomyosarcoma
D. Endometrial stromal tumors

Ans: B

60. Which of the following sarcomas are mixed tumors demonstrating both malignant epithelial and malignant stromal components?

A. Adenosarcomas
B. Carcinosarcomas
C. Leiomyosarcomas
D. Endometrial stromal sarcomas

Ans: B

61. Which of the following is not a suspected risk factor for Sarcomas?

A. African-American race
B. Oral contraceptive use
C. Prior pelvic radiation
D. Excess estrogen exposure or tamoxifen use

Ans: B

62. True regarding pathogenesis of leiomyosarcomas is: (NEET SS PATTERN)

A. Share molecular pathways with normal myometrium
B. Arise from preexisting benign leiomyomas
C. Monoclonal origin
D. Rarely found in close proximity to benign leiomyomas

Ans: C

63. Most leiomyosarcomas are diagnosed at what FIGO stage? (AIIMS SS PATTERN)

A. Stage I
B. Stage II
C. Stage III
D. Stage IV

Ans: A

64. Nodal metastasis propensity is more with which type of sarcoma? (NEET SS PATTERN)

A. Adenosarcoma
B. Carcinosarcoma
C. Leiomyosarcoma
D. Endometrial stromal tumors

Ans: B

65. Poorest prognosis among the following is: (AIIMS SS PATTERN)

A. Adenosarcoma

B. Carcinosarcoma

C. Leiomyosarcoma

D. Endometrial stromal sarcoma

Ans: C

66. Sarcoma that is confined to uterus has highest cure with: (NEET SS PATTERN)

A. Chemotherapy

B. Complete surgical resection

C. Whole-pelvis radiation therapy

D. Intracavitary radiation therapy

Ans: B

CERVICAL CANCER

67. Metastasis to pelvic nodes occurs in stage 1b carcinoma cervix:

A. 12-20%

B. 0.5-2%

C. 3-5%

D. 25-30%

Ans: A

INCIDENCE OF LYMPH NODE METASTASIS IN CERVICAL CANCER

Stage	Pelvic	Para-Aortic
IA1	0	
IA2	4.8	<1
IB	15.9	2.2
IIA	24.5	11
IIB	31.4	19
III	44.8	30
IVA	55	40

68. Surprise finding in Hysterectomy specimen revealing carcinoma cervix stage IA2, management is:

A. Evaluate for metastasis

B. Post op chemotherapy

C. Radical surgery with lymphadenectomy

D. Post op radiotherapy with or without chemotherapy

Ans: C

STAGE IA2 MANAGEMENT:

- Standard surgical treatment for stage IB and IIA cervical cancer is radical hysterectomy and bilateral pelvic lymphadenectomy.
- For stage IA2, modified radical hysterectomy with pelvic lymphadenectomy/radical trachelectomy is treatment of choice.

69. High grade Squamous Intraepithelial lesion includes all except:

A. Moderate dysplasia

B. Severe dysplasia

C. HPV Changes

D. CIS

Ans: C

CERVICAL INTRAEPITHELIAL NEOPLASIA:

LSIL	HSIL
Mild/low grade dysplasia HPV Changes	Moderate/severe dysplasia CIS
Low risk HPV types	High risk HPV types
Low likelihood of progressing to invasive cancers.	High likelihood of progressing to invasive cancers.

70. What % of women with CIN will resolve in 2 yrs:

A. 10%

B. 25%

C. 50%

D. 75%

Ans: D

LIFE CYCLE-UNSTABLE CERVICAL EPITHELIUM:

- More than 60% of the cases regress to normal in patients with CIN I.

Cervical epithelium	CIN I	CIN II	CIN III/CIS
Regression to normal %	60	40	30
Persistence %	30	35	50
Progression to CIN/CIS	10	20	-
Progression to cancer	**<1%**	**5%**	**22%**
Duration of progression	CIN I,II – 5yrs	CIN III/CIS-10 yrs	Invasive- 20 yrs
Age of the patient	25-30 yrs	30-35 yrs	40-45 yrs

71. Treatment of choice for CA CERVIX stage IA1 in 55 yr old lady:

A. Type III Radical hysterectomy with pelvic lymphadenectomy

B. Type II Radical hysterectomy with pelvic lymphadenectomy

C. Primary chemoradiation

D. Primary chemotherapy+/-radiation

Ans: B

MANAGEMENT OF INVASIVE CANCER CERVIX:

Stage	Invasion	Surgery
IA1	<3mm invasion, no LVSI	Conization/type 1 hysterectomy
	<3mm invasion, LVSI	Radical trachelectomy/type 2 radical hysterectomy with pelvic lymphadenectomy
IA2	3-5mm invasion	Radical trachelectomy/type 2 radical hysterectomy with pelvic lymphadenectomy
IB1	5mm-2cm invasion	Radical trachelectomy/type 3 radical hysterectomy with pelvic lymphadenectomy
	2cm to 4cm invasion	Type 3 radical hysterectomy with pelvic lymphadenectomy
IB2	>4cm	Type 3 radical hysterectomy with pelvic and para-aortic lymphadenectomy/primary chemoradiation
IIA	Type 3 radical hysterectomy with pelvic and para-aortic lymphadenectomy/primary chemoradiation	
IIB,IIIA,IIIB	Primary chemoradiation	
IVA	Primary chemoradiation/Primary exenteration	
IVB	Primary chemotherapy+/-radiation	

72. Therapeutic conisation is indicated in:

A. Microinvasive carcinoma
B. Unsatisfactory colposcopy with cervical dysplasia
C. CIN III
D. Cervical metaplasia

Ans: A

CONISATION:

- Performed with cold knife/laser
- Preferred for treatment of young patients with Microinvasive carcinoma 1a1 stage for young patients who wants to retain uterus.

73. CIN I progresses to cancer cervix in:

A. 15%
B. 60%
C. 30%
D. <2%

Ans: D

LIFE CYCLE OF UNSTABLE CERVICAL EPITHELIUM:

CERVICAL EPITHELIUM	CIN I	CIN II	CIN III/CIS
Regression to normal %	60	40	30
Persistence %	30	35	50
Progression to CIN/CIS	10	20	-
Progression to cancer	<1%	5%	22%
Duration of progression	CIN I,II – 5yrs	CIN III/CIS-10 yrs	Invasive- 20yrs
Age of the patient	25-30 yrs	30-35 yrs	40-45 yrs

74. All are newer markers used in diagnosis of cervical cancer except:

A. Serum squamous cell carcinoma antigen level
B. HPV genotype
C. Microvessel density
D. CEA

Ans: C

- SCC antigen is most commonly used serum marker for squamous cell cervical carcinoma
- ***Serum SCC level also proved to be an independent predictor of response to neoadjuvant chemotherapy in locally advanced cervical cancer patients who received neoadjuvant chemotherapy and radical surgery.***
- Microvessel Density as Prognostic Factor in women with Breast & prostate cancer.

SERUM BIOMARKERS FOR EARLY DETECTION OF GYNECOLOGIC CANCERS:

Types	Serum Markers
SCC	Management of advanced cervical cancer
CYFRA 21-1	Cytokeratin 19 fragments
CA 125	Cancer antigen-125
CA 19-9 ; CA 15-3	Adjuvant therapy needed (CA 19-9àDeep myometrial involvement ; cervical involvement
CEA	Cancer embryonic antigen
IAP	Immunosuppressive acidic protein
M-CSF	Macrophage colony stimulating factor
YKL-40	CHI3L1-Human cartilage glycoprotein-39
sFas	Serum soluble Fas
VEGF	Vascular endothelial growth factor
TK	Thymidine kinase

75. Colposcopic criterias in Reid colposcopic index are all except:

A. Margin of lesion

B. Color of acetowhite

C. Iodine staining

D. Leukoplakia

Ans: D

REID COLPOSCOPIC INDEX:

- Reid's Colposcopic Index (RCI) is a systematic, objective method of colposcopically grading the severity of premalignant cervical lesions.

Colposcopic sign	**0**	**1**	**2**
Colour	Pale aceto whitening ; Shiny snow white	Shiny grey	Dull, opaque, oyster white
Margin of lesion & surface configuration	Condylomas ; Micropapillary areas ;pale acetowhitening; Satellite lesion and acetowhitening extending beyond transformation zone,	Regular smooth, straight outlines	Rolled, peeling edges ; internal demarcation areas of different appearances.
Vessels	Fine caliber vessels	Absent vessels	Define punctuation and mosaicism
Iodine staining	Positive staining/minor iodine negativity	Partial iodine uptake	Negative staining

76. Pap smear is useful in all of following except:

A. Gonorrhea

B. Trichomonas

C. HPV

D. Inflammatory changes

Ans: A

PAP SMEAR:

- Screening test for diagnosis of CIN
- **Others:** Trichomonas; Candidiasis; HSV; HPV; Actinomycosis
- Also useful in Inflammatory changes; Atrophy, Cellular changes associated with radiation, Cellular changes associated with intrauterine devices, Glandular cell status post hysterectomy.

77. Following solutions are applied on cervix during colposcopy except:

A. Toluidine blue

B. Normal saline

C. 3-5% Acetic acid

D. Lugol's iodine

Ans: A

COLPOSCOPY AGENTS

- Lugol's iodine
- Normal saline
- 3-5% acetic acid

78. Mean transition time from normal to carcinoma in situ in the cervix is about:

A. 2 yrs

B. 4.5 yrs

C. 10 yrs

D. 6.5 yrs

Ans: C

79. A 47-year-old woman G4P4 has a Pap smear which shows HSIL. Colposcopy is performed which is adequate, and reveals CIN III. An endocervical curettage is negative. Patient also has menorrhagia caused by uterine fibroids. Thus, the patient undergoes total abdominal hysterectomy, including removal of the cervix. Patient asks whether Pap smears need to be performed now that her cervix has been surgically removed. Which of the following is the most accurate statement?

A. Patient should continue to have annual Pap smears of Vaginal cuff

B. Patient should have Pap smears every 2 to 3 years, which may be discontinued if negative after 10 years

C. Patient does not need Pap smears any longer

D. Patient should have HPV vaccine

Ans: A

- When the patient has a history of cervical dysplasia, even after total hysterectomy (removal of uterine corpus and cervix), annual Pap smears should be performed of vaginal cuff.
- This is because vaginal cancer may arise.
- In contrast, when total hysterectomy is performed for benign reasons, and no history of cervical dysplasia, then no further Pap smears need to be performed.

80. A 33-year-old woman has a Pap smear showing moderately severe cervical dysplasia(HSIL). She denies smoking history and does not recall having any sexually transmitted infections. Which of following is best next step?

A. Repeat Pap smear in 3 months

B. Conization of the cervix

C. Colposcopy-directed biopsies

D. Radical hysterectomy

Ans: C

- Colposcopic examination with directed biopsies is next step to evaluate abnormal cytology on Pap smear.

81. A 40-year-old woman is referred for a Pap smear showing high-grade squamous intraepithelial lesions. Which of the following statements is most accurate?

A. If HPV subtyping reveals no high-risk virus present,then routine cytology is done

B. If colposcopy shows entire transformation zone, then no further analysis is needed.

C. If curettage shows cervical dysplasia, then excisional procedure of cervix is appropriate

D. Cervical cancer is highly unlikely due to the Pap smear revealing only HSIL.

Ans: C

- A cervical excisional procedure (loop electrosurgical excisional procedure) or cone biopsy is indicated when there is the possibility of endocervical disease.
- H PV typing has a role in triaging atypical cells of undetermined significance, but not HSIL.
- ***Demonstration of entire transformation zone during colposcopy allows biopsy of worst area.***

82. HPV subtype is most strongly associated with adenocarcinoma of cervix?

A. HPV 6

B. HPV 16

C. HPV 18

D. HPV 31

Ans: C

83. True regarding smoking and cervical cancer relation is:

A. Women who smoke are less likely to clear high-risk HPV infection.

B. Passive smoking increases risk of cervical cancer.

C. Smoking alters viral oncoprotein expression.

D. All of the above

Ans: D

84. HPV oncogene E6 binds to _____ and gets inactivated finally leading to immortalization of cell?

A. RB

B. p16

C. p53

D. Cyclin D1

Ans: C

- HPV oncogene E6 binds to p53 and gets inactivated
- This finally leads to immortalization of cell.

85. Cervical cancer histologic subtype associated with Peutz-Jeghers syndrome?

A. Adenoma malignum

B. Clear cell adenocarcinoma

C. Glassy cell adenocarcinoma

D. Villoglandular adenocarcinoma

Ans: A

86. Not used for staging in cervical cancer according to FIGO is:

A. Cystcscopy

B. Chest radiograph

C. Intravenous pyelogram

D. Computed tomography scan

Ans: D

87. A 45-year-old woman has a 6 cm adenocarcinoma cervix. She has +ve paraaortic nodes found on PET scan and during IVP. Stage to which belongs is

A. IB2

B. 1lB2

C. IIIB

D. IVB

Ans: C

88. Most commonly used radiation sensitizer for the treatment of cervical cancer is:

A. Cisplatin

B. Paclitaxel

C. Carboplatin

D. 5-Fluorouracil

Ans: A

89. For brachytherapy in case of cervical cancer, Point A is defined by:

A. 2 cm lateral and 2 cm superior to the external os

B. 5 cm lateral and 2 cm superior to the external os

C. 2 cm lateral and 5 cm superior to the external os

D. 5 cm lateral and 2 cm superior to the internal os

Ans: A

90. Patient with stage IB1 SCC recurs at Vagina after a radical hysterectomy and pelvic lymph node dissection. Most appropriate treatment will be?

A. Chemoradiation

B. Radiation alone

C. Systemic chemotherapy

D. Total pelvic exenteration

Ans: A

91. Site at which uterine artery is ligated during Type 3 Radical hysterectomy?

A. At uterine isthmus

B. At level of ureter

C. At origin of uterine artery

D. At level of uterosacral ligament

Ans: C

OVARIAN CANCERS

92. What is the 5 year survival of patients with epithelial ovarian cancer stage I?

A. About 90%

B. 50%

C. 35%

D. 70%

Ans: A

5 YEAR SURVIVAL RATE:

STAGE	PERCENTAGE
I	85-90%
II	60%
III	30%
IV	10%

93. Adjuvant chemotherapy for epithelial ovarian cancer is indicated for all except:

A. Stage IA grade I

B. Stage IA grade III

C. Stage IIA grade I

D. Stage IIIA grade I

Ans: A

ROLE OF CHEMOTHERAPY IN EPITHELIAL OVARIAN TUMOURS:

- No adjuvant therapy is usually required for low risk patients-stage I.
- But indicated in stage I grade III high risk patients.
- Adjuvant chemotherapy is given in almost all rest of the stages.

94. Premenarchal girls with ovarian tumours should have karyotyping done if dysgerminoma is suspected in order to assist decision making about removal of both gonads in following conditions except

A. Gonadal dysgenesis 46XY – bilateral streak gonads

B. Mixed gonadal dysgenesis 45X/46XY – unilateral streak gonads,contralateral testis.

C. Androgen insensitivity syndrome 46XY – testicular feminization

D. Dysgerminoma 46XX.

Ans: D

DYSGERMINOMAS IN PHENOTYPIC FEMALES WITH ABNORMAL GONADS:

- **Pure gonadal dysgenesis**→46XY; Klinefelter syndrome

- **Mixed gonadal dysgenesis**→45XO/46XY;
- **Androgen insensitivity syndrome** 46XY
- For patients in whom karyotype reveals **Y chromosome**

95. Reinke crystals are present in:

A. Steroid cell tumours
B. Leydig cell tumours
C. Germ cell tumors
D. Teratoma

Ans: B

- Rienke crystals are rod like inclusions which are found in Leydig cell tumors, they are rare in normal testis.

OVARIAN TUMOURS	
Call exner bodies	Granulosa cell tumor
Schiller duval bodies	Endodermal sinus tumor
Rienke crystals	Leydig(Hilus) cell tumor
Psammoma bodies	Serous epithelial tumors
Walthard cell nest	Brenner tumour
Signet ring cells	Krukenberg tumor

96. Type 1 ovarian cancers include following except:

A. High grade serous tumors that are likely to arise from tube
B. Low grade serous
C. Low grade mucinous
D. Low grade endometrioid

Ans: A

TYPE 1 OVARIAN TUMORS	TYPE 2 OVARIAN TUMORS
Generally indolent, present in stage I (tumor confined to the ovary)	Highly aggressive, present in advanced stage
Low-grade serous, low-grade endometrioid, clear cell and mucinous carcinomas, and Brenner tumors	High-grade serous, high-grade endometrioid, malignant mixed mesodermal tumors (carcinosarcomas), and undifferentiated carcinomas
Specific mutations, including KRAS, BRAF, ERBB2, CTNNB1, PTEN, PIK3CA, ARID1A, and PPP2R1A, which target specific cell signaling pathways	High frequency of TP53 mutations, highly unstable
Arise from precursor lesions in ovary	De-novo
Platinum Insensitive	Platinum sensitive

97. Aggressive ovarian tumours express which of the genes:

A. CXCL 12, CCL 21
B. MMP-2,MMP-9
C. TGF-Beta 1 & 2
D. TP53,P16

Ans: D

- Type 2 ovarian tumours are highly aggressive and they express TP53, P16.

98. HOB NAILS are seen in:

A. Hilus cell tumor
B. Clear cell Carcinoma
C. Dysgerminoma
D. Arrhenoblastoma

Ans: B

OVARIAN TUMOURS	
Call exner bodies	Granulosa cell tumour
Schiller duval bodies	Endodermal sinus tumour
Rienke crystals	Hilus cell tumour
Psommoma bodies	Serous epithelial tumours
Walthard cell nest	Brenner tumour
Signet ring cells	Krukenberg tumour

99. Percentage of protection of OCP against ovarian cancer when used for 5 yrs:

A. 75%

B. 25%

C. 50%

D. 80%

Ans: C

PROTECTION AGAINST OVARIAN CANCER:

- OCP decrease risk by 50% for usage of 5yrs/longer
- Pregnancy reduces risk of 13-19% per pregnancy
- Breast feeding, Chronic anovulation, Multiparity, Tubal ligation & Hysterectomy also protect from ovarian cancer

100. Following are true except for:

A. Cervical Cancer arises as a result of viral inactivation of TP53 and RB tumor suppressor genes by HPV E6 & E7 respectively.

B. HPV negative cervical cancers exhibit overexpression of mutant p53 protein

C. Endometrial cancer is associated with mutations in PTEN gene, inactivation of TP53, HER 2/neu overexpression.

D. Complete moles are characterized by extra haploid set of one set of chromosomes

Ans: D

- Partial moles are characterized by extra haploid set of chromosomes characterized by 69 XXX, 69XXY, 69XYY.
- Complete mole is characterized by 49XX, 49XY-entirely from paternal chromosomes because of fertilization of an empty ovum by a single spermatozum.

101. Genetic mutation associated with the highest risk of developing ovarian cancer?

A. PTEN

B. MLH1

C. BRCA1

D. BRCA2

Ans: C

102. Worst prognostic feature associated with low-malignant-potential tumors?

A. Advanced stage

B. Invasive implants

C. Mucinous histology

D. Stromal microinvasion

Ans: B

103. Which conditions can cause an elevated cancer antigen 125 level?

A. Leiomyomata

B. Menstruation

C. Endometriosis

D. All of the above

Ans: D

104. Ovarian cancer NOT associated with endometriosis is:

A. Clear cell
B. Endometrioid
C. Papillary serous
D. All of the above

Ans: C

105. Not a characteristic of Krukenberg tumors?

A. Almost always bilateral.
B. Usually arise from primary gastric tumors.
C. Usually only site of metastatic disease.
D. Composed of mucinous and signet ring adenocarcinoma cells.

Ans: C

106. Not a risk factor for ovarian cancer?

A. Nulliparity
B. Late menopause
C. Oral contraceptive pills
D. Hereditary Nonvpolyposis Colorectal Cancer (HNPCC).

Ans: C

107. Main difference between low-malignant-potential tumor & epithelial ovarian cancer in histologically is?

A. Stromal invasion
B. Mitotic activity
C. Degree of nuclear atypia
D. Nuclear to cytoplasmic ratio

Ans: A

108. Not a positive prognostic factor for ovarian cancer is?

A. Younger age
B. Clear cell type
C. Absence of ascites
D. Debulking to no gross residual

Ans: B

109. Appropriate chemotherapy regimen for treatment of platinum sensitive ovarian cancer

A. Carboplatin with paclitaxel
B. Carboplatin with gemcitabine
C. Carboplatin with pegylated liposomal doxorubicin
D. Any of the above

Ans: D

110. Most common presenting symptom of a sex cord-stromal tumor in a prepubescent girl is

A. Hirsutism
B. Abdominal pain
C. Primary amenorrhea
D. Isosexual precocious puberty

Ans: D

111. Which of the following tumors is hormonally active and most often secretes estrogen?

A. Thecoma
B. Fibroma
C. Sertoli-Leydig tumor
D. None of the above

Ans: D

112. A woman undergoes exploratory laparotomy, total abdominal hysterectomy, and bilateral salpingo-oophorectomy for a solid pelvic mass, ascites, and an elevated serum cancer antigen 125 level. Her preoperative chest radiograph shows pleural effusion. Frozen section demonstrates a benign ovarian neoplasm. What is the most likely diagnosis?

A. Meigs syndrome

B. Benign ovarian neoplasm with cirrhosis

C. Metastatic cancer with a benign adnexal mass

D. Ovarian cancer with an inaccurate frozen section diagnosis

Ans: A

113. A 30-year-old woman with Peutz-Jeghers syndrome is found to have a sex cord-stromal tumor. Which of the following is FALSE?

A. Her sex cord-stromal tumor is malignant.

B. Her sex cord-stromal tumor is likely bilateral.

C. She probably has hamartomatous polyps in her colon.

D. She has a 15-percent chance of developing adenoma malignum.

Ans: A

114. A 35-year-old nulligravida who desires uterine fertility is found to have a granulosa cell tumor during frozen section analysis of a right salpingo-oophorectomy specimen. What is the appropriate surgical management of this patient?

A. RSO alone

B. RSO, omentectomy, multiple peritoneal biopsies; consider pelvic & paraaortic LN dissection

C. RSO, omentectomy, multiple peritoneal biopsies; consider pelvic and paraaortic LN dissection and dilatation and curettage of endometrial cavity

D. Total abdominal hysterectomy, bilateral salpingooophorectomy, omentectomy, multiple peritoneal biopsies; consider pelvic and paraaortic lymph node dissection

Ans: C

115. Routine surveillance of malignant sex cord-stromal tumors includes all the following EXCEPT:

A. Inhibin levels

B. History and physical examination at regular intervals

C. Routine abdominopelvic computed tomography every 6 months

D. Imaging as clinically indicated based on physical examination findings and tumor marker levels

Ans: C

116. Which of the following is NOT an appropriate adjuvant treatment for a patient with a stage III granulosa cell tumor?

A. Whole pelvic radiotherapy

B. Carboplatin and paclitaxel

C. Bleomycin-etoposide-cisplatin chemotherapy

D. All of the above are appropriate treatment options.

Ans: A

117. A 52-year-old woman with a history of granulosa cell tumor has a rising inhibin level. CT reveals an isolated pelvic mass. What is the next most appropriate treatment?

A. Surgical resection

B. Carboplatin and paclitaxel

C. Medroxyprogesterone acetate

D. Bleomycin-etoposide-cisplatin chemotherapy

Ans: A

118. Which of the following is a prognostic factor for sex cord-stromal tumors?

A. Age
B. Stage
C. Amount of residual disease
D. All of the above

Ans: D

119. NOT true about sex cord stromal tumors diagnosed during pregnancy?

A. Granulosa cell tumors are most common.
B. Chemotherapy, if indicated, should be given during pregnancy.
C. A third of these cases are diagnosed incidentally at the time of cesarean delivery.
D. Surgery should consist of unilateral salpingooophorectomy, omentectomy & peritoneal biopsies.

Ans: B

120. Which invasive cancer is most commonly diagnosed in women during their 20s?

A. Germ cell tumors
B. Sex cord-stromal tumors
C. Epithelial ovarian cancer
D. All of these occur with equal frequency.

Ans: C

121. Most common presenting symptom in a woman with a germ cell tumor is:

A. Bloating
B. Abdominal pain
C. Abdominal distention
D. Menstrual abnormality

Ans: B

122. NOT a tumor marker for germ cell tumors is:

A. Inhibin
B. Alpha-fetoprotein
C. Lactate dehydrogenase
D. Human chorionic gonadotropin

Ans: A

123. An 18-year-old woman presents with severe, acute abdominal pain. She is found to have a large pelvic mass, and torsion of an enlarged ovary is suspecteD. During the ensuing surgery, frozen section reveals dysgerminoma. There is no gynecologic oncologist at your hospital. What is the most appropriate next step?

A. Perform a bilateral salpingo-oophorectomy and close
B. Perform a unilateral salpingo-oophorectomy and close
C. Close her abdomen and refer her to a gynecologic oncologist
D. Perform a unilateral salpingo-oophorectomy, obtain peritoneal washings, carefully palpate the abdomen for metastases, and perform biopsies as indicated.

Ans: B

124. Most commonly diagnosed ovarian malignancy during pregnancy is:

A. Dysgerminoma
B. Choriocarcinoma
C. Immature teratoma
D. Granulosa cell tumor

Ans: A

125. Not a protective factor against the development of a sex cord-stromal tumor?

A. Smoking
B. Obesity
C. Multiparity
D. Combination oral contraceptive pills

Ans: B

126. A 19-year-old female nulligravid college student is found to have a pelvic mass and an elevated LDH level. She was amenorrheic until she started taking combination oral contraceptive pills at age 17. She undergoes surgical exploration, and frozen section analysis of the surgical specimen reveals ovarian dysgerminoma, Which of the following is FALSE?

A. Her karyotype is most likely 46,XX.

B. Regardless of stage, she has an excellent prognosis.

C. Her other ovary may contain a gonadoblastoma & should be removed.

D. She should undergo complete surgical staging, but her uterus may be preserved.

Ans: A

127. What percentage of gonadoblastomas undergoes malignant transformation?

A. 0.1 percent
B. 10 percent
C. 40 percent
D. 80 percent

Ans: C

128. Which germ cell tumor is most likely to be bilateral?

A. Dysgerminoma
B. Mature teratoma
C. Immature teratoma
D. Embryonal carcinoma

Ans: A

129. Which of the following malignant germ cell tumors has the worst prognosis?

A. Dysgerminoma
B. Yolk sac tumor
C. Immature teratoma
D. Nongestational choriocarcinoma

Ans: B

130. Which of the following is true regarding mixed germ cell tumors of the ovary?

A. Dysgerminoma is the most common component.

B. Treatment is based on the dysgerminoma component.

C. Women with a presumed pure dysgerminoma and an elevated AFP level are likely to have component of immature teratoma.

D. All of the above

Ans: A

131. Most common germ cell tumor of the ovary is:

A. Dysgerminoma
B. Yolk sac tumor
C. Choriocarcinoma
D. Teratoma

Ans: D

132. Which of the following characteristics is primarily used to grade immature teratomas?

A. Amount of solid component present
B. Amount of immature elements present
C. Amount of immature neural tissue present
D. None of the above

Ans: C

133. An 18-year-old adolescent has a history of a stage IC grade 3 immature teratoma. She received adjuvant chemotherapy with bleomycin, etoposide, and cisplatin(BEP). At her 6-month follow-up, she is found to have a pelvic mass. Which of the following is the most appropriate management?

A. Chemotherapy
B. Radiation therapy
C. Continued observation
D. Exploratory laparotomy with removal of masses found

Ans: D

134. Most common cancer found in a mature teratoma is:

A. Struma ovarii
B. Basal cell carcinoma
C. Neuroectodermal tumors
D. Squamous cell carcinoma

Ans: D

135. Which of the following patients does NOT need adjuvant chemotherapy after unilateral Salpingo- oophorectomy with surgical staging?

A. Stage Ia dysgerminoma
B. Stage IA yolk sac tumor
C. Stage IA grade 3 immature teratoma
D. All of the above

Ans: A

136. Most common chemotherapy regimen used to treat malignant germ cell ovarian cancers?

A. Carboplatin and etoposide
B. Carboplatin and paclitaxel
C. Bleomycin, etoposide, and cisplatin
D. Bleomycin, etoposide, and paclitaxel

Ans: C

137. Which of the following is a prognostic factor for malignant ovarian germ cell cancers?

A. Stage
B. Histologic subtype
C. Amount of residual tumor
D. All of the above

Ans: D

VAGINAL CANCER

138. Most common primary vaginal cancers is of ______ histologic type:

A. Leiomyosarcoma
B. Squamous cell carcinoma
C. Clear cell adenocarcinoma
D. Endometrioid adenocarcinoma

Ans: B

139. Most common mechanism by which primary vaginal cancer spreads is:

A. Lymphatic
B. Localized (No spread)
C. Hematogenous
D. Transperitoneal

Ans: A

140. Factor which is most commonly linked with primary SCC vagina is?

A. BRCA1 mutation
B. Diethylstilbestrol exposure
C. HPV
D. HNPCC

Ans: C

141. Not a known risk factor for primary vaginal cancer?

A. Cigarette smoking
B. Early age of 1st intercourse
C. History of vulvar or cervical cancer
D. Hormonal therapy use for menopausal symptoms for >5 years

Ans: D

142. Most common presenting complaint in primary vaginal cancer women is?

A. Bleeding
B. Vaginal mass
C. Constipation
D. Urinary retention

Ans: A

143. Vaginal cancers mostly develop in which part of vagina?

A. Upper third
B. Middle third
C. Lower third
D. At the hymeneal ring

Ans: A

144. Which of the following is associated with poorer prognosis for survival with primary vaginal cancer?

A. Nulliparity
B. Younger age
C. Adenocarcinoma cell type
D. All of the above

Ans: C

145. Chemotherapeutic agent is used as an adjunct to radiotherapy for treatment of locally advanced vaginal cancer?

A. Cisplatin
B. Doxorubicin
C. Vincristine
D. Methotrexate

Ans: A

146. Which suggests pelvic side wall disease during surveillance for recurrent disease?

A. Sciatica
B. Lymphedema
C. Hydronephrosis
D. All of the above

Ans: D

147. A woman presents with postmenopausal spotting and pelvic pain and is diagnosed with adenocarcinoma of Vagina. Which of the following most commonly gives rise to this histologic type of vaginal cancer?

A. Vaginal adenosis
B. Wolfian duct remnant
C. Endometriosis implant
D. Metastases from upper genital tract

Ans: D

148. Most common malignancy of the vagina in infants and children?

A. Melanoma
B. Chondrosarcoma
C. Leiomyosarcoma
D. Embryonal rhabdomyosarcoma

Ans: D

149. Expoure to ______ leads to clear cell adenocarcinoma of vagina in young woman:

A. Thalidomide
B. Alkylating agents
C. Diethylstilbestrol
D. Ionizing radiation

Ans: C

150. Symptom that is most typical for sarcoma botryoides is?

A. Pain
B. Hemoptysis
C. Vaginal bleeding
D. Ureteral obstruction

Ans: C

151. Which melanoma staging system is not applicable for vaginal melanoma?

A. Clark
B. Chung
C. Breslow
D. All of the above

Ans: A

- Both Clark & Breslow systems have been shown to correlate with prognosis in patients with cutaneous melanoma.
- **Chung argued that Clark micro staging was inappropriate for the vulva and labia,** which lack a well-defined papillary dermis, and substituted measurement of tumor thickness as a multiple of 1 mm for the middle three Clark levels.

152. Preferred primary therapy for Vaginal leiomyosarcoma is (NEET SS PATTERN)?

A. Radiotherapy alone
B. Chemotherapy alone
C. Radical pelvic exenteration
D. Surgical resection with negative margins

Ans: D

153. True about Vaginal melanoma is?

A. Carries good prognosis.
B. Most frequently found in distal vagina.
C. Most common site for reproductive tract melanoma.
D. Often diagnosed early

Ans: B

154. Most frequent malignant neoplasm of vagina:

A. SCC
B. Melanoma
C. Adenocarcinoma
D. Secondary from cervix

Ans: A

- 80-90% of vaginal malignancies are SCC.
- 5-10% are adenocarcinomas.
- Vaginal melanomas are 3% of primary vaginal tumors and <20% of genital melanomas.
- *Distal one third of vagina is most commonly affected.*
- Poor prognosis than vulvar melanomas.

VULVAR CANCERS

155. Not a risk factor for vulvar cancer: (NEET SS PATTERN)

A. Lichen planus
B. Tobacco abuse
C. Lichen sclerosis
D. Human papillomavirus infection

Ans: A

156. What is the second most common histologic type of vulval cancer:

A. Sarcoma
B. Melanoma
C. Basal cell
D. Adenocarcinoma

Ans: B

157. What percentage of all vulval cancers is positive for human papilloma virus?

A. 5 percent
B. 30 percent
C. 60 percent
D. 90 percent

Ans: C

158. A 39-year-old woman came to the OPD with painful vulvar mass measuring 3 cm. Biopsy of the mass reveals invasive squamous cell carcinoma. Which of the following tests should be performed prior to definitive surgery?

A. Vulvoscopy
B. Cervical cytology
C. Human immunodeficiency virus assay
D. All of the above

Ans: D

159. A 68-year-old woman came to the OPD for annual examination and complains vulvar pruritus. Thickened, white plaque is noted on vulvar skin. Most appropriate next step?

A. Biopsy of the lesion
B. Prescribe clobetasol cream and re-evaluate in 3 months
C. Prescribe estrogen cream and re-evaluate in 3 months
D. Perform wide local excision

Ans: A

160. A 5 cm invasive squamous cell carcinoma of the vulva involving lower third of vagina that has undergone radical vulvectomy with bilateral inguino-femoral lymph node is subjected to histopathology. Specimen shows excision margins and lymph nodes are negative for tumor involvement. Clinical stage of lesion is?

A. I
B. II
C. III
D. IVA

Ans: B

161. Vulvar lesion that is associated with a primary cancer at distant site: (AIIMS SS PATTERN)

A. Lichen planus
B. Paget disease
C. Lichen sclerosis
D. Basal cell carcinoma

Ans: B

162. A 55-year-old woman presents with dyspareunia and vulvar mass. She is a suspect of Bartholin gland carcinoma. What is the most appropriate management step?

A. Antibiotics
B. Radical vulvectomy
C. Incision and drainage along with biopsy of cyst wall
D. Radical vulvectomy with inguinofemoral lymphadenectomy

Ans: C

- This is a case of Bartholin gland carcinoma

163. Most appropriate treatment for a 3 cm right vulvar basal cell carcinoma that lies 2 cm from midline and that lacks associated inguinal lymphadenopathy?

A. Lmiquimod
B. Primary radiation
C. Radical partial vulvectomy
D. Radical vulvectomy with bilateral inguinofemoral lymph node dissection

Ans: C

- This is a case of Basal cell carcinoma which is locally aggressive
- Treatment is Radical partial vulvectomy

164. Which mutation has a targeted agent for treatment of metastatic melanoma?

A. p53
B. BRAF
C. IFN gamma
D. CTLA-4

Ans: B

165. A 75 yr old woman undergoes pelvic CT after presenting with a large vulvar mass and grossly enlarged groin nodes. Biopsy of vulvar mass revealed poorly differentiated SCC. CT scan reveals right pelvic lymphadenopathy. Stage of the cancer if pelvic lymph nodes are involved?

A. IIIB
B. IIIC
C. IVA
D. IVB

Ans: D

166. Most important prognostic factor in vulvar cancer (NEET SS PATTERN)

A. Grade
B. Tumor size
C. Depth of invasion
D. Lymph node metastasis

Ans: D

167. Which factor does not increase the risk of lymph node metastasis in vulvar melanoma?

A. Lesion diameter
B. Tumor thickness
C. High mitotic rate
D. Lesion ulceration

Ans: A

168. Not associated with an increased risk of lymph node metastasis in vulval cancer:

A. Clitoral lesion
B. Depth of invasion
C. Increasing tumor diameter
D. Lymphovascular space invasion

Ans: A

169. Not true regarding vulvar melanoma is:

A. Occurs in elderly patients.
B. Most commonly arises from labia
C. Dysplastic Nevus syndrome can predispose to melanoma
D. More common in African-Americans and other racial groups than in white women.

Ans: D

170. A 60 yr old woman presents with 4 cm cauliflower-like mass on vulva located within 1 cm of midline. Biopsy reveals verrucous carcinoma. Most appropriate treatment is:

A. Wide local excision with 1-cm margin
B. Radical partial vulvectomy with sentinel node biopsy
C. Wide local excision with 1-cm margin and sentinel node biopsy
D. Radical partial vulvectomy with bilateral inguinofemoral lymphadenectomy

Ans: A

171. Most common complication of an inguinofemoral lymph node dissection?

A. Lymphocele
B. Groin infection
C. Lymphedema
D. Wound dehiscence

Ans: C

172. If cribriform fascia is left intact rate of which of the following complication is reduced?

A. Infection
B. Lymphedema
C. Wound breakdown
D. All of the above

Ans: D

173. Not an appropriate candidate for a sentinel lymph node biopsy?

A. 2.5 cm lesion with 1 mm depth of invasion
B. 3 cm midline lesion with 4 mm depth of invasion
C. 1.4 cm lesion with 0.6 mm depth of invasion
D. 3 cm lesion located 1 cm from the midline

Ans: C

174. A 65 yr old woman has history of stage IIIA squamous cell carcinoma vulva treated by radical partial vulvectomy with bilateral inguinofemoral lymphadenectomy. She develops a 1 cm recurrence on right vulva. Most appropriate treatment is?

A. Radiation
B. Chemoradiation
C. Systemic chemotherapy
D. Radical partial vulvectomy

Ans: D

175. Vulvar carcinoma in situ tends to be:

A. Multifocal in old women

B. Higher risk of invasion in young women

C. Multifocal with high risk of invasion in young women

D. Unifocal with high risk of invasion in old women

Ans: C

VULVAR CARCINOMA IN SITU:

- Associated with STD and viral infections such as HPV(70-80%), HSV-2.
- Obesity, DM, Chronic pruritis and dermatosis are associated with it.
- Mean age for invasive vulvar cancer is 65-70 yrs.
- But mean age for VIN is 45-50 yrs.
- 80 to 90% of VIN lesions contain HPV- 16→multifocal and invasive.
- Common in young women

176. Premalignant lesion of vulva is:

A. Krausosis

B. Leukoplakia

C. Condylomata

D. Localised scleroderma

Ans: C

- Post-menopausal woman, Nulliparous
- Obese, DM, HTN,
- Associated with chronic vulvar dystrophy, HPV 16,18, Syphilis, LGV
- CONDYLOMATA is caused by HPV infection.

177. Bowen's disease of vulva best treated by:

A. Simple vulvectomy

B. Chemotherapy

C. Radiotherapy

D. Cryotherapy

Ans: A

BOWEN'S DISEASE OF VULVA:

- Intraepithelial carcinoma of vulva. Slow growing.
- Pruritis is main complaint.
- Presence of giant cells and corps round are characteristic of the lesion.
- Biopsy reveals prickle cells invading epidermis.
- Simple vulvectomy is treatment of choice.

178. In vulvar cancer most commonly involved nodes are:

A. Femoral

B. Superficial inguinal

C. External iliac

D. Internal iliac

Ans: B

VULVAR CARCINOMA:

- Most common route of spread is lymphatics.
- For most lesions, initial regional metastasis is to inguinal lymph nodes that are superficial to camper's fascia.

- From here secondary metastasis occurs to deep inguinal nodes.
- Most common site of hematogenous spread is to lungs.

179. Treatment of choice for early invasive vulvar cancer is:

A. Radical vulvectomy with lymphadenectomy
B. Interstitial radium implantation followed by lymphadenectomy
C. Vulvectomy & external radiation
D. Multi drug CT

Ans: A

TREATMENT OF VULVAR CANCER:

- Stage 1- less than 2 cm with margin 3 cm beyond growth responds to partial vulvectomy with inguinal node dissection.
- Stage 2- 2 to 4 cm requires total vulvectomy and bilateral lymph node dissection.
- Stage 3- megavoltage therapy
- Stage 4- chemoradiotherapy

180. Vulvar melanoma all are true except:

A. 5-10% of vulvar cancers
B. 3-5% malignant melanoma in women
C. More common in asian womwn
D. Constitute 2-3% of vulvar cancer

Ans: B

VULVAR MELANOMA:

- Malignant melanoma of vulva account for approximately 2-4% of primary vulvar malignancies and 1-3% of melanomas arising in women.
- Most frequently in women older than 60 yrs
- Most common variety is mucosal lentigenous type
- Poor prognosis - Older age group, Clinical amelanosis, Ulceration.
- Nearly 8% are malignant melanoma

181. Basal cell carcinoma vulva all are true except:

A. Average age at diagnosis is 65
B. Most commonly occurs in labia majora
C. Treatment is vulvectomy with lymphadenectomy
D. Constitute 2-3% of vulvar cancers

Ans: C

BASAL CELL CARCINOMA:

- Constitute about <1% of all BCC and 2-5% of vulvar cancers.
- Mean age of presentation is 65 yrs.
- Most common site is labia majora.
- Risk factors - exposure to ultraviolet radiation, arsenic, hereditary skin conditions such as xeroderma pigmentosum and nevoid basal cell carcinoma syndrome and immunosuppressive states
- Treatment of BCC is wide local excision with pathologically-proven clear margins of approximately 1 cm.

182. Ca vulva as per FIGO staging, tumor of any size with adjacent spread to lower urethra

A. Stage IV

B. Stage II

C. Stage IIA

D. Stage III

Ans: C

CARCINOMA VULVA:

Table: Staging of vulval cancer	
State I	Tumour confined to the vulva
IA	Lesion ≤ 2 cm in size, fonfined to the vulva or perineum and with stromal invasion ≤ 1.0 mm*, no nodal metastasis
IB	Lesions > 2 cm in size or with stromal invasion > 1.0 mm*, confined to the vulva or perineum, with negative nodes
Stage II	Tumour of any size with extension to adjacent perineal structures (1/3 lower urethra, 1/3 lower vagina, anus) with negative nodes
Stage III	Tumour or any size with or without extenion to adjacent perineal structures (1/3 lower urethra, 1/3 lower vagina, anus) with positive inguino-femoral lymph nodes
III A	(i) With 1 lymph node metastasis (≥ 5 mm), or (ii) 1–2 lymph node metastatis (es) (< 5 mm)
III B	(i) With 2 or more lymph node metastases (≥ 5 mm), or (ii) 3 or more ly mph node metastases (<5 mm)
III C	With positive nodes with extracapsular spread
Stage IV	Tumour invades other regional (2/3 upper urethra, 2/3 upper vagina), or distant structures.
IVA	Tumour invades any of the following: (i) Upper urethral and/or vaginal mucosa, bladder mucosa, rectal mucosa, or fixed to pelvic bone, or (ii) Fixed or ulcerated inguino–femoral lymph nodes
IVB	Any distant metastasis including pelvic lymph nodes